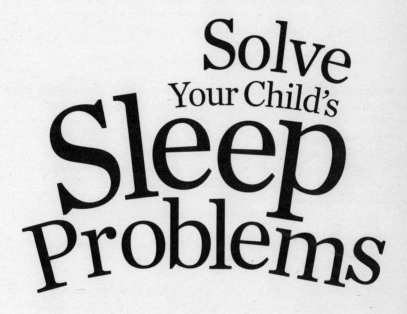

Solve Your Child's Sleep Problems

The world's bestselling guide to helping
your child sleep through the night

Dr Richard Ferber

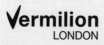

Vermilion
LONDON

1 3 5 7 9 10 8 6 4 2

First published in 2013 by Vermilion, an imprint of Ebury Publishing
A Random House Group company
First published in the USA by Simon and Schuster in 1985
This revised edition published in the USA by Fireside,
an imprint of Simon and Schuster in 2006

The Random House Group Limited Reg. No. 954009

Addresses for companies within the Random House Group can be found at
www.randomhouse.co.uk

The Random House Group Limited supports The Forest Stewardship Council
(FSC®), the leading international forest certification organisation. Our books
carrying the FSC label are printed on FSC® certified paper. FSC is the only
forest certification scheme endorsed by the leading environmental organisations,
including Greenpeace. Our paper procurement policy can be found at
www.randomhouse.co.uk/environment

Printed in the UK by CPI Group (UK) Ltd, Croydon, CR0 4YY

ISBN 9780091948092

To buy books by your favourite authors and register for offers visit
www.randomhouse.co.uk

Solve
Your Child's
Sleep
Problems

To my sons, Matthias and Thaddeus.
As children, they taught me how to be a parent.
As adults, they have taught me to remember being a child.

Acknowledgements

I have gone to great effort to make the material in this book clear but not simplistic, rational but not dogmatic, and comprehensive but not encyclopedic. In so doing, I have had the great joy of working closely with my son Matthias. Matthias has taken these goals as his own and devoted considerable energies to the project with an ability far greater than mine. I can say for certain that if you find this book easy to read and understand, clear in its formulations and consistent in its approaches, resistant to misunderstanding, and straightforward to apply, then it is because of his efforts. Any mistakes in content remain my own.

Contents

Acknowledgements   *vii*
List of Figures   *xv*
Preface to the Second Edition   *xvii*

PART I

YOUR CHILD'S SLEEP

CHAPTER 1   At the End of Your Tether   *3*
     Can a Child Just Be a 'Poor Sleeper'?   *6*
     How to Tell Whether Your Child Has a
        Sleep Problem   *8*
     Starting with a Basic Understanding of Sleep   *13*

CHAPTER 2   What We Know About Sleep   *14*
     Non-REM Sleep   *15*
     REM Sleep   *18*
     How Sleep Stages Develop in Children   *21*
     Children's Sleep Cycles   *23*
     Sleep and Waking Patterns   *28*
     The Importance of Biological Rhythms   *31*

CHAPTER 3   Helping Your Child to Develop Good
Sleep Practices   *33*
     The Importance of Your Child's
        Bedtime Routines   *34*

'Back to Sleep': Reducing the Risk of SIDS   37
Should Your Child Sleep in Your Bed?   41
Specific Issues Related to Co-sleeping   44
The Sleep Challenges of Multiples:
    Twins and Triplets   49
The Special Toy or Favourite Blanket   52
Developing Good Schedules   53

PART II

THE SLEEPLESS CHILD

CHAPTER 4   Sleep Associations: A Key Problem   61
             A Typical Sleep Association Problem   63
             Why Sleep Associations Matter   65
             Wrong Sleep Associations   67
             How to Solve the Problem:
                 The Progressive-Waiting Approach   72
             Making the Changes in One Step or Several 83
             Associations to the Breast, Bottle or Dummy 85
             Co-sleeping and Related Considerations   87
             If Things Are Not Getting Better   92
             General Observations   95

CHAPTER 5   The Problem of Limit-Setting   105
             Who's in Charge?   106
             Difficulty Setting Limits   108
             Limits, Associations, Feedings, Schedules
                 and Fears   111
             Setting Limits at Night   112
             Limit-Setting Problems: Some Examples   129

CHAPTER 6   Feedings During the Night: Another Major
             Cause of Trouble   136
             Is Your Child's Sleep Problem Caused by
                 Night-time Feedings?   139
             How to Solve the Problem   140

Other Points to Keep in Mind   148
Medical Considerations   149

CHAPTER 7 Night-time Fears   151
The Anxious Child   151
Bedtime Fears   153
Evaluating Your Child's Fears   156
How to Cope with Night-time Fears   165
Techniques to Help a Child Feel Less
    Frightened and Fall Asleep Quickly   167
Final Considerations   177

CHAPTER 8 Colic and Other Medical Causes of Poor Sleep   178
Colic   178
Chronic Illness   181
Nocturnal Pain   182
Medication   184
Abnormal Brain Function and a
    True Inability to Sleep Well   188

PART III

SCHEDULES AND SLEEP RHYTHM
DISTURBANCES

CHAPTER 9 Schedules and Rhythms   195
Sleep Phases   199
The Circadian System and the Forbidden
    Zone for Sleep: Why You Can Stay Awake
    Until Bedtime – and Sleep Until Morning   200
Setting the Biological Clock: How Do You
    Know What Time Zone You Are In?   204
Individual Differences: Are You a Lark
    or an Owl?   206
Society, Sleep Deprivation and the Adolescent 207
Specific Sleep Problems Affecting Different
    Parts of the Sleep Cycle: A Summary   211

CHAPTER 10   Schedule Disorders I: Sleep Phase Problems   214
                  Sleep Phases   214
                  Sleep Phase Shifts   219
                  Sleep Phase Shifts in the Adolescent   230

CHAPTER 11   Schedule Disorders II: Other Common
                  Schedule Problems   241
                  Problems in Regular Schedules   241
                  Irregular and Inconsistent Sleep-Wake
                      Schedules   255
                  Travel   260

CHAPTER 12   Naps   264
                  Problems with the Length and Timing of
                      Naps   267
                  Trouble Giving Up a Nap: Transition
                      Problems   280
                  Nap-time Sleep Association Problems   281
                  Napping (or Not) at Home and at Day Care   282
                  You May Have to Accept What Works   283

PART·IV

INTERRUPTIONS DURING SLEEP

CHAPTER 13   Partial Wakings: Sleep-Talking, Sleepwalking,
                  Confusional Arousals and Sleep Terrors   287

             I. What They Are and Why They Happen   287
                  The Normal Transition from Deep (Stage IV)
                      Sleep Towards Waking   289
                  More Intense Transitions: A Spectrum of
                      Confusional Events   291
                  What a Confusional Event Feels Like   296
                  Why Confusional Events Happen:
                      The Balance Between Sleep and Waking   297

The Variability of Arousals over Time   *311*
Evaluating Confusional Events: When to
   Take Action   *312*

II. Treatment   *315*
What You Should Do and What Else
   to Consider   *315*
How We Helped the Children Described
   Earlier   *322*

CHAPTER 14 Nightmares   *333*
What Nightmares Are and Why They
   Occur   *333*
How to Help Your Child If He Is Having
   Nightmares   *337*
Nightmares and Confusional Events   *341*
Nightmares or '"No"-mares'?:
   'I had a bad dream'   *345*

CHAPTER 15 Bed-wetting   *347*
The Impact of Enuresis   *348*
What Causes Enuresis?   *350*
Approaches to Treating Enuresis   *355*
Final Words   *367*

CHAPTER 16 Head-Banging, Body-Rocking and
Head-Rolling   *368*
When Do These Behaviours Occur?   *369*
What Do These Behaviours Look Like?   *370*
Is Head-Banging Dangerous?   *371*
When Should You Be Concerned?   *371*
What Causes Rhythmic Behaviours?   *372*
Treating the Problem   *378*
Outcomes   *382*

PART V

THE SLEEPY CHILD

CHAPTER 17 Noisy Breathing, Snoring and Obstructive
            Sleep Apnoea   387
              What Happens in Sleep Apnoea   388
              What Causes the Obstruction   392
              Treating Sleep Apnoea   396
              Some Words of Caution   401
              Getting Your Child the Help She Needs   403

CHAPTER 18 Narcolepsy and Other Causes of Sleepiness   406
              Is Your Child Abnormally Sleepy?   408
              Causes of Sleepiness Other Than Narcolepsy 409
              Treating Simpler Causes of Sleepiness   410
              Evaluation at a Sleep Disorders Centre   411
              Narcolepsy   414
              The Cause of Narcolepsy   424
              The Treatment of Narcolepsy   426
              Future Treatments   430

Index   431

List of Figures

FIGURE 1 Typical Sleep Requirements in Childhood 10
FIGURE 2 Brain Wave Patterns in Waking and in Sleep 17
FIGURE 3 Typical Sleep Stage Progression in the Young Child 25
FIGURE 4 Helping Your Child Learn to Fall Asleep with the Proper Associations: The Progressive-Waiting Approach 74
FIGURE 5 Sleep Chart for Parents to Use 77
FIGURE 6 Betsy's Sleep Chart 81
FIGURE 7 Helping Your Child Learn to Stay in His Room 121
FIGURE 8 Eliminating Extra Feedings at Sleep Times 143
FIGURE 9 Sleepiness and Alertness Across the Day and Night – Homeostatic and Circadian Drives 203
FIGURE 10 Common Causes of Sleep Problems at Different Times of the Day and Night 211
FIGURE 11 Sleep Phase Shifts 223
FIGURE 12 Too Long in Bed: Potential Sleep Problems 244
FIGURE 13 Drifting Nap Patterns 279
FIGURE 14 Spectrum of Behaviour in Children at the End of a Period of Stage IV Sleep 295
FIGURE 15 Partial Wakings: A Summary of the Major Patterns Across Childhood and General Recommendations for Management 330

FIGURE 16 Nightmares Versus Sleep Terrors 343
FIGURE 17 Your Child's Urinary System 358
FIGURE 18 Obstructive Sleep Apnoea 390
FIGURE 19 Use of CPAP 399
FIGURE 20 How to Tell Whether Your Child Has
Sleep Apnoea 404

Preface to the Second Edition

When the first edition of this book appeared in 1985, the medical field devoted to the treatment of sleep disorders in children was new. Still, over the years, the basic information I presented on the nature of sleep and sleep problems in children has remained sound, and the techniques I described to help children with sleep problems have proven to be well conceived and practical. The value of these approaches has been confirmed repeatedly, not only at our sleep disorders centre in Boston, USA, but at many others – and by many different professionals – around the world. Most of the comments I have received from families who carefully read and then applied the techniques outlined in the first edition have expressed gratitude, with parents thanking me for helping them to find a solution to a sleep problem that had been going on for months or years.

So why did I see the need, twenty years later, for this revised and considerably expanded edition? There are three main reasons.

The first reason is to correct some widespread misconceptions regarding my methods and their application. My goals have always been to help parents to understand the nature of sleep and of childhood sleep problems, determine the causes of their own child's sleep difficulties and choose or design an appropriate treatment programme that fits their own philosophy of child-rearing. I have always believed that the more you understand about your child's sleep problems, the more humane and effective you can be in solving them. A child may cry repeatedly each night, for example, but until parents understand why that is happening and institute proper treatment, they may be unable to resolve it in a way they find satisfactory.

Despite my efforts in the first edition to communicate these goals, it became clear that they were not always understood as I had intended. Many people thought I recommended a single method to treat all sleep problems, regardless of the nature of the problems, their causes or the parenting styles and wishes of the family. Even worse, the particular method they refer to (only one of many approaches described in this book) has sometimes been incorrectly described as the same 'cry it out' method that my suggested techniques were meant to counter. Simply leaving a child in a cot to cry for long periods alone until he falls asleep, no matter how long it takes, is not an approach I approve of. On the contrary, many of the approaches I recommend are designed specifically to avoid unnecessary crying. Most of the sleep problems discussed in this book can be corrected without any crying at all or, if the child is already crying at night, by rapidly reducing it. In the one case where some crying may be necessary – when undesirable nightly practices or habits must be changed – crying can be kept to a minimum.

In this edition I have attempted to make it much clearer that there are many different sleep problems, that apparently identical sleep problems may have different causes in different children and that a single sleep problem may have multiple contributing causes. To properly choose a treatment, one must take all these factors into account. Each problem and cause may require a different treatment (what works well for one problem may be inappropriate for another), and all component causes may have to be treated (a partial solution is no solution at all). In addition, often a number of treatment options are available, some of which fit a particular child's needs or personality and his or her parents' desires better than others. I have tried to present more of these choices so that you, the reader, can find an approach you believe appropriate and are comfortable with, whether you live in a big home or small, sleep separately or together or have one child or many; and whether your child is nervous or confident, co-operative or difficult, outgoing or shy.

The second reason for this new edition is to better address topics that were discussed inadequately in the original. Questions from parents have helped me to identify topics that needed to be expanded, such as co-sleeping, naps, sleep problems in twins and travel to different time zones. (The omission of co-sleeping from the original version, apart from a regrettably brief reference that only repeated the conventional attitude of the day, was unfortunate, given the importance of the issue to many parents.) This edition covers such topics in the detail they deserve.

Finally, in this revision I have added new information drawn from the last twenty years' experience, study and scientific discoveries. We now have more accurate information than we did in 1985 about children's sleep requirements, and we know more about the biological clock and its effects on sleep and alertness, about sleep terrors and related problems and about medical issues such as bedwetting, sleep apnoea and narcolepsy. Through my work with thousands of families, I can now offer a number of new methods for treating a variety of common sleep problems.

How to Use This Book

Sleep problems are rather complex by nature, and to understand and treat them, you need to know a little bit about how sleep works. Although you may be tempted to skip directly to the chapters describing a particular problem of interest to you, I suggest that you begin – regardless of the type of sleep problem you hope to solve – by reading the four general introductory chapters on sleep and sleep rhythms: the three chapters in Part I and Chapter 9, 'Schedules and Rhythms' in Part III. These chapters give you the background information you will need to understand most of what appears in other chapters.

You will be best equipped to understand *any* problem if you also read through most of the remaining chapters. At least skim through them quickly and go back for a closer read once you've identified the most relevant material. Many children have more than one sleep problem, and sleep problems are often interconnected.

For instance, although the most common cause of sleeplessness in young children – poor sleep associations – is addressed in a single chapter, you may not be able to treat it successfully unless you take into account material from the chapters on limit-setting, fears, schedules or partial wakings. If your child has sleep terrors, you may need to understand the impact of habits and schedules on your child's symptoms before you can help effectively. And you cannot always deal properly with a problem of limit-setting unless you also take into account your child's anxiety or an inappropriate bedtime.

Some more specific suggestions follow.

For a sleepless child (including a child who exhibits sleepwalking, sleep terrors or head-banging):

- In addition to the introductory chapters, read over much of the material from Parts II, III and IV before deciding what the problem is and embarking on a treatment programme. At a minimum, read Chapters 4 and 5 on sleep associations and limit-setting, Chapters 10 and 11 on schedule disorders and Chapters 13 and 14 on partial wakings and nightmares.
- If your child is still feeding at night, also read Chapter 6.
- If your child is frightened at night, also read Chapter 7.
- If your child is colicky or has another underlying medical problem, read Chapter 8.
- If your child is still napping, or should be but isn't, read Chapter 12.
- If your child rocks or bangs his head at night, read Chapter 16.
- If your child snores, read Chapter 17.

For a child who is sleepy during the day:

- Since sleepiness is most commonly caused by insufficient sleep or an inappropriate schedule, start by reading through the same chapters suggested above for dealing with a sleepless child.

- In addition, read Part V.

For a child who wets the bed:

- Focus on Chapter 15.

For a child whose main problem is snoring:

- Focus on Chapter 17.

If you base your interventions on the contents of a single chapter and then find that the problems do not resolve quickly, you should stop what you are doing and finish reading the chapters suggested before you proceed any further.

COMMENT ON CASE HISTORIES

As in the first edition, many examples are presented using actual patient histories. Many new ones are included in this edition. Some of the original stories have been retained from the first edition, sometimes with modifications, with some of the names changed to fit contemporary usage. A few of the patients described are composites of several children; however, all descriptions are based on real patients.

Richard Ferber

PART I

YOUR CHILD'S SLEEP

CHAPTER I

At the End of Your Tether

The most frequent calls I receive at the Center for Pediatric Sleep Disorders at Children's Hospital Boston, USA, are from parents whose children are sleeping poorly. When the parent on the phone begins by saying, 'I am at the end of my tether' or 'We are at our wits' end', I can almost always predict what will be said next.

Typically, the couple or single parent has a young child (often their first) who is between five months and four years old. The child does not fall asleep readily at night or wakes repeatedly during the night, or both. The parents are tired, frustrated and often angry. Their own relationship has become tense, and they are wondering whether there is something inherently wrong with their child and whether they are unfit parents.

In most cases the parents have had lots of advice from friends, relatives and even their paediatrician on how to handle the situation. 'Let him cry; you're just spoiling him', they are told, or 'That's just a phase; wait until she outgrows it'. They don't want to wait, but they are beginning to wonder if they will have to, since despite all their efforts and strategies, the sleep problem persists. Often, the more the parents do to try and solve the problem, the worse it gets.

Sooner or later they ask themselves, 'How long do I let my child cry – *all night*?' And if the child gets up four, five or six times a night, 'Will this phase pass before we collapse from exhaustion?'

Everything seems pretty hopeless at first. If your child isn't sleeping well or has other problems that worry and frustrate you – such as sleep terrors, bed-wetting, nightmares or loud snoring – it won't take long for you to feel as if you're at the end of your tether, too.

Let me assure you that there is hope. With almost all of these children, we are able at least to reduce the sleep disturbance significantly, and usually we can eliminate the problem entirely. The information in this book will help you to identify the type and cause of your child's particular disturbance, and it will give you a variety of practical ways of solving the problem.

When a family visits the Sleep Center, I meet with the parents and child together and learn all I can about the child's problem. How often does it arise, and how long has it lasted? What are the episodes like? How do the parents handle the child at bedtime and during the night-time wakings? Is there a family history of sleep problems, and are there social factors that might be contributing to the problem? Given this detailed history, a physical examination and, in certain cases, laboratory study, it is usually possible to identify the disorder and its causes. At that point I can begin to work with the family to help them to solve their child's sleep problem.

At the Sleep Center, our methods of treatment for the 'sleepless child' rarely include medication. Instead, I work with the family to set up new schedules, routines and ways of handling their child. Often the child's biological rhythms may need normalising, or at least his sleep-wake schedule may need to be changed. He may have to learn to associate new conditions with falling asleep or get used to fewer and smaller night-time feedings. The family may have to learn how to set appropriate limits on the child's behaviour, and the child may need an incentive to co-operate. And any anxiety in the child (or parent) must be taken into account. I always negotiate the specifics of the plan with the family. It is important that they agree with the approach and feel confident that they will be able to follow through consistently. As much as possible, I offer choices. The *best* solution frequently differs considerably from family to family, and from one culture or social group to another. If the child is old enough, we include him in the negotiations. Thus, we use a consistent and firm but fair technique tailored to the particular sleep problem and to the needs and desires of the child and family.

Sleep problems are rarely the result of poor parenting. Nor (with a few exceptions) are they part of a 'normal phase' that must be waited (and waited, and waited) out. Finally, there is usually nothing physically or mentally wrong with the child himself. Most parents are immensely reassured to know that sleep problems are common in all types of family and social environments and that most children with such problems respond well to treatment.

In certain cases, such as in sleep apnoea or, less often, in bed-wetting, medical factors may be involved, and our intervention may include medication or surgery. Emotional factors may play a role in other instances, such as in the sleepiness of depression, recurrent nightmares in an anxious child, sleep terrors in the adolescent and extreme night-time fears. Here it is important to identify the source of these feelings and to deal with them satisfactorily so the sleep problems can resolve. Sometimes professional counselling is recommended.

How well your child sleeps from the early months affects not only his behaviour during the day but also your feelings about him. I have often heard parents say, 'He is such a good baby. We even have to wake him for feedings'. Although the parents are really just commenting on the baby's ability to sleep, they may start thinking that their baby is 'good' in the moral sense.

It is easy to see how this distinction can influence the way you relate to your child. If your child does not sleep well, he may well be making your life miserable. It isn't hard to think of such a child as a 'bad' baby. You will probably feel enormously frustrated, helpless, worried and angry if you have to listen to crying every night, get up repeatedly and lose a great deal of your own much-needed sleep. If your child's sleep disturbance is severe enough, your frustration and fatigue will carry over into your daytime activities, and you are bound to feel increasingly tense with your child, partner, family and friends. If this is the case in your home, you will be pleased to learn that your child is almost certainly capable of sleeping much better than he is now, letting you get a good night's sleep yourself. To make that happen, you need to learn how to identify your child's problem; then you can begin to solve it.

The case studies in this book are based on my experience at the Sleep Center. The discussions of these cases, along with descriptions of the underlying sleep disorders and explanations of the methods of solving them, will help you to identify, understand and deal with your own child's sleep problem.

Can a Child Just Be a 'Poor Sleeper'?

Parents often believe that if their child is a restless sleeper or can't seem to settle down at night, it's because he is by nature a poor sleeper or doesn't need as much sleep as other children of the same age. These beliefs are almost never true. Virtually all children without major medical or neurological disorders have the ability to sleep well. They can go to bed at an appropriate time, fall asleep within minutes and stay asleep until a reasonable hour in the morning. And while it is normal for a child (or an adult) to wake briefly a few times during the night, these arousals should last only a few seconds or minutes and the child should go back to sleep easily on his own.

In fact, the mistaken belief that your child is unable to sleep normally can have a strong influence on how his sleep pattern develops from the day you bring him home from hospital. I have seen many parents who were told by the nurse in the maternity unit, 'Your baby hardly sleeps at all. You're in for trouble!' Because parents like these are led to believe their child is a poor sleeper and there isn't anything they can do about it, they allow him to develop poor sleep habits; they don't think it is possible for him to develop good ones. As a result, the whole family suffers terribly. Yet almost all of these children are potentially fine sleepers, and with just a little intervention they can learn to sleep well.

It is true that children differ in their ability to sleep. Some children are excellent sleepers from birth. In the early weeks they may have to be wakened for feedings. As they grow older, not only do they continue to sleep well, but it becomes difficult to wake them even if one tries. They sleep soundly at night in a variety of situations: bright or dark, quiet or noisy, calm or chaotic. They can tolerate an occasional disruption of their sleep schedules, and they sleep well even during periods of emotional stress.

Other children seem inherently more susceptible to having their sleep patterns disrupted. Any change in bedtime routines – an illness, a hospitalisation or the presence of houseguests – can cause their sleep patterns to worsen. Even when these children have always been considered 'non-sleepers', we usually find that they, too, can sleep quite satisfactorily once we have made appropriate changes in their routines, schedules, surroundings or interactions within the family. Such children may still have occasional nights of poor sleep, but if the new routines are followed consistently, normal patterns will return quickly.

There are, of course, children who sleep very poorly for reasons we have as yet been unable to identify; however, these problems are extremely uncommon and account for only a tiny percentage of the children we see with difficulty sleeping. For these few, our usual behavioural treatments may help very little or not at all, and medication may even be required. If your child is up a great deal in the night, it may be tempting to assume that he is one of these genuinely poor sleepers. But that is almost certainly not the case. Such instances of truly poor sleep ability are quite rare among otherwise normal young children. In all probability your child's sleep problem can be solved. He almost certainly has a normal *inherent* ability to fall asleep and remain asleep. This is true even if he has a sleep disturbance such as sleepwalking or bed-wetting. These problems, occurring during sleep or partial waking, are sometimes bigger management challenges than is sleeplessness, but with the appropriate intervention, they too can usually be decreased significantly if not resolved completely.

How to Tell Whether Your Child
Has a Sleep Problem

If your child's sleep patterns cause a problem for you or for him, then he has a sleep problem, whether this problem is just an undesirable expression of normal function or a reflection of an actual underlying emotional or physical 'disorder' in the sense of a true psychological disturbance or a physiological abnormality of body function. Sometimes it is easy to see that such a problem exists. Other times sleep problems may be less obvious and easier to miss.

It is usually clear that a problem exists, for example, if your child commonly complains that he can't fall asleep, or if you find you must be up with him repeatedly during the night. In fact, the most common problems are easy to recognise. They are: frequent difficulty falling asleep at bedtime; waking during the night with an inability to go right back to sleep without parental support or intervention; waking too early or too late in the morning; falling asleep too early or too late in the evening; difficulty getting up for school or day care; and being excessively sleepy during the day. Sleep terrors, sleepwalking and bed-wetting are also readily apparent and quite easy to identify.

Your child could also have a sleep problem that you do not recognise. You may not be able to tell if your child routinely gets too little sleep at night to function normally during the day or if by sleeping late on weekend mornings he decreases his ability to learn during the week. You (and his teacher) may think that when he falls asleep every day in school and on the bus it is because he is bored or unmotivated; in fact, he may not be getting enough sleep, his sleep may be of poor quality or he may even have a disorder, such as narcolepsy, that leaves him unable to stay awake during the day no matter how much sleep he gets and regardless of his motivation. You may see him as lazy or irritable, not recognising that his behaviours are a reflection of poor sleep or of a sleep disorder. You may know he snores loudly every night, but not realise that the snoring is a sign that he might not be breathing satisfactorily, a problem that can interfere with his sleep and leave him overtired and irritable during the day.

It is important to remember that poor sleep affects daytime mood, behaviour and learning. At the same time, you should also know that sleep problems don't explain all daytime problems. If you don't know enough about normal sleep patterns, you may fail to recognise sleep problems as the cause of your child's behavioural or learning difficulties, or you may be tempted to blame these difficulties on poor sleep even when your child's sleep is perfectly 'normal'.

One of the least obvious problems of sleep is simply not getting enough of it. There is no absolute way to judge from numbers alone whether the amount of sleep your child gets per day is appropriate. Figure 1 on page 10 shows the average amount of sleep children get at various ages during the night and at nap times. Most children will fall within about one hour of the times on that chart. After the very early months, total sleep time per twenty-four-hour period drops to about eleven or twelve hours, diminishing only very gradually after that. The total amount of sleep differs surprisingly little among children, although the way they choose to distribute it may differ. One nine-month-old may sleep nine hours at night and take two solid ninety-minute naps. Another may sleep close to twelve hours at night and nap only briefly during the day.

Children should fall asleep quickly, sleep well at night, wake spontaneously (or at least easily) in the morning and nap only as appropriate for their age. If they do all these things and function well during the daytime, then they are probably getting enough sleep. If it's always hard to wake them, or if they sleep an extra hour or two on weekends, then they are almost certainly not getting enough sleep. This is especially likely if they also sleep inappropriately (or at least get very sleepy) during the day, or if their behaviour and ability to concentrate deteriorate markedly, typically in the mid- to late afternoon. But each child is different.

We can watch a child's behaviour during the day closely to see if he seems excessively sleepy or grumpy, but the symptoms of

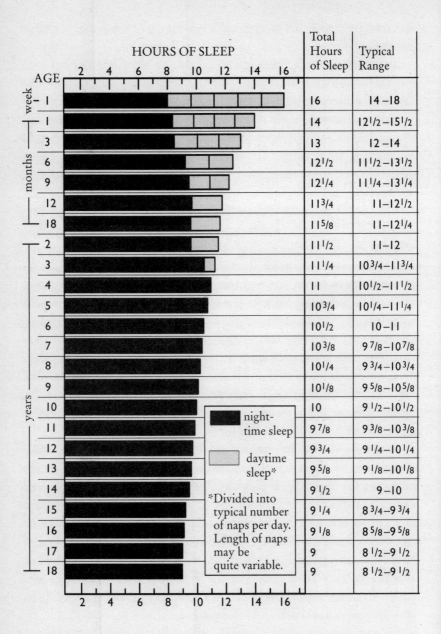

FIGURE 1. TYPICAL SLEEP REQUIREMENTS IN CHILDHOOD

AGE		Total Hours of Sleep	Night Sleep	Day Sleep	No. of Naps (¹/₂–2 Hrs)
week	1	16	Varied	Varied	Varied
months	1	14	Varied	Varied	Varied
	3	13	8 1/2	4 1/2	3 – 4
	6	12 1/2	9 1/4	3 1/4	2 – 3
	9	12 1/4	9 1/2	2 3/4	2
	12	11 3/4	9 1/4 – 10 1/4	1 1/2 – 2 1/2	1 – 2
	18	11 5/8	9 5/8	2	1
years	2	11 1/2	9 5/8	1 7/8	1
	3	11 1/4	9 3/4 – 11 1/4	0 – 1 1/2	0 – 1
	4	11	10 – 11	0 – 1	0 – 1
	5	10 3/4	10 3/4	0	0
	6	10 1/2	10 1/2	0	0
	7	10 3/8	10 3/8	0	0
	8	10 1/4	10 1/4	0	0
	9	10 1/8	10 1/8	0	0
	10	10	10	0	0
	11	9 7/8	9 7/8	0	0
	12	9 3/4	9 3/4	0	0
	13	9 5/8	9 5/8	0	0
	14	9 1/2	9 1/2	0	0
	15	9 1/4	9 1/4	0	0
	16	9 1/8	9 1/8	0	0
	17	9	9	0	0
	18	9	9	0	0

insufficient sleep in a young child can be very subtle. If your two-year-old sleeps only eight hours at night but seems happy and functions well during the day, it is tempting to assume he doesn't need more sleep. But eight hours is rarely enough sleep for a two-year-old. If you can find out why he sleeps so little and make appropriate changes, he will probably sleep an hour or two longer every night. You may begin to notice an improvement in his general behaviour, and only then will you be aware of the more subtle symptoms of inadequate sleep that were actually present before you adjusted his sleep schedule. Your child will probably be happier in the daytime, a bit less irritable, more able to concentrate at play and less inclined to have tantrums, accidents and arguments.

Adolescents almost never get enough sleep. Teenagers are not likely to wake spontaneously on school days, and they almost always sleep late on weekends (at least one hour later than on weekdays and often three to five hours later). When adolescents have the opportunity to sleep as much as they like every night, they average about nine to ten hours per night, and that is probably closer to the optimal level for their age.

Night-time wakings are another potential problem that can be difficult to recognise as 'abnormal'. A young child (between six months and three years old, say) may be getting adequate amounts of sleep at night even though he wakes several times during the night and has to be helped back to sleep. Parents say to me, 'Tell me if this is normal. If it is, I will continue getting up; but if it is not, then we would like to *do* something about it!' I assure them that most healthy full-term infants are sleeping through the night (which really means that they go back to sleep on their own after normal night-time wakings) by three or four months of age. Certainly by six months, all healthy babies can do so.

If your baby does not start sleeping through the night on his own by five or six months at the latest, or if he begins waking again after weeks or months of sleeping well, then something is interfering with the continuity of his sleep. He should be able to sleep better, and in all likelihood the disruption can be corrected.

STARTING WITH A BASIC UNDERSTANDING OF SLEEP

Before we begin to discuss specific problems and their solutions, you will need some background information about sleep itself, which is covered in Chapter 2. Although you don't need to be familiar with all the scientific research on sleep, it will be helpful for you to have some understanding of what sleep really is, how normal sleep patterns develop during childhood and what can go wrong. Then you will be better able to recognise abnormal patterns as they begin to develop, to correct problems that have become established and to prevent other problems from occurring.

Although the information on sleep in Chapter 2 is not overly technical, you may be eager to read the later chapters to learn about specific sleep disorders and their treatments. If that is the case, I suggest that you scan the next chapter first and then come back to read it more closely once you have identified your own child's sleep problem. Most people find the information interesting, and it is especially important for parents who want to help a child sleep better at night.

CHAPTER 2

What We Know About Sleep

Although our knowledge remains incomplete, a great deal has been discovered about what happens in the brain during sleep: what areas of the brain become active or quiescent, how cellular activity changes and which neurotransmitters (chemicals that carry signals between nerve cells) are released or blocked. Much has also been learned about the so-called biological clock, a small group of cells that keeps our sleep-wake cycle running on about a twenty-four-hour rhythm. This clock controls not only sleep but also variation in just about every other physiological system throughout the day. The cells that constitute it lie in a primitive area of the brain (the *hypothalamus*) that also controls many other important automatic functions such as hunger, thirst, temperature and hormone levels.

Nevertheless, we do not fully understand why we need to sleep, what causes us to sleep and what purposes sleep serves. There can be no single answer to these questions, in any case, because how you answer them depends on the level at which you approach sleep and waking. At the most basic level, that of neurophysiology, we can say we sleep (and wake) because of changes in the brain's chemical environment and in its cellular and electrical activity. On a

higher level, that of function and behaviour, we can say we sleep because sleep serves a restorative function for our bodies and perhaps
our minds. Sleep certainly is necessary for us to function properly
during the day: if we don't get enough of it we feel 'sleepy', and this
feeling can only be relieved by sleep. Finally, from an evolutionary
perspective, the purpose of sleep lies in the benefits it provides for
our survival. We can say, as various researchers have, that the purpose of sleep is to protect us from nocturnal predators, to rest the
body, to maximise our alertness during the day or to allow us to
process memories. If we turn the whole question round and ask,
'Why do we ever *stop* sleeping and wake up?' we could also answer
in terms of physiology (because of chemical and electrical changes
in the brain) or of function, behaviour and evolution (we need to be
awake to eat, procreate and care for our young).

Until the 1950s, doctors and other researchers believed that sleep
was a single state distinguishable only from waking. However, we
now know that sleep itself is divided into two distinctly different
states: REM (pronounced as a single word, 'rem'), or 'rapid-eye-
movement' sleep, and non-REM sleep. During non-REM sleep you
lie quietly, with a regular heart rate and breathing pattern; it is probably closest to what we usually think of as 'sleep', and it provides
most of sleep's restorative properties. There is very little dreaming
in this state, if any, although thought-like processes may continue.
In REM sleep physiological systems are much more active, and it is
in this state that we do nearly all of our dreaming. During the night
you cycle back and forth between periods of non-REM and REM
sleep as well as having the (usually brief) occasional waking.

NON-REM SLEEP

After the earliest months of life, non-REM sleep divides further into
four distinct stages. These stages range progressively from drowsiness to very deep sleep, and they can be identified in the laboratory
by monitoring brain waves, eye movements and muscle tone.

As you begin to fall asleep, you enter Stage I, the state of
drowsiness. Although you are unaware of it, your eyes move about

slowly under your closed eyelids. Your awareness of the external world begins to diminish as well. You have no doubt had the experience of becoming drowsy in a lecture or meeting. As you nod off, you miss some of the speaker's comments, yet you will jerk awake instantly if your name is called or if your head bends so far forward that you are about to fall off the chair. You might think you hadn't been asleep at all if it weren't for your lapse of awareness. On waking from this drowsy state, you might remember some thoughts of the kind usually described as 'daydreams.' Some people report seeing or hearing things more like the true dreams that occur during REM sleep, except that they are shorter, less well formed and less bizarre.

If you allow yourself to continue the transition through drowsiness toward deeper sleep, you may notice a sudden jerk of your whole body that actually wakes you briefly and interrupts your descent into sleep. This 'hypnagogic startle' is quite normal, although it does not happen every time we fall asleep.

Drowsiness really represents a transitional state between wakefulness and the more fully established stages of non-REM sleep, but we can only identify the arrival of the next stages for certain if we monitor the brain's electrical activity or 'brain waves'. At the onset of Stage II, short bursts of very rapid activity (called 'sleep spindles') and large, slow waves ('K-complexes') begin to appear (see Figure 2 on page 17). You can still be awakened easily from this stage, but you may not believe that you had really been asleep, depending on how long you had been in Stage II, how deep into this stage you were at the time of waking and, as always, on variations between individuals. As in a waking from Stage I, you would probably not report any odd dream images, but you might describe some thoughts or daydreams.

As you fall into still deeper sleep, you enter Stage III and finally Stage IV (similar stages that together can be thought of as your deep sleep). The smaller and faster brain waves of waking and light sleep disappear, replaced predominantly by large, slow 'delta' waves. Your breathing and heart rate become very regular, you may sweat profusely and you will be very difficult to wake. Someone calling

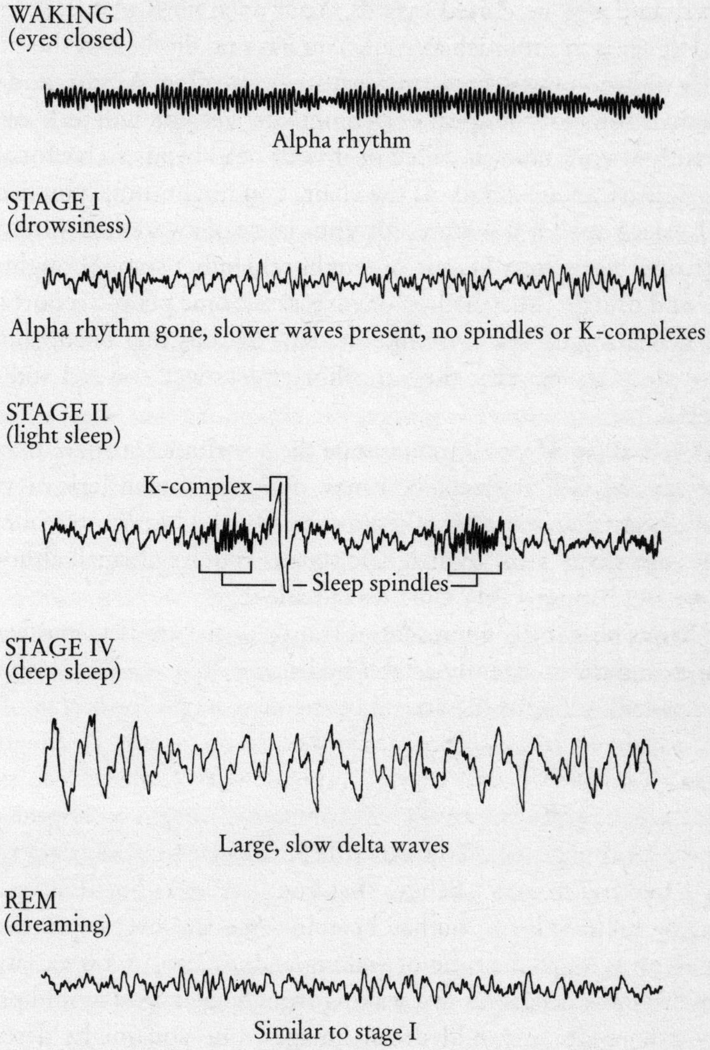

WAKING
(eyes closed)

Alpha rhythm

STAGE I
(drowsiness)

Alpha rhythm gone, slower waves present, no spindles or K-complexes

STAGE II
(light sleep)

K-complex

— Sleep spindles —

STAGE IV
(deep sleep)

Large, slow delta waves

REM
(dreaming)

Similar to stage I

FIGURE 2. BRAIN WAVE PATTERNS IN WAKING AND IN SLEEP

your name will no longer easily rouse you, as they would from Stage II sleep; instead, you may be oblivious to the sound.

However, if a stimulus is important enough, you will likely wake even from Stage IV. Apparently, even in the deepest sleep our minds can still process some outside information. For example, although it may be difficult to wake you when it is your turn to get up and feed the baby, shouts of 'Fire!' or a child's screams of pain will rouse you promptly. Yet even though you will wake in these emergencies, you will initially be confused. You may be aware that you need to take quick action, but you will have trouble 'clearing the cobwebs' from your head so that you can think clearly and sort out what to do. The difficulty one has making the transition from Stage IV sleep to alert waking is very significant in several sleep disorders in children, as you will learn when we discuss sleep terrors, confusional arousals and sleepwalking (Chapter 13).

In non-REM sleep your muscles are more relaxed than when you are awake. You are able to move (unlike in REM sleep, as we will see), but you lie still because your brain is not sending movement signals to most of your muscles. Disorders such as sleepwalking and sleep-associated head-banging are exceptions to this rule.

REM SLEEP

After one or two periods of non-REM sleep you cycle into REM sleep, a different state entirely. Breathing and heart rate become irregular. Your reflexes, kidney function and patterns of hormone release change. Your body's temperature regulation systems are impaired, so you do not sweat or shiver. Males have penile erections in this state; females undergo clitoral engorgement and an increase in vaginal blood flow. The significance of these genital changes is not known.

REM sleep is an active state. Your body uses more oxygen than it does in non-REM sleep, a sign that you are expending more energy. More blood flows to your brain, your brain's temperature increases and your brain waves become busy again, resembling a mixture of waking and drowsy patterns. The mind now 'wakes up', but the wakefulness of the dream state is quite unlike that of true waking: you respond mainly to signals originating within your own body instead of those coming from the world about you, and you accept without question the bizarre nature of your dreams.

In this state your muscles have very poor tone, especially in the head and neck, and you become profoundly relaxed. Most nerve impulses that would otherwise pass down the spinal cord and out to the muscles are blocked within the spinal cord, so that not only are your muscles relaxed but much of your body is effectively paralysed: signals to move may still be sent out from your brain, but they do not reach your muscles. Only the muscles controlling eye movements, respiration and hearing are spared. Because this blockade is not complete, some of the stronger signals still get through to the muscles, causing frequent small twitches of the hands, legs or face. So although REM sleep is very active in terms of metabolic and brain function, you remain fairly still.

(In babies, the blockade of motor impulses is not fully developed: more impulses get through to the muscles than in an older child or adult. As a result, a young infant in REM sleep will jerk, grimace, twitch, kick and even make sounds. Of course, a newborn cannot get up, walk around and get into trouble. The inhibitory system and the baby mature together, so that by six to twelve months of age – that is, by the time the baby can crawl or walk – most motor impulses are blocked and she stays safely in place.)

The most striking feature of REM sleep is its characteristic bursts of rapid eye movements. During these bursts, the heart rate, blood pressure, respiratory rate and blood flow to the brain all increase and fluctuate irregularly. If you are awakened during one of these bursts, you will almost certainly report that you were having a dream, and the length of the dream you describe will correspond roughly to the time you had been in that state. Children as young as two have described dreams after such wakings. As for younger children, who lack sufficient language to describe dreams, we cannot know for certain that they do dream or what they dream about. However, since all the other features of REM sleep are in place at birth, it is reasonable to presume that even newborns dream. The first dreams are probably very simple repetitions of daily experiences (sounds, smells, sights); dreams then become more and more complex as higher brain centres and language develop.

We cannot say for sure whether your pattern of eye movements indicates that you were actually 'watching' your dream occur. We suspect that this is partly true and that at least some of the muscle-twitching corresponds to the actions taking place in the dream. Fortunately, because only a few of the signals to move actually reach your muscles, you merely twitch a little now and then, rather than getting up and moving about, dangerously acting out a dream. One thing this tells us is that sleepwalking and sleep terrors do not result from dreams or nightmares: such complex body movements simply cannot occur during REM sleep.

Some researchers believe that REM sleep has important psychological functions. Their research suggests that REM dreaming allows us to process daytime emotional experiences and transfer recent memories into longer-term storage. Such theories remain unproven. Certainly dreams have emotional significance, but their ultimate importance to the dreamer remains a mystery. REM sleep must serve some purpose, since we all dream every night – even those of us who think we don't – and if we are deprived of REM sleep for several nights in a row we compensate by getting more REM sleep than usual the next night. Yet, when people are deprived of most of their REM sleep for long periods of time, as a side effect of medication, for example, they don't seem to show any major ill effects. (Humans cannot be totally deprived of REM sleep, at least not easily. Such studies have been done in animals; complete elimination of REM sleep led to withering and even death.)

Waking a person from REM sleep can be easy or difficult, depending on how important the waking stimulus is to her and how involved she is in her dream. So the clock-radio may not wake you immediately from a really interesting dream; you may even incorporate something you hear on the radio into your dream. On the other hand, an important stimulus such as a burglar alarm will wake you easily and, unlike someone awakened from Stage IV sleep, you will become alert quickly.

To sum up, we seem to live in three distinct states. In the waking state we are rational and we can take care of ourselves and meet our survival needs. In non-REM sleep the body rests and restores itself while the mind rests. And in REM sleep the mind is again active, but it is not rational and it is 'disconnected' from the body; major body movements do not take place even though the brain does send out signals to move.

One theory suggests that over the course of evolution REM sleep developed as an intermediate state between non-REM and waking, in which the mind would 'wake up' before being 'connected' to the body. An animal in non-REM sleep, lying quiet and still except for soft regular breathing, would be relatively safe from predators, but a sudden waking would leave the animal physically active yet confused and disorientated, and thus vulnerable to attack. An animal that first switched into REM sleep would become more alert, but with its brain still disconnected from its muscles it could not make any movement or sound that might alert a predator. Once it was sufficiently alert, the animal could wake fully; the muscle paralysis would disappear, and it could react appropriately to danger. This capacity to check for danger may still be important to humans. We all tend to wake up briefly after an episode of dreaming, and at that moment we are sensitive to anything amiss in our environment: the smell of smoke, footsteps downstairs or quiet sobbing from the next room. If all seems well, we simply return to sleep, and in the morning we probably won't remember waking up at all. Young children often cannot return to sleep quickly after these normal arousals because something seems 'wrong' to them – in one typical situation, it feels 'wrong' that they are alone in their cot instead of in a parent's arms. This common problem is discussed in detail in Chapter 4.

How Sleep Stages Develop in Children

Sleep patterns begin to develop in babies even before birth. REM sleep appears in the foetus at about six or seven months' gestation, and non-REM sleep follows a month or so later. In the foetus and infant, REM sleep is referred to as 'active sleep' and non-REM as 'quiet sleep'. By the end of the eighth month of gestation, both states are well established.

In the newborn, active sleep is easy to identify because the baby twitches and breathes irregularly and you can see her eyes dart about under her thin eyelids. Sometimes you may also see her smile briefly. In quiet sleep she breathes deeply and lies very still; occasionally you may see fast sucking motions, and now and then a sudden body jerk or 'startle'.

Quiet sleep is still somewhat different from the non-REM sleep of older children and adults. For one thing, it is undifferentiated: the division into separate, distinguishable stages comes later. The brain waves in quiet sleep show large slow waves occurring in bursts rather than in a continuous flow. During the first month of life the non-REM brain waves become continuous and startles disappear. By the time a baby is a month old, sleep spindles begin to appear, and over the next month or two we can begin to separate non-REM sleep into lighter and deeper stages. K-complex waves (see Figure 2), characteristic of mature non-REM sleep, do not appear until a baby is about six months old, although precursors appear earlier.

REM sleep is the earliest stage to form. Premature babies spend 80 per cent of their sleep time in this state; in full-term infants it makes up half of their sleep. We do not fully understand why REM sleep is so prominent in the early stages of development. We do know that quiet sleep requires a certain degree of brain maturation, so one would expect to see less of that stage in newborns. In REM sleep, the higher centres of the brain receive stimulation from deeper, more primitive areas. Impulses come up the same sensory pathways that are used for sight and sound, and perhaps touch, smell and taste. Later on, such stimuli are probably incorporated by the brain into dream imagery. While we can know nothing of infants' 'dreams', this state might allow the baby's developing brain to receive sensory input – to 'see' and to 'hear' – even before birth. This input might be important to the development of the higher brain centres.

We also know that the baby in the uterus makes no breathing

motions in non-REM sleep. If respiratory movements were never practised, the child would be born with no experience at all in using these muscles that are so vital to survival. However, respiratory motions *do* occur in REM sleep, and it may be that the baby is also practising other kinds of motor activity. Muscular impulses in a foetus are not blocked as completely as they are in children and adults, so the foetus has some ability to practise actual body movements in REM sleep. Fortunately for the mother, there is still *some* blockage of motor impulses during REM sleep, or the baby might never be still!

It may be, then, that REM sleep is most important in the early months as the foetus and baby develops, and progressively less so with increasing age. In fact, although at birth a full-term baby spends half of her sleep time in the REM state, only one-third of her sleep will be REM by age three, and she will reach the adult level of 25 per cent by later childhood or adolescence.

CHILDREN'S SLEEP CYCLES

During a period of sleep, children (and adults) cycle back and forth between REM and non-REM sleep. Once non-REM sleep has developed four distinct stages and most of the baby's sleep time has consolidated into a single night-time sleep period, the sequence of sleep stages settles into a cyclical pattern that remains fairly constant throughout life. It is important to know something about these sleep cycles if you are to understand the development of normal sleep patterns in your child and the nature of any sleep problems that may occur.

As a child grows from a newborn to an adolescent, the length of the sleep cycle increases from fifty to ninety minutes; also, the total amount of REM sleep and the percentage of sleep time spent in REM decrease until they too reach adult values. The total amount of Stage IV non-REM sleep also decreases throughout childhood and adolescence as total sleep decreases, but it continues to account for about a quarter of the child's total sleep.

A newborn enters REM sleep immediately after falling asleep.

By about three months of age she will enter non-REM first, a pattern that will continue for the rest of her life. Unlike adults, who achieve deep sleep only gradually at the start of the night, young children usually plunge through drowsiness and the lighter stages of non-REM sleep into Stage IV within a few minutes (see Figure 3 on page 25). In youngsters Stage IV is an extremely deep sleep, and waking a child from that stage may be almost impossible. For example, if your child falls into Stage IV sleep at night in the car, you can probably carry her into the house, change her into her pyjamas and put her in bed with only the slightest sign of movement or arousal. Even a child who always seems to wake when put into her cot after being rocked to sleep will remain asleep as long as she is not placed into the cot until she has reached Stage IV. And if you wake your child from Stage IV sleep to go to the toilet, she may do so in a semi-awake state and then return to sleep instantly without any recollection of the arousal in the morning. This partial arousal is very similar to what happens during sleepwalking and sleep terrors (see Chapter 13).

A child remains in Stage IV for about an hour or two. After that she undergoes a brief arousal. This partial waking may last for only a few seconds or up to several minutes. Her brain waves change abruptly, showing a mixture of patterns from deep sleep, light sleep, drowsiness and waking. She will probably move about, perhaps rubbing her face, chewing, turning over, crying a little or speaking unintelligibly. She may even open her eyes for a moment with a blank stare or sit up briefly before returning to sleep. Occasionally, and briefly, she may even wake fully before the progression of sleep stages continues.

There is actually a spectrum of behaviours that can occur during these arousals. The mild ones just described are quite normal. More dramatic behaviours may also occur at these times, including sleepwalking, sleep terrors and confused thrashing. These events all occur during partial waking from deep non-REM sleep, and in all of them the child shows features of both sleeping and waking at the same time. We will discuss these behaviours at length in later chapters, but for now remember that they are *not* stimulated by a dream.

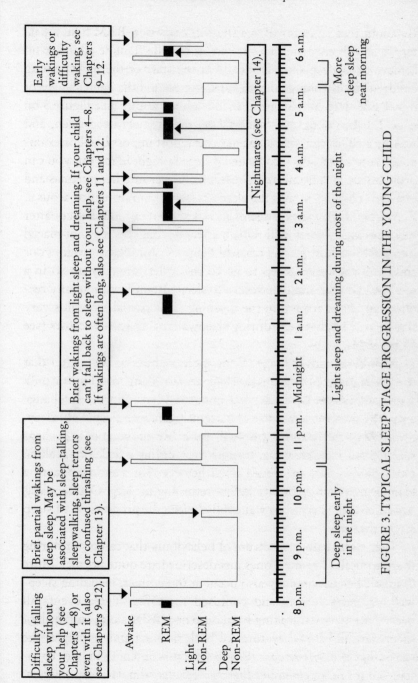

FIGURE 3. TYPICAL SLEEP STAGE PROGRESSION IN THE YOUNG CHILD

As noted above, true dreams, including nightmares, occur only during the REM state.

After the brief arousal, there follows a period of a few minutes resembling drowsiness or, perhaps, the beginnings of REM sleep. There may actually be a short REM episode at this point, especially in adolescents and adults, but young children tend to skip it. The first REM episode, whenever it appears, tends to be relatively short – five to ten minutes – and not very intense. There are not many eye movements, and the child's breathing and heart rates remain fairly stable.

Following this episode of REM or 'almost-REM', the child enters another cycle of deep non-REM sleep. In young children, the descent back into Stage IV sleep will probably be quite rapid, although not as rapid as it was in the first cycle. This period of deep sleep lasts between thirty minutes and two hours (depending, somewhat, on the child's age), and the arousal that follows it marks the end of the deep sleep period that characterises the first third of the night. Thus, in children, the first three or four hours of the night are spent mainly in very deep sleep from which the child is not easily roused. Parents are often aware of this fact, because the period of lighter sleep that follows, with more frequent wakings, may well begin at about the time they are going to sleep themselves.

The arousal that ends the initial three or four hours of deep sleep will almost certainly be followed by a REM episode lasting five to twenty minutes. This period of REM sleep may be interrupted by several brief wakings, each followed by a rapid return to sleep. (In babies, REM sleep is particularly unstable, interrupted fairly frequently by brief movements and wakings; however, by the time the baby is around six months old, the inhibition of motor activity is more complete and REM sleep becomes more continuous.)

The REM episode ends with another brief arousal, and the child moves about, adjusts her position, subconsciously checks to see that everything is normal, then goes back to sleep. This momentary awakening has several functions. Changing position is important for the health of skin, muscles and joints, and the child can check to see that things are the same as when she went to sleep. It is important to be aware that these wakings occur in all children and adults and are quite normal. Parents often perceive them as abnormal, especially if the child cannot return to sleep afterwards because the conditions she associates with falling asleep – such as being rocked or patted – are no longer present. This problem of sleep associations will be discussed more fully in Chapter 4.

The middle part of the night, after the first REM episode, begins with another period of non-REM sleep followed by another arousal and a longer and more intense REM episode. Throughout this part of the night, usually lasting about four hours, the child alternates between progressively longer and more intense periods of REM and relatively light periods of non-REM sleep. It is during these hours of light sleep, particularly at the transitions between REM and non-REM sleep, that wakings are most common. Normally these wakings are brief, but it is also at these times that problems of sleeplessness tend to be most severe. Even adolescents and adults may notice that they seem to wake more easily in the middle of the night (to go to the toilet, perhaps) than they do in the morning when their alarm goes off for the day (see Chapter 9). Some children who are kept in bed too long at night sleep only at the beginning and the end, and this middle period of light sleep becomes one of full waking (see Chapter 11).

As morning approaches, children descend once more into fairly deep Stage IV sleep before the final waking; thus the last one or two hours of the night are often quiet, regardless of what came before. Children who tend to wake for the day directly out of this Stage IV period may seem to wake unhappy or crying every morning. The crankiness usually lasts only about ten minutes, and although it may seem worrisome, it is not a cause for concern. Other children, who re-enter lighter Stage II or REM sleep before waking, are more likely to wake in good spirits. There is nothing you can do to change the sleep state out of which a child wakes spontaneously.

The very deep sleep that children experience at the end of the night is uncommon at older ages. This isn't because the capacity for such sleep is lost, but because adults rarely sleep long enough to allow it to emerge. An adult who sleeps eleven hours or so, or an adolescent who sleeps late at the weekend, may show the same end-of-the-night deep sleep typical of young children. A need for deep sleep built up during the day presumably explains why there is deep sleep at the start of the night, but it does not explain why there is more deep sleep at the end. The return to deep sleep near morning is an inherent feature of our sleep cycling system, one controlled by our biological clock (see Chapter 9).

This overview should give you an idea of what is actually happening to your child during the different stages of sleep during the night. It will also help you decide what state your child is in, based on when she fell asleep and what her sleep behaviour is like at a given time. These observations will be important as you try to understand what sort of sleep problem your child has and how to deal with it.

SLEEP AND WAKING PATTERNS

As you read through this section, keep in mind that the sleep requirements described are only approximate and are not the same for all children.

A newborn baby sleeps about sixteen hours a day, but for no more than a few hours at a time. She goes through about seven sleeping and waking periods distributed fairly evenly throughout the day and night. These episodes, which vary from twenty minutes to five or six hours in length, begin with a period of REM sleep, and, depending on the length of the sleep time, they show several REM/non-REM cycles. Even when your baby sleeps well for a few hours, you can usually observe brief arousals. In the early weeks there may seem to be no pattern to the sleep cycle – shorter and longer periods of sleep and waking are scattered over each twenty-four-hour period and vary from day to day.

When the baby is around three months old, daytime sleep settles into a three-nap pattern, with the main naps in the mid-morning and mid-afternoon and, generally, a brief nap in the early evening. (Naps are further discussed overleaf and in Chapter 12.) By the age of three or four months, your baby still sleeps about thirteen hours a day, but now her sleep pattern has consolidated into about four or five regular and predictable sleep periods, with two-thirds of her sleep occurring at night. By now there should be a clear and appropriate differentiation between day and night. At this age most infants have 'settled', which means they are now sleeping through most of the night, at least from a feeding late at night to one in the early morning.

By six months almost all infants have settled, and the periods of continuous night-time sleep have grown longer. The pattern of settling varies with each child, of course, and your baby's night-time wakings may diminish very gradually, or she may settle quickly, as if suddenly forgetting the remaining night-time feedings. Some babies settle very erratically. In any case, at some point between three and six months, your baby should be sleeping well at night. A typical six-month-old baby sleeps about twelve or thirteen hours in total. Night-time sleep typically lasts about nine and a quarter hours (and as long as eleven hours if daytime naps are short) with only occasional brief wakings. In addition, she will take two one- to two-hour naps each day, one in mid-morning and a second in the afternoon. (The evening nap is usually dropped at around this age.) On most schedules, the morning nap will start between 9.30 and 10.30 a.m., and the afternoon nap between 2.00 and 3.00 p.m.

At one year, most children are still sleeping close to twelve hours, with nine or ten of these hours occurring at night. Most youngsters give up their morning nap at this point or within a few months. The single nap that remains generally follows lunch and occurs at 12.30 or 1.00 p.m., between the times where the two naps had previously been. At the transition to a single-nap schedule you may see other, related changes. Since the child now stays awake for longer stretches, sleep may come more easily both at nap time and at night. (This is often particularly noticeable if there were problems before.) Also, although the second nap may have been dropped, total sleep time generally does not change: either the remaining nap or the night-time sleep lengthens.

By age two, your child should still sleep about nine to ten hours at night, with a one- to two-hour nap after lunch – about eleven and a half hours in total. She will probably continue her afternoon nap until at least age three; some children stop by age two, and others continue napping up to age five. The dropping of the final nap is the least predictable of all the developmental changes in napping in the first five years. However, most children stop napping somewhere between their third and fourth birthdays. Those who tend to sleep longer at night, perhaps eleven hours, may simply not be able to sleep during the day. A child who develops this sleep pattern too early may not make it through the day functioning well. Cutting back that child's night-time sleep to nine or ten hours may allow the nap to re-emerge (see Chapter 12). Some children continue napping when the circumstances are especially conducive to sleep (for example, in the car) or at day care or nursery (where there is strong pressure to lie quietly during a prescribed rest period) but refuse to nap at home or at the weekends.

From age three to adolescence, children need gradually less and less sleep, but the decrease is smaller and far more gradual than was previously thought. Once children are past the toddler age they rarely nap, and they slowly begin to sleep less at night, dropping from about eleven hours in the nursery years to about ten hours in preadolescence. The years from five to twelve years of age are really the most wakeful in a child's life. Children between those ages generally sleep well at night and 'wake well' during the day. The ability to nap in the afternoon is mostly lost (even in siesta cultures); occasional naps may suggest illness. A child who naps most days, especially in school, may have a sleep disorder such as narcolepsy (but, as discussed in Chapter 18, even narcoleptic children at this age may only nap occasionally). Chronic sleep loss at night can cause napping, but that pattern is unusual in the school-aged child; instead, the more common consequence of insufficient sleep is behavioural change during the day.

During the four years of puberty rapid changes occur in the child's body, but the total sleep requirement stays about the same. Children aged fourteen to seventeen still need at least nine hours of sleep for optimal functioning, but few actually get that much, at least on school nights.

Remember, sleep requirements vary among children and families.

However, if your child is getting one to two hours more or less sleep than the amount shown for her age in Figure 1 on page 10, you should at least suspect that her sleep may need adjustment. I hope that the remaining chapters will help you to decide whether she has a problem and, if she does, to identify the cause and correct it.

The Importance of Biological Rhythms

To understand certain childhood sleep problems, we need to look beyond the sleep patterns themselves to the biological systems that control them. The term *circadian rhythms* refers to biological cycles that repeat about every twenty-four hours. All of us have many such rhythms. They include patterns of sleeping and waking, activity and rest, and hunger and eating, as well as fluctuations in body temperature and hormone-release. These cycles must be in harmony if we are to have a sense of well-being during the day. Our ability to fall asleep and stay asleep is closely tied to the timing of these cycles. Typically we fall asleep as our body temperature is dropping towards a daily minimum, and we wake up as it starts rising towards a peak. If we have to wake up at a time when our temperature level is low, we do so only with great difficulty. Similarly, we have trouble falling asleep when our body temperature is still high and has not yet begun to fall.

It is important to know that, in all of us, these cycles are inherently somewhat longer than twenty-four hours. The difference is a matter of only a few minutes. However, exposure to artificial light in the evening, after sunset, and to artificial darkness in our bedrooms in the morning, after sunrise, makes the internal clock run still slower, functioning as if its inherent cycle length were closer to twenty-five hours. We re-set the clock's timing each day through exposure to light in the morning and darkness at night. However, at weekends or on holiday, when our schedules are more flexible, many of us begin to operate on this twenty-five-hour day: we go to bed later and get up later. Then we have great difficulty re-adjusting to the earlier schedule when we return to work or school. This problem, called a *sleep phase delay,* is discussed in Chapter 10.

Although it is not difficult for us to stay on a twenty-four-hour cycle if we keep to it regularly, problems arise when our routines are irregular or when we try to sleep at times that conflict with our sleep-wake rhythms. Shift workers and adolescents, both of whom tend to sleep different hours at weekdays and weekends, as well as people who travel across time zones, all suffer the malaise, sleep difficulties and lack of well-being commonly referred to as 'jet lag'.

So do children whose sleep cycles have been disrupted or shifted or whose sleep schedules are variable, inconsistent or otherwise inappropriate. These children may sleep poorly at night, and they may be sleepy or behave badly during the day. It is important to understand this effect, because treatments for problems related to sleep schedule abnormalities are very different from those for other sleep disorders. Besides, even when sleep schedule abnormalities are not the primary problem, their existence often complicates other sleep problems and must be taken into consideration when planning treatment.

The biological rhythms controlling sleep, the ways they can be affected by inappropriate sleep schedules, the various sleep problems that can result and the ways these sleep problems can be treated are discussed in greater detail in Chapters 9 through 12. For now, remember that normal circadian rhythm function is necessary for normal sleep and optimal daytime function and that many abnormalities having to do with circadian rhythms are quite simple to identify and correct.

CHAPTER 3

Helping Your Child to Develop Good Sleep Practices

We all have our own ways of interacting with our children at sleep times as well as different means of shaping their sleep habits. These differences occur among families, ethnic groups and cultures. The sleeping child may be swaddled, lightly clothed or naked; he may sleep in his own room or share a room with brothers and sisters, or the entire family may sleep in a single room, even in the same bed. The child may sleep on his stomach, side or back, in a room that is dark, dimly lit or brightly illuminated. It may be quiet, or there may be noise: constant sounds from a humidifier or air conditioner; intermittent sounds from a radio, television or traffic outside; or occasional noises from aeroplanes, sirens and other children. He may fall asleep nursing at the breast, sucking on a bottle or dummy, rocking in a chair or lying alone in bed. He may say good night downstairs and go to bed by himself, or fall asleep only after having a story read to him, saying his prayers, playing a quiet game or discussing the day's events. A child may go to bed at different times every night with no set routine, or he may follow exactly the same routine each night.

Considerable variation among routines exists, but not all routines work equally well.

THE IMPORTANCE OF YOUR CHILD'S BEDTIME ROUTINES

Although I do believe some bedtime rituals are better than others, there are few absolute rules regarding sleep behaviour. If your routine is working – if you and your child are happy with it, if he falls asleep easily and night wakings are infrequent, if he is getting enough sleep and if his daytime behaviour is appropriate – then whatever you are doing is probably fine.

However, it is important to keep in mind that some routines and approaches are more likely to help your child to develop good sleep patterns now and avoid problems as he gets older. For example, if you are in the habit of rocking your child to sleep (or rubbing his back, or any similar custom) for twenty to thirty minutes each night, and you need to repeat the ritual once or twice in the middle of the night to get him back to sleep, you may actually be interfering with his sleep and delaying his ability to sleep through the night. Even if you 'don't mind' waking up, I suspect you would be happier if you could simply put him down easily at bedtime and have him sleep through the night as well. Whether or not you mind having your own sleep disrupted, you should still be aware that it is in your child's best interests to sleep through the night without interruptions. The kinds of bedtime ritual and routine to consider include all the activities that take place as your child prepares for bed and while he falls asleep. If he is an infant, you probably change his nappy and then hold him until he falls asleep. Perhaps you rock him and nurse him until sleep comes, then move him to the cradle, cot or bed. Or your infant may still be awake when you put him down, so that he falls asleep on his own. Generally any one of these patterns is fine in the first few months, when you cannot expect your baby to sleep through the night anyway. But by about three months of age most full-term healthy infants are able to sleep through most of the night. If your baby still has more than one or two nightly wakings at that age, or if he still hasn't 'settled' (started sleeping through the entire night) by five or six months, then you should take a close look at his bedtime routines. If your child is always nursed or rocked to sleep, he may have difficulty going back to sleep alone after normal night-time arousals. To help him sleep better at night, you may have to change some of his routines. For instance, it is very important for some children to be put down awake so that they can learn to settle themselves and fall asleep alone both at bedtime and after night-time wakings (see Chapter 4).

As your child gets older, bedtime routines remain important. If bedtime is pleasant, your child will look forward to it instead of becoming fussy when the time approaches. Bedtime rituals differ, of course, and you should choose a routine that suits your family, but make sure you always allow enough time to spend with your child each night. Follow the routine as consistently as you can. Your child should know when he has to change into his pyjamas, brush his teeth and go to bed. He should know what bedtime activities are planned and how much time will be spent on them, or how many stories will be read.

Bedtime is often a time of separation that can be difficult for many children, especially young ones. Simply sending a toddler or young child off to bed alone is not fair to him, and he may even find it scary. It also means you will miss out on what could be one of the best times of the day. So set aside ten to thirty minutes to do something special with your child before bed. The final routine should take place in the room where your child sleeps so he will learn to look forward to going there. If it takes place elsewhere, then he'll learn that he must leave that pleasant place to go to bed, and the bed or bedroom can take on negative associations, signalling the end of that happy interactive period and perhaps the start of a separation. If a child is to fall asleep alone, it should be the parents who leave: he should stay where he just had an enjoyable time. Avoid teasing, scary stories and anything else that will excite your child at this time – save the wrestling and tussling for other times of the day. You might both enjoy a discussion, quiet play or story-reading.

But let your child know that your special time together will not extend beyond the time you have agreed on and then stick to those limits. It's a good idea to tell your child when the time is almost up or when you have only two or three more pages to read. Don't give in to demands for an extra story: your child will learn the rules only if you enforce them. If both you and he know exactly what is going to happen, you'll avoid the arguments and tension that can arise when there is uncertainty (see Chapter 5).

Paul is a four-year-old boy. His father leaves for work early in the morning and doesn't see Paul until dinner-time. He likes to be the one to put his son to bed; if he weren't, the two would not have any time together until the weekend. So the period from seven o'clock to 8.00 each night is special for both of them.

At seven, they play together with Paul's racing cars or Lego set for about twenty-five minutes; in warm weather they sometimes play outside. Paul's father tells him when it is about 7.25, and then the bedtime routine begins. Paul has a bath and his father helps him to put on his pyjamas. Often they read a pleasant children's novel, one chapter each night. Both Paul and his father look forward to the night's reading, and Paul enjoys the bedtime routine rather than resisting it. Paul's father warns him when only a few pages remain in the chapter. When the reading is over for the evening, the light goes off and the night light is turned on. Paul kisses his father good night, curls up with his stuffed monkey, lets his father leave the room and goes to sleep.

In later years, your child will still appreciate having some time with you before he goes to sleep. He needs close, warm, personal time, something that simply watching television together, for instance, will not provide: even if the shows are not exciting or scary – which is unlikely – and even if you are sitting next to him, the lack of direct personal interaction makes this bedtime routine a poor one. Instead, use the time to discuss school events, plans for the weekend, football, dance class, after-school programmes or music lessons. It might also be helpful to talk about any worries your child may have, so he will be less likely to brood over them in bed. (Use common sense, however: in some cases, it may be better to have that discussion during the day, to avoid giving him something new to worry about at bedtime.) As your child gets older, you can begin to vary the bedtime ritual from night to night. Some nights you may enjoy a walk outside, a trip for ice cream, a board game, ping-pong (if it isn't too exciting) or helping with homework.

An eleven- or twelve-year-old may already want privacy as he readies himself for bed: he may want to read, listen to music or spend time on a hobby before he turns out the light. But do stop in to say good night and chat for a while. A final routine before bed is still important, even though he can now handle everything himself. He should see that you still enjoy that time with him, that you remain available to help with problems or concerns and that ultimately you are still the one in charge, preventing his routines from going too long or otherwise becoming inappropriate.

Emily, eleven, has a good bedtime routine. After dinner she finishes her homework, practises piano and sometimes calls a friend on the telephone. She and her mother, a single parent, then spend some time together. They like to build things – a birdhouse or a picture frame – and they are currently working on a giant jigsaw puzzle. While they work, they get a chance to talk. At about nine o'clock, Emily changes for bed and begins to read while listening to music. Her mother stops in for a few minutes to discuss plans for the next day, and at 9.30 Emily turns off the light and the stereo and goes to sleep.

Of course, not all nights in Paul's and Emily's homes are quiet and pleasant, but most are, and major disruptions at bedtime are rare. If bedtimes in your home are usually unpleasant and full of struggle, the solution may be to establish more pleasant and consistent routines. At first that may not seem easy to do, and your child may resist for a while. But if you persist, both you and your child will grow to enjoy the bedtime routines, and the struggles will be over. It is certainly worth the effort.

'BACK TO SLEEP': REDUCING THE RISK OF SIDS

Because of the relationship between sudden death in infants and features of sleep position and environment, this chapter's discussion of good sleep practices must include a discussion of sudden infant death syndrome, or SIDS, and related conditions. SIDS, also know as cot death, is the most common cause of death in babies between one month and twelve months old. The term SIDS is defined as the sudden death of an infant younger than one year of age that remains unexplained despite thorough medical investigation. We presume that breathing stops (although we don't know why), and eventually so does the heart. Nine out of ten cases occur in the first six months, with a peak between two and four months. Although no single cause has yet been determined, we do know of some practices and circumstances that can affect the level of risk. Among the factors known to increase the risk of SIDS are late or nonexistent pre-natal care, prematurity and low birth weight and maternal smoking during pregnancy. Some ethnic groups are particularly vulnerable, and boys are affected more often than girls. Some studies suggest that breastfeeding offers some protection against SIDS, but the effect is slight if it is even present at all; not all studies confirm this finding – although most agree that breast-feeding is beneficial for other reasons – and the apparent effect, when present, may be due to other factors such as less smoking among women who breastfeed.

Sleeping in the prone (face-down) position, however, has been shown to increase risk significantly. So, unless your doctor specifically tells you to do otherwise, always place your baby on his back to sleep. Placing him on his side is better than face-down, but it is best for him to lie on his back. The Foundation for the Study of Infant Deaths (FSID) along with the Department of Health established their 'Reduce the Risk of Cot Death' campaign in the UK in 1991 (and, in the United States, the American Academy of Pediatrics, along with other groups, began their 'Back to Sleep' campaign in 1994). Since then the proportion of infants in these locations sleeping face-down has decreased dramatically and the incidence of SIDS has decreased by more than 70% in the UK (and more than 40% in the US) – a truly dramatic improvement for such a simple change.

At first, some parents and paediatricians feared that babies who slept on their back might choke if they vomited, but this has proved not to be a problem. A temporary flattening of the back of the head can occur, particularly if the child always sleeps with his head in the same position. To avoid it, place the baby's head so that he sometimes faces a little one way and sometimes a little the other, and turn the baby or cot so that the door or light is not always in the same direction. In any case, SIDS is a much more serious risk, and this flattening is generally harmless and usually corrects itself over time.

Supine positioning is only important when the baby is asleep. During the daytime while awake, prone periods ('tummy time') and periods held upright ('cuddle time', as opposed to excessive time in car seats and 'bouncers') are important for upper-body motor development and to further avoid flattening of the back of the head.

By around five or six months of age, most babies can turn from their backs to their stomachs (they should have learned to turn from their stomachs to their backs a few weeks earlier). After this point, you can no longer assure supine sleep, but by this time the risk of SIDS is low anyway.

Other aspects of the infant's sleep environment can also pose a risk to the baby. It's dangerous to allow a baby to sleep on a surface not designed for infant sleep, especially extremely soft ones – a soft chair or sofa, a waterbed, a pillow, a duvet, a quilt or a sheepskin. Such soft surfaces under a baby, or loosely tucked-in bedding over a baby, pose a risk of suffocation. Poorly chosen places for the infant to sleep can create a risk of *entrapment*, in which the baby's face is caught between a mattress and a wall or bed frame, or between cushions. Sleeping together with a parent, particularly one who is overweight or whose own ability to wake is impaired by drugs or alcohol, not only increases the risk of entrapment against the parent but also adds the danger of 'overlying', where the sleeping parent rolls on top of the infant. The more people in bed with the infant, the less room there is for the baby and the greater the risk. Improper bed surfaces and bedding, bed placement and adjacent walls and furniture, common in a parent's bedroom, may increase the risk further.

Cigarette-smoking in the home, especially in the same room as the baby, can double or triple the likelihood of death from SIDS.

Overheating, another risk factor, can be avoided by clothing the infant properly for sleep, keeping the room temperature at a level comfortable for a lightly clothed adult and avoiding inappropriate bedding. If a baby is clothed properly and the room kept at a comfortable temperature, blankets can often be avoided altogether. 'Overbundling' in clothes and bedding, and subsequent overheating, may be one reason why SIDS is more common in the colder months. (Seasonal increases in respiratory infections may be another.)

Finally, based on a small number of studies reporting decreases in SIDS among infants who fall asleep with a dummy, FSID and the Department of Health suggest that parents consider offering their infants a dummy at bedtime and nap times. The specific recommendations in their 2009 'Reduce the Risk of Cot Death' campaign guidelines are:

- 'It is possible that using a dummy at the start of any sleep period reduces the risk of cot death.'
- 'Don't worry if the dummy falls out while your baby is asleep and don't force him to take it if he doesn't want it.'
- 'Never coat a dummy in anything sweet.'
- 'Do not begin to give a dummy until breastfeeding is well established, usually when the baby is around one month old.'
- 'Stop giving the dummy when the baby is between 6 and 12 months old.'

Additional studies should clarify the value of these recommendations (you can always check the FSID's website, www.fsid.org.uk, for the complete and newest guidelines). The period from two to six months of age is the most important, since after that the risk from SIDS is quite low and the likelihood of dummy-related middle-ear infections increases. It's not clear how dummies protect against

---

* 'Reduce the Risk of Cot Death', FSID and the Department of Health, produced by COI for the Department of Health, Crown copyright 2009.

SIDS, if the effect is even real. It could be that dummies keep the mouth clear of soft bedding. Or the protective effect could be due to the increase in wakings known to occur among babies using dummies – in other words, the increase in safety may come at the expense of worsened sleep. Dummy-caused sleep problems are described in Chapter 4.

SHOULD YOUR CHILD SLEEP IN YOUR BED?

The practice of 'co-sleeping', where the child sleeps in bed with his parents, is probably the single most controversial topic related to paediatric sleep. Some argue that it is always best for the child, while others argue that it is never appropriate. Each camp warns that the other's position threatens psychological and even physical harm to the child.

Over the more than twenty-five years I've spent working with families and children with sleep problems, I've come to the conclusion that children can sleep quite well under a surprisingly wide range of conditions. As long as the children are sleeping well, there is little evidence that any of these ways is inherently better for them psychologically than the others. Children do not grow up insecure just because they sleep alone or with other siblings, away from their parents; and they are not prevented from learning to separate, or from developing their own sense of individuality, simply because they sleep with their parents. Whatever you want to do, whatever you feel comfortable doing, is the right thing to do, *as long as it works.* I do not presume to dictate parents' child-rearing philosophies. As long as they don't choose a path that I think will be harmful to their youngster, I will work with them according to their choice. The techniques may vary somewhat, but most problems can be solved regardless of the philosophical approach chosen. No choice is irreversible: parents are free to try one approach, and then change their minds if they find it did not work as well as they had hoped. If the path chosen is working well for everyone involved, it is probably fine; but if anyone is unhappy or not sleeping well, then the choice should probably be re-thought.

Much importance has been attached by some to the fact that some form of co-sleeping predominated as our species evolved and persists in those cultures that remain socially and economically most 'primitive'. Although this is perhaps an interesting fact, it tells us little about how children should sleep in modern cultures. Certainly we should not return to the circumstances of our early ancestors (where most infants died before their first birthday) and move our children out of heated homes into caves, have them sleep on the ground or on floors or mats instead of on mattresses and eliminate medical care, sanitation and most clothing. Clearly, premodern practices are not always the best ones.

Furthermore, in many co-sleeping communities, custom dictates that women and young children sleep together, older boys and men elsewhere. Privacy needs are different as well, since sexual encounters in these communities are usually not activities for the bedroom but, instead, routinely take place in the fields. Few Westerners, if any, would advocate either of these practices today.

We live in very different circumstances from those that existed when our species first evolved. That does not mean we should always do the opposite of what was done in the Stone Age, but it does mean that there are other factors to consider, including how we live now. Basically, as this applies to children's sleep, it means you are free to choose the way that best suits you and your philosophy of parenting.

Children generally fall asleep quickly and sleep soundly at night, regardless of where they sleep. In the absence of any problems, most are asleep 98 to 99 per cent of the time from lights out to final waking – that is, they are awake only a tiny fraction of that time, perhaps five to ten minutes during the night in all. Even during those five or ten minutes, they are drowsy, usually barely aware of anything other than the need to find a comfortable position and return to sleep. Thus, for most of the night children are not conscious of where they are or of who else is or is not with them.

But they are awake and aware most of the daytime: it is then that they need loving and nurturing adults constantly available. They need to know that their parents will be nearby, taking care of them, while they sleep, so they won't get anxious at each waking.

But when they are asleep, they are oblivious to their parents' whereabouts, which is why many parents respond to their children's wakeful crying at night but sneak away when the child is asleep again.

The majority of the families I work with have chosen to have their children sleep alone. Many parents who co-sleep would prefer not to but do so because of financial or space constraints, or because co-sleeping seems to be the only way they can get any sleep themselves. Still others choose the partial alternative to co-sleeping of keeping a bassinet or cot, designed for infant sleep and safety, in parents' rooms in the early months. But I have also had the pleasure of working with many families who chose co-sleeping for sound philosophical reasons, and most have been quite happy with their choice.

Before you make this decision, there are certain considerations you should take into account. The decision should be yours, made by the parent or parents, and based on your own personal philosophies, not on pressure from your child or from anyone else. Another family's good or bad experience with co-sleeping or sleeping separately should not influence your decision: your child is not theirs, and your family is not the same. Finally, and very important, if you choose co-sleeping, you must plan when and how to stop. Far too many families start co-sleeping early, assuming it will stop on its own at some point, and then find themselves years later with a five-, seven-, ten- or twelve-year-old that they 'can't get out of' their bed. The parents are unhappy and the child is embarrassed, feeling 'different' and unable to host or attend sleepovers. At that point most children want to leave their parents' bed even more than the parents want them to go.

If one parent favours co-sleeping and the other is against it, either choice can lead to anger and frustration. If neither of you prefers to co-sleep but you do so because your child 'demands' it, then you are probably making a poor choice for the long run. If your child sleeps with one of you and the other parent sleeps elsewhere, all of you may feel that the child has forced a separation and has replaced one parent as the other parent's partner. Whether the decision was made out of compassion or out of desperation, it can lead to anger towards your partner and towards your child. When you are angry and tired, it is difficult to nurture your child during the day and difficult to make rational decisions at night. I have worked with many such families who tell me that they will continue co-sleeping if that is the only 'solution', but that they will not consider having more children.

SPECIFIC ISSUES RELATED TO CO-SLEEPING

Advantages and Disadvantages

Co-sleeping provides several potential benefits:
1. Constant closeness whenever the child is awake. Children may like this, and many parents enjoy this feeling as well.
2. Immediate support for any night-time separation concerns or other anxieties or difficulties.
3. The ability to nurse, and to respond to other night-time wakings, quickly and without getting up.
4. More time to spend with the child.
5. Possibly better sleep for both the child and the parents, if the child was sleeping poorly to begin with.

Co-sleeping also has potential drawbacks:
1. There may be a slight increase in the risk to the infant from SIDS and related causes.
2. Parents may sleep poorly if their children are restless sleepers.
3. Parents may end up sleeping in separate rooms, and they may become angry at their child or with each other.
4. Children's and adults' sleep cycles do not coincide.
5. Parents may have to go to bed at a very early hour, with their children, and be left with little time for their own evening activities and unable to use a babysitter for even the occasional night out.

6. Certain sleep problems that arise (namely those based on patterns of parent-child interaction) may be more difficult to correct.
7. Parents have little privacy.

Since it is the drawbacks of co-sleeping that can lead to problems, the potential difficulties bear discussing in more detail.

Co-sleeping with an infant in the kinds of bedding typically used in Western societies (soft mattresses, fluffy pillows and plush duvets – as opposed to mats on the ground and thin pillows and blankets) does increase the risk of SIDS and suffocation slightly (available studies do not always make a clear distinction between the two). An overweight parent or one impaired by alcohol or other drugs or medications poses additional risks.

Some people claim that co-sleeping actually protects against SIDS, possibly because babies (and parents) experience more arousals during the night when they co-sleep than when they sleep alone. However, the scientific evidence regarding the safety of co-sleeping is mainly to the contrary, at least in the Western countries where most studies were done. But these studies are generally looking at the risk of unexpected sudden death from any cause (not specifically SIDS). Since this risk is increased when more people share the bed, and with inappropriate bedding, exposed places of entrapment (between bed and wall) and parental alcohol consumption and obesity, it seems that the increased risk may be mainly for suffocation. Furthermore, the SIDS rate in different countries where co-sleeping is the norm may be high or low, and where it is high it often at least partly reflects related environmental and socio-economic factors, such as smoking and poor prenatal and post-natal care, more than it does co-sleeping itself.

If you choose to co-sleep, you can take steps to minimise or eliminate most of these risk factors. Most important is to take the precautions discussed in the section on SIDS and to be sure that the infant sleeps on his back and that smoking does not occur in the house, especially not in the bedroom. To reduce the risk even further, move the bed away from the wall and other furniture, be sure the sleeping surface is firm and flat, avoid loose, soft bedding and covers, limit the number of others in the bed to one or both parents and avoid alcohol and other drugs that impair arousal. The safest way to assure that these precautions are always met while still keeping your infant close by, according to FSID (www.fsid.org.uk) in their 2009 guidelines, is to keep your infant in your room but in a separate cot, bassinet or cradle with a firm mattress and proper bedding.

If your child is to share your bed after the early months, be aware that young children are frequently very restless sleepers. During normal night-time arousals, they often kick, roll, moan and thrash. Not uncommonly, they complete several full head-to-toe rotations before the night is done. They sleep well, but the parents may not. Or an H pattern may develop in the bed, with the child sleeping across the middle of the bed and the parents teetering on the very edges, the child's head against one of them, his feet against the other. The size of a bed is a constraint that was not present for most of human evolution. In primitive or poor societies where people sleep on the floor or on the ground, and in societies that use futons, parents can give a restless toddler the sleeping space he needs without running out of space themselves. Some co-sleeping advocates suggest converting a single bedroom for sleep, with mattresses covering the entire floor, and setting up a separate room for intimate relations. This approach can work, but many families consider it impractical.

Because of a child's restless sleep, some parents take turns sleeping in another room so that at least one of them will get some rest. This habit may not be good for the parents' relationship. If this is happening in your home, examine your motivations for this choice of sleep patterns carefully. Do you and your partner want to sleep together? If so, you should. Or do you really want to sleep separately? If so, you may be blaming your child for your night-time separation instead of admitting your problems and exploring their significance.

A child's sleep cycles never coincide perfectly with those of his parents – they cannot, since adult cycles are longer than a child's.

Each person's normal, periodic arousals disrupt the sleep of the others in the bed; the more people, the more disruption. This generally affects the parents' sleep more than the child's, since adults sleep less deeply and often have more difficulty returning to sleep.

If your child not only sleeps in your bed but can fall asleep only when you are present, then you must be prepared to go to sleep when he does. If that means seven o'clock, so be it. You may or may not be able to sneak out later once he is asleep – but as will be discussed in Chapter 4, routinely sneaking away from a sleeping child is never a good idea anyway. You will not be able to leave him with a babysitter unless he's already asleep, and if he wakes before you return, he will not be able to go back to sleep. (Going out to the cinema once in a while was not a consideration for our cave-dwelling ancestors.)

When parents and children share a bed, it is more difficult to set limits or change habitual sleep patterns. For instance, if you want your nine-month-old to stop nursing hourly all night long, or if you want to get your eighteen-month-old to stop twisting your hair, rubbing your face or lying on top of you when he goes to sleep, you can make these changes more easily if you and your child are not in the same bed.

Keeping a separate room for sex is unworkable for most families. Waiting until your child seems to be asleep and then having sex 'quietly' is not a good idea. He may wake to find you having intercourse – not the worst thing that can happen, but it may be misunderstood and confusing.

If the parents agree philosophically about co-sleeping, many of these potential problems can be addressed. Those caused by a child's restless sleep may be unsolvable if he sleeps in your bed, but a solution would be to allow him to sleep in your room in a separate bed, on the floor or in a cot. Also, a child can be taught to go to sleep alone in your bed, where you will join him later. Limits on inappropriate demands and behaviours can be set even if you sleep in the same bed. We will return to these points in later chapters.

Co-sleeping: The Endgame

Recommendations about when co-sleeping should stop are quite varied. Some people suggest ending it by the time the child is six months old, before separation anxiety becomes an issue; others suggest waiting until he is a year old. Some recommend stopping when he is weaned. Few child care specialists recommend co-sleeping much past the age of three. Again, the choice is yours, but when you begin co-sleeping, you should have a plan in mind of how and when you will stop. Unless housing and financial limitations dictate otherwise, in most cases I would agree that it makes sense to move a youngster out of the parental bed at least by age three. It is quite easy to do at six months. At one year a child with little previous experience of being in a cot is unlikely to adapt to one very easily, if at all, and he may have to continue sleeping in a bed or on a mattress on the floor. But since he is already quite mobile, other boundaries such as gates will be necessary, for his protection if for no other reason. At age three, a child is able to be resistant and, now, verbally demanding for a longer time at bedtime, since the ability to stay awake and protest increases with age. Finally, a child who still needs to sleep with his parents by the start of school faces embarrassment, sometimes even shame, because almost all of his peers will be sleeping in their own beds. The older a child gets, the harder it becomes to change his sleeping location against his will, because as he grows, enforcement becomes more difficult.

Some specialists recommend a transitional approach, getting your child used to sleeping in a cot or a separate bed in your room, even in a sleeping bag on your floor, before he makes the move to his own room. That approach is fine if it works smoothly, but it is difficult to enforce if the child resists (at least if he is out of a cot and continues to try to get into your bed). Even if you are successful getting him to sleep in another location in your room, you still have the job left of eventually moving him into his own room. A more consistently workable approach, I find, is to temporarily move into the child's room with him as the first step, but to insist that he sleep in his own bed, with you sleeping in a separate bed or on a mattress on the floor. (This separation is easier to enforce in his room, using a gate or door as necessary, as described in Chapters 5 and 7.) Get him accustomed to sleeping in his room and in his bed before asking him to sleep in the room alone. It is not too difficult to enforce a plan of sleeping in separate beds in the same room; then, gradually (within days or weeks, depending upon the child's needs and desires), the parent can begin leaving the room at bedtime, initially briefly, then longer, gradually helping the child to get used to being in the room and falling asleep alone. At first the parent would return and sleep there the rest of the night. Then, as another step, the child could be left to sleep alone the whole night. The techniques to do this are the same ones used to combat night-time fears in an anxious child with difficulty sleeping alone and are discussed in detail in Chapter 7. The specifics depend upon the child's age and personality, and they may include gradual desensitisation, negotiation, limit-setting and positive reinforcement. It is too much to expect a child to move out voluntarily or to move out completely in one night if he has always slept with his parents.

The Sleep Challenges of Multiples: Twins and Triplets

Multiple births are relatively common nowadays. Approximately 1 in every 300 births produces a set of identical twins. Nonidentical, or fraternal, twins are born about three times as often (this rate differs considerably from country to country and culture to culture). The incidence of nonidentical twins has increased in recent years because of fertility treatments such as in vitro fertilisation.

Parents of multiples often assume that their children's sleep problems are different, or at least need to be treated differently, from those that occur in other children. In reality, the sleep and sleep problems of multiples are no different from those that affect other children, and the situations that arise are the same as those seen in any home, particularly in homes with two or more children close to the same age. Even though twins may do everything together all day, especially when they are young, the process of falling asleep is a task that each twin needs to learn for himself.

Even so, some specific considerations do need to be taken into account. Coming home from hospital with a single child is hard enough; the challenges are even greater with multiples. If you have other children already, the work seems to increase exponentially, especially since two new children seem to require more than twice as much work as one. Children who are exactly the same age may have all the same needs at the same time: feeding, changing, toilet-training, starting school. Even with help, the task for a parent may seem almost overwhelming. There is work to be done all day long. - It's not easy to work all night long as well.

Twins are almost always put in the same room, even if other rooms are available. Some families initially place twin newborns in the same cot. Regardless, twins are almost always expected to go to bed, wake up, nap and eat on the same schedule. Parents do not usually have such expectations of siblings who are merely close to the same age. Most of the sleep problems that families perceive as specific to twins are actually due to these habits.

Putting infants into the same cot to sleep offers little benefit, especially after the first few weeks. Remember, although twins may often be together during the day, they are physically apart much of the time. They may share a pram, but not the same seat. They ride in separate car seats, and they eat in separate high chairs. There is no reason why they should not also be physically apart at night. If they are sleeping properly, they will not even be conscious of whether they are in the same cot for most of the night and nap times, and the rest of their time in the cot they should be too sleepy to care. Sharing a cot can even be detrimental: neither child will learn to fall asleep without the other one there, and each child's movements will wake the other one.

Although identical twins commonly have very similar sleep requirements and are often able to adapt to very similar schedules, they will not match perfectly every day, any more than a single child will sleep and wake at exactly the same times every day. The divergence between nonidentical twins' schedules may be much more striking. No parents should try to force a new baby to follow the exact schedule their first child was on at the same point in his life, but many families effectively do just that for their twins.

Every child, twin or not, has particular abilities and needs, and the parents need to learn to recognise them and respond properly. One child may sleep more hours; the other may give up middle-of-the-night feedings sooner. One may play quietly when awake at night; the other may do everything he can to wake his twin (not to mention the rest of the house).

In short, twins or triplets, sleeping in separate cots or beds in the same room, can have the same problems that any set of siblings sharing a room might have, and they should be handled in the same ways. For example, if one twin, who needs to sleep ten hours, is regularly awakened early by his sibling, who only requires nine hours, you have the same choices you would have for any two children. You can put the shorter-sleeping twin to bed an hour later than the other (the fact that they are twins does not mean they have to share a bedtime), or they can have the same bedtime, as long as you are prepared to get the early riser out of the room before he wakes the other. Or you may be able to shorten nap times a bit for the one who sleeps less at night (especially if he takes long naps), hoping that his night-time sleep will lengthen to match that of his brother. You might get the nightly sleeping times to match, but possibly at the expense of differing nap times.

If one twin is sleeping well at night but the other needs frequent interventions, you may find it works best to separate them, at least temporarily. Then you can focus on normalising the sleep of the wakeful twin (as described in later chapters) while allowing the other twin to sleep uninterrupted. Depending in part on the location of bedrooms, other sleep location options and the severity of the problem to be addressed, sometimes it is best to move the twin who is having sleep problems, and sometimes it is better to move the other one. Even if both twins are having problems, it may be easier to work with them separately, in separate rooms, and then consider putting them back together once the problems have been addressed. You can always start to work on the problems with the twins in the same room, but be prepared to separate them if that isn't working. Sometimes just being in sight of each other is enough to keep twins from quieting down and going to sleep; in that case, being in separate rooms may be the easiest way for them to start to sleep well. If only one twin gets excited, you may be able to keep them in the same room, but you might have to wait until the excitable one is asleep before you can put the other one to bed. The situation is no different here than when, for example, a three-year-old and a six-month-old share a room. It may be necessary to move the cot to another room, or to put the toddler in another bed temporarily, until matters are resolved. When the children are put back in the same room, they will very likely have different bedtimes.

The idea that multiples might have separate bedtimes or separate bedrooms, even temporarily, often seems wrong to parents. But failing to take the children's individual needs into account does not do them justice. There is no reason the child with the shorter sleep requirement should stay in bed longer than he needs to, for example, just because his brother sleeps later. If one twin needs to go to bed before the other, he will quickly learn to fall asleep in a room by himself, just as he would if you had to take the other one out to deal with an illness.

Having multiples to care for is a difficult job. But don't let the sleep needs of one dictate how you manage the others.

THE SPECIAL TOY OR FAVOURITE BLANKET

If your older infant or toddler needs to have something or someone in the bed with him to fall asleep, better that it be a 'transitional object' – a stuffed animal, a doll, a toy, a special blanket – than that it be you (even if you share a bed). This item can help him to prepare for and accept his night-time separation from you, and it can be a source of reassurance and comfort when he is alone. It will give him a sense of control over his world, because the toy or blanket can be with him whenever he wants, something he cannot expect from you. His toy won't get up and leave when he falls asleep, and his special blanket will be there whenever he wakes. Even if he sleeps in your bed, his reliance on a special object will help give you the freedom to pick your own bedtime and the ability to leave him with a babysitter.

A child will often choose such a special object early in the toddler years, typically at twelve to eighteen months, and he may continue to rely on it, or on other objects, for several more years. If your child does not have anything special that he likes to keep with him, it is reasonable to offer him things that you think might take on this role. However, he will always be the one to make the final choice, and you cannot make him attach to any particular toy that you think appropriate. More important is that you avoid playing this role yourself. If you always allow yourself to be used like a special toy – if you lie with him, nurse him or rock him, or let him cuddle you, caress you or twirl your hair whenever he wants and for as long as he wants, particularly whenever he wants to fall asleep – he will never take on a transitional object, because he won't need to.

If your child begins to favour a particular stuffed toy or doll, include it in his bedtime rituals. Have him tuck it in, or let it 'listen to' the story. If he has a special blanket, make sure it is close at hand when he gets into bed. The comfort that these special objects provide will make the final good night that much easier.

DEVELOPING GOOD SCHEDULES

As you may recall from Chapter 2, newborn infants do not have regular sleep patterns, and it usually takes between six and ten weeks for them to develop a consistent twenty-four-hour schedule with the longest period of sleep at night. Your baby's sleep patterns during the first few days after birth are not an indication of things to come. Whether he sleeps well or fitfully in the hospital, and whether the nurses assure you that he is 'extremely good' or warn you that they have never seen a baby who 'sleeps so little', things are likely to change considerably once you leave hospital. If problems appear to develop after you get home, you might blame yourself and assume that your inexperience as a parent was to blame, but you would almost certainly be wrong. If you are too quick to believe a nurse's warning about problems ahead, it can all too easily become a self-fulfilling prophecy.

In most babies, a sleep pattern emerges over the first two weeks, with many naps, some brief and some longer, distributed across the day and night. Some infants do sleep unusually well from the beginning, even having to be wakened for some feedings, but this is the exception rather than the rule. Try not to feel frustrated if your child takes a while to fall into a reasonable, easy-to-follow schedule.

Some babies seem to have their days and nights reversed, with the longest period of sleep falling during the day and the longest period of wakefulness occurring at night. This, too, will change. It is actually impressive that a child so young can show such a consistent (if inverted) pattern, since he has had little time to develop regular twenty-four-hour rhythms, and even less of a chance to learn day from night. This night-day reversal is not abnormal; it is, rather, an indication that the child has already developed a regular and predictable schedule. Most children correct this schedule reversal by themselves. But it will be easy to re-adjust their schedules if they don't (as you will see below and in Chapters 10, 11 and 12).

Although most infants will develop a regular twenty-four-hour sleep schedule regardless of anything we do or don't do, parents can assist the process considerably. You should use approaches that take into account your baby's schedules, habits, learned associations and nutritional and emotional needs, and avoid approaches that could interfere with the development of normal rhythms.

Feeding patterns are an important part of an infant's daily schedule. Few paediatricians still urge parents to put their babies on a precise four-hour feeding schedule from the beginning. Instead, they generally recommend that you follow your infant's cues. A newborn baby usually needs to be fed every two to six hours. Only if your baby was premature, or if he has medical problems, feeding difficulties or poor weight gain, will you have to follow a more rigid feeding schedule.

There are two problems to watch for when feeding on demand. First, not all cries are hunger cries, and it will take you a little time to learn to recognise which sounds mean your child is hungry. Second, you should take care to impose reasonable limits. A newborn obviously needs to be fed more than twice a day, even if he seems to cry for feedings only every twelve hours. But it may be less apparent that a full-term, healthy infant does not need hourly feedings, even if he seems hungry at these times and nurses when you offer the breast or bottle. Hourly feeding is exhausting for the parent and painful for the mother if she is breastfeeding. It is unnecessary for the baby, and it interferes with the development of healthier sleep-wake and feeding patterns.

Of course, you want to show your baby that he has been born into a good and caring world, so you respond when he cries, and you try to do whatever it takes to soothe him. But helping him to develop good sleep schedules is also an important part of his care, and to do that, you may have to tolerate some crying or find ways to calm him other than feeding him. Babies often stop crying if they are walked, rocked or stroked for a while, and sometimes these are useful temporary measures to help you accustom your baby to falling asleep without an unnecessary feeding. (If these measures become troublesome habits of their own, they too can easily be eliminated later, as discussed in Chapter 4.)

If your baby has been feeding every hour, begin to increase the time between feedings by an amount you feel comfortable with – perhaps fifteen minutes a day – until he is being fed every two hours, then every two and a half or three hours. He will adapt to the better schedule, the hourly crying will cease and he will begin to develop the good sleeping and eating rhythms that should be forming over the first three months.

You can also start to make changes in your baby's sleep schedule. For example, if he is sleeping six hours at a time during the day but is awake much of the night, and if this pattern persists past the early weeks, you can begin waking him earlier and earlier from the long sleep period, so that he will start to treat it as a nap and move the longer sleep segment into the night-time hours. Although you are following your child's cues up to a point, in this way you can still help to structure his sleep-wake schedule.

Over the first three months, most infants begin to respond on their own to the external cues of darkness, quiet and inactivity at night and light, noise and activity during the day. By three or four months of age they will be getting most of their sleep at night, usually including an unbroken stretch of five to nine hours. They will continue to nap at three or four fairly predictable times during the day, and the time during the day when they are awake the longest will become predictable as well. At this point you should begin working with your baby to improve his schedule further, to stabilise it and to make changes in it as he grows. You will be doing both of you a favour, because as your baby settles into an appropriate schedule, you will be able to make better use of your own time and enjoy him more when he is awake.

As you begin to observe your baby's periods of waking, activity, feeding and sleep, you will learn to anticipate his needs and know when to play with him, feed him or put him to sleep. Even if your baby is not crying for a feeding at the expected time, he may be ready to eat and will nurse eagerly. Similarly, he may be ready for his nap before he starts to yawn and become fussy. Although you can't tie your child's feedings, play and sleep precisely to the clock, if you are aware of his emerging schedule you can encourage him to eat and sleep at reasonable and consistent times. That, in turn, will help him to stabilise his developing twenty-four-hour cycles.

By the time your baby is three months old and has developed a fairly predictable twenty-four-hour pattern, it becomes more important for you to provide increasingly consistent structure. If you do your best to establish a reasonable and consistent daily routine and keep to it as much as possible, then it is likely that your child will continue to develop good patterns. If instead you allow the times of your child's feedings, playtimes, baths and other activities to change constantly, chances are his sleep will become irregular as well. Remember from Chapter 2 that when there is no schedule, people (including children) tend to run on a twenty-five-hour day. So if you don't stick to a schedule for your child's sleep, a pattern might emerge that would surprise you (although it wouldn't surprise a sleep scientist).

I have worked with many families who had this problem. Typically, their child was functioning on a regular pattern, but one lasting twenty-five or twenty-six hours instead of twenty-four. As a result, the parents were following their child around the clock, letting him stay up later and later at night and getting up with him one or two hours later each morning. At times, most of the child's sleep was occurring during the day. These children were normal, but since their biological clock was not being re-set to a twenty-four-hour day by a regular schedule and, especially, by consistent exposure to light at appropriate times (see Chapter 9), their rhythms were allowed to drift.

It is equally important to help our children maintain consistent schedules through infancy, childhood and adolescence. In fact, all of us, regardless of age, function best when we keep regular schedules. Studies on adults have shown that irregular sleep-wake patterns cause significant changes in our moods and sense of well-being and undermine our ability to sleep at desired times. The same is true of young children. So don't let your two- or three-year-old decide what time he should go to bed – many would wait until they were so sleepy they could not stay awake any longer. Before long his schedule would be disrupted, becoming inconsistent and unpredictable. He might fall asleep early one night and late the next; he might nap some days and not others; and when he did nap it could be in the morning, afternoon or early evening. With even more disruption, his mealtimes would also fluctuate. He might have breakfast anywhere from 7.00 to 10.00 a.m.; he would want lunch and dinner at odd hours and might skip meals altogether. Children on uncontrolled schedules like that can develop major sleep problems. Behaviour problems may follow as well, though they can be subtle at first.

Instead, establish a reasonable daytime schedule in your baby's first three months and maintain consistency as much as possible throughout his childhood. Your child cannot be expected to keep to a schedule on his own; you will have to set one for him and then be willing to enforce it. Of course, some flexibility is called for. Some children need more sleep than others, and some are better able to tolerate variations in their day-to-day routines. You will have to learn from experience with your child what schedule is best and how closely it needs to be followed.

Consistent schedules are especially important in treating sleep disorders. Regardless of a child's age (at least after the early weeks

of life) or the cause of his disorder, a regular and appropriate schedule will help the treatment to succeed and may even be a cure in itself. So if you are beginning to address a sleep problem in your
child, be sure to set up a firm schedule and stick to it rigorously for
several weeks after your child has begun sleeping well again. At that
point you will be able to relax the schedule somewhat without the
problem recurring. You might skip an occasional nap for a special
outing, or take your child out with you in the afternoon even
though he may fall asleep in the car at an unaccustomed time.

Once a baby has settled into a good sleep-wake pattern, it is still
subject to disruption. Teething, an illness, a trip or an upset in the
family can interfere with his sleep pattern. The disruption can continue for months unless you intervene. You may need to re-establish
your child's schedule, help him unlearn bad habits, address his
anxieties and be firmer in setting limits. We will discuss all of these
approaches in detail throughout this book.

PART II

THE SLEEPLESS CHILD

CHAPTER 4

Sleep Associations: A Key Problem

Many infants and toddlers are unable to settle themselves and fall asleep without their parents' help at night. If your child has this problem, you might have to hold him, rock him, rub his back or talk to him to get him to fall asleep. He might wake several times during the night, crying, calling out or (if he sleeps in your bed) reaching for you, and each time you might have to repeat the whole process before he can go back to sleep. You're tired and frustrated, and you're probably angry at your child because your own sleep is so badly disrupted. That, in turn, may leave you feeling guilty: you want to do what's best for your child, and if that means less sleep for you, then perhaps you must learn to accept it. Maybe you've been told that his behaviour is a normal phase some children go through and that there's nothing you can do but wait until he outgrows it. Still, you may wonder, 'Is it really normal and do I really have to wait it out, and for how long?'

It's true that this behaviour is not abnormal, but neither is it something you have to put up with. You certainly don't need to wait for it to change on its own: it's almost always possible to identify the causes of these sleep disturbances and treat them successfully. If your child is not sleeping through the night by three or four months of age, when most full-term infants have 'settled', it may be time to start thinking about what could be causing the problem and, perhaps, to begin to correct it; if more than occasional wakings are still happening when your child reaches five or six months of age, you not only can but probably should take definite steps to address them. If you do nothing, his sleep will eventually improve on its own, but the process could take months or even years. If you can figure out why your child is sleeping poorly and make the necessary changes, he should be sleeping well much sooner – usually within a few days, two weeks at the most.

The root of the problem often lies in your child's sleep associations. All children learn to connect certain conditions with falling asleep. For most children, that means being in a particular bedroom, lying in a particular cot or bed and perhaps holding a favourite stuffed animal or a special blanket. When they wake periodically during the night, as all children do between sleep cycles, most will promptly fall back to sleep, because the conditions they associate with falling asleep are still present. But if the conditions have changed, such children may not be able to fall asleep again without help re-establishing them.

As you read this chapter, remember that not all children become dependent enough on particular conditions to cause trouble. If you always rock your child to sleep at night, say, but he sleeps through the night without needing your help to return to sleep after normal brief wakings, then there is no problem and you certainly shouldn't feel compelled to stop rocking him at bedtime. If he does develop a problem associated with the rocking later, you can treat it then. (See 'General Observations' later in this chapter for more discussion on how sleep associations can vary in different locations and at different times.) But if his bedtimes and night-time wakings are longer and more troublesome, as with the children described in this chapter, you should make changes so he won't have to deal with nightly surprises.

The same principles apply whether your child has his own bed or cot or sleeps in bed with you, although if you share a bed, you may find it a little harder to refuse to rub his back when he wakes, or to delay or refuse an unneeded nursing. Either way, he should generally go to sleep in the place where he will be spending the rest of the night.

A Typical Sleep Association Problem

Betsy was causing her parents much distress. Although she had started sleeping through the night at the age of three months, soon after that she had begun waking repeatedly during the night. When I saw her, now ten months old, she still fought being put into her cot, and she was still waking several times every night. In the evening, she would not fall asleep without her mother or father rocking her and rubbing her back for around twenty minutes. She seemed to be trying to stay awake, her parents told me: she would begin to doze off, then suddenly she would open her eyes and look around before starting to nod off again. Once she had been fast asleep for fifteen minutes her parents could move her into the cot, but any sooner and she would wake up and start crying again, and they would have to start over. It was difficult to tell when she was sleeping deeply enough to be moved. Sometimes her parents could get away with rubbing her back as she lay in the cot instead of rocking her, but again, if they stopped too soon, she would wake and cry.

Once Betsy was so deeply asleep that she could be placed or left in her cot without waking, she would stay asleep for several hours. Then, several times between midnight and 4.00 a.m., she would wake crying vigorously. She would not settle on her own, but she did not seem to be in pain; when her mother or father began to rock her, she would promptly quiet down and return to sleep. As at bedtime, she had to be deeply asleep before she could be returned to the cot, but at these times that rarely took longer than five minutes. From 4.00 a.m. to 6.00 a.m. she slept well, but she usually woke crying in the morning. She had two daily naps, one in the morning and one in the afternoon, and she had to be rocked to sleep for both, just as at bedtime.

Betsy's parents had tried everything they could think of. A few times they had let her cry for fifteen or twenty minutes before rocking her to sleep, but it hadn't helped. Once, at their doctor's suggestion, they had tried to let her cry until she fell asleep on her own. But Betsy only cried harder and harder and showed no signs of settling down; after an hour and a half her parents decided they were being cruel and couldn't bear it anymore, so they went in, comforted her and rocked her to sleep as usual. Finally, they asked the doctor for medication. He prescribed an antihistamine, which Betsy took for a week. During that week she feel asleep a bit more quickly at bedtime, but night-time wakings and nap-time difficulties remained as troublesome as ever.

Problems like Betsy's are extremely common, and they can be quite frustrating for parents. Yet, once you understand the nature of the problems, they are usually fairly easy to correct. What most parents do not realise is that in most cases the 'abnormal' wakings at night are actually quite normal – children always wake from time to time at night, between sleep cycles. In fact, in their attempts to treat their child's 'abnormal' wakings by helping him to go back to sleep, the parents are actually *causing* the disturbances, or at least reinforcing them.

The problem with Betsy was that she was used to falling asleep while being held and rocked and having her back rubbed. During her normal night-time arousals, she found herself lying in her cot alone with none of these familiar conditions present. She could not simply go back to sleep by herself: she did not know how to. And by giving in and rocking her back to sleep, whether after fifteen minutes or ninety, her parents were unknowingly preventing her from learning how.

For a child like Betsy, normal night-time arousals are prolonged because the conditions the child associates with falling asleep are no longer present. From the child's point of view, something is wrong. Instead of going back to sleep, he wakes more fully and begins to cry. The wakings during the night are not the problem; rather, the problem is that the child *cannot fall back asleep* after these normal wakings, because of his particular associations with falling asleep.

Why Sleep Associations Matter

Sleep associations play a role in the sleep of adults as well as children, and it's easiest to understand how they can become problems in children by considering the sleep associations we all have. As adults, we take for granted our own associations with falling asleep, but they are very important to us. We all learn to fall asleep under a certain set of conditions: on a certain side of the bed, with a hard or soft pillow, with a heavy or light blanket or even while watching the news, listening to the radio or reading. Some of us are more able than others to tolerate changes in our bedtime routines, but we are all affected to some extent.

Recall from Chapter 2 that we spend the first few hours of the night mostly in deep, nondreaming sleep (Stage IV, non-REM), and during the rest of the night we alternate between lighter sleep (Stage II) and dreaming (REM). (Unlike our children, we adults usually - don't sleep long enough to fit in another period of deep sleep near morning.) We all wake briefly from time to time, especially during the transitions between non-REM and REM sleep. During these arousals we change position and briefly check our environment to make sure everything is in order. Typically, we turn over, straighten the blanket and re-position the pillow. If all is well, we return to sleep promptly, usually without remembering the waking in the morning. But if something feels wrong – if we hear strange noises or smell worrisome odors, for example – we wake more fully to investigate. There doesn't need to be actual danger: if anything has changed from the way it was when we went to sleep, we may notice the change, feel that something isn't right and become fully alert.

Perhaps you've had the experience of waking during the night just enough to notice your pillow missing. Most likely, instead of going straight back to sleep, you wakened a little more, enough to find the pillow on the floor and pull it back into bed before returning to sleep. But if you couldn't find it right away, you probably - wouldn't be able to ignore it and go back to sleep. Instead, you'd become more fully awake so you could look round for it. If you still couldn't find it, eventually you might turn on the light, get out of bed and begin searching the room. You might get angry and perhaps curse – showing the same kind of frustration that a child shows by crying.

Even if your pillow falls out of your bed once or twice every night, it will hardly disturb your sleep: retrieving the pillow from the floor doesn't require you to wake up very much or for very long. But suppose that you are physically unable to get the pillow yourself, and you have to call someone else – perhaps a nurse – to come into the room to replace it whenever you wake up and find it missing. The nurse will soon learn that once you have your pillow back you'll fall asleep quickly, but your frequent wakings during the night might still seem abnormal to him or her.

To stretch the analogy a bit further, suppose you discover that someone has been sneaking into your room each night and stealing your pillow. Once you know that, you might have trouble falling asleep at bedtime for fear that the pillow will be taken away as soon as you're asleep. Whenever you catch yourself starting to drop off to sleep, you might wake yourself up again to make sure the pillow is still there.

Now imagine that this person, instead of just taking your pillow, actually moves you from your bed to another room, without waking you. Every night you go to sleep in your bed with everything just as you like it, only to wake after your first sleep cycle on, say, the floor of the living room. Unless you're an exceptionally tolerant sleeper, you won't even try to go back to sleep right there; you'll get up and head back to your bedroom. But now suppose you find your bedroom door locked from the other side. Now there's nothing you can do but wake someone who can unlock the door for you. Once that's been done, you can at last get back into bed and get your pillow and blanket arranged properly, thereby re-establishing the conditions that were present at bedtime. Once you calm down, you will fall back to sleep – but some ninety minutes later you'll wake up again, back on the living room floor and again locked out of your bedroom.

If that happens throughout the night every night, you will not be sleeping at all well, and neither will the person who has to keep getting up to unlock your door. Soon you might be resisting sleep in hopes of identifying the person who keeps moving you; in other words, you might have trouble falling asleep even in your own bed because you know that you'll be moved once you fall asleep. If that happened to you every night, you would not be very happy.

As you have probably recognised, this last scenario describes what actually happens to many children every night. They fall asleep in one place, maybe being held and rocked in the living room with the television and a small light on. But whenever they wake up they find themselves in a different place under different conditions, perhaps alone in their cot in a dark, quiet room, not being held and not being rocked. Someone has stealthily moved them. They cannot re-establish the conditions that were present when they fell asleep, so they must cry and yell until someone comes in and does it for them. They must be picked up, brought back to the rocker, maybe even taken back to the living room and the television; and no sooner are they asleep than someone moves them again. Soon, these children start resisting sleep, and each time they wake they find that the change happened anyway.

Wrong Sleep Associations

This is the situation Betsy was in. She could fall asleep fairly easily when rocked, and if the rocking could continue all night her sleep would be continuous as well (she would stir occasionally at her normal wakings, but she would fall back asleep quickly without crying). It was difficult to place Betsy in the cot without waking her until she was very deeply asleep, because she had learned to be constantly on guard against being moved. Once deeply asleep, she slept well until her first spontaneous waking, when, finding her surroundings 'wrong', she became frustrated and showed that frustration by crying until one of her parents came in and began rocking her, re-establishing the conditions that she associated with falling asleep.

In fact, the last thing Betsy remembered when she fell asleep at night was being held and rocked, and the first thing she noticed when she woke up was that everything had changed. She did not remember being moved to the cot – or being in the cot at all – and she did not remember being asleep. It was as if she had suddenly been transported out of her parent's arms into her cot, her parent had suddenly disappeared from her room and the rocking had suddenly stopped. She did not even have to open her eyes to find that out. And since she had learned that her parents did the same thing to her over and over, night after night, as soon as she started to arouse she forced herself to wake fully to check. Of course she became frustrated.

Betsy's ability to fall asleep quickly in her parents' arms proved that she had no actual sleep impairment: no inherent abnormality would allow a child to fall asleep quickly in a parent's arms but not alone in her cot. Betsy's inability to settle in her cot was due only to her inexperience falling asleep that way; that is, the sleep associations she had learned were different ones.

Most children will sleep well only if there are no surprises, no changes after they are asleep, and no need for them to check where they are and where their parents are every time they stir. In particular, there should be no sneaking about. Sneaking away from a child at night does not foster trust, and a sense of trust is important for good sleep.

Problems like Betsy's occur most commonly in infants and toddlers because, unlike older children, they have little control over the conditions in which they sleep and are more likely to need your participation. However, similar problems can occur in older children as well. A child of four, five or six may need to be moved to his own bed each night after falling asleep in the living room or in your bed. Or he can become dependent on other conditions for going to sleep: he may need you sitting in his room, or he may have to have music playing or the television on. When he wakes up, you may have to return and sit with him, lie down with him or let him into your room; or he may have to turn on the light or the television before returning to sleep.

William's difficulties were typical. He was a three-and-a-half-year-old who had always had trouble settling at bedtime and during the night. Six months before I saw him he had moved from a cot into a bed, and his bedtime rituals had changed: instead of rocking him to sleep, his parents would lie down with him for a while. He usually fell asleep fairly quickly, although if his parents tried to leave his bed too soon he would wake up. Once he was deeply asleep, they could quietly sneak away. William would sleep for three or four hours, then wake up and call for his parents. He sometimes complained about being scared or seeing monsters, but he never seemed truly frightened. If his parents didn't answer his calls, he grew more demanding; sometimes he went to their room and refused to return to his bed. William's parents, concerned about what they interpreted as night-time anxiety, always took him back to his bed and lay down with him, knowing he would go back to sleep in five or ten minutes and then they could sneak away again. Usually he would wake up one or two more times and repeat the whole routine. But occasionally one of the parents fell asleep in William's bed, and when that happened, William slept through the rest of the night without difficulty.

William's problem, like Betsy's, was not abnormal wakings but inappropriate associations: he could not fall asleep unless one of his parents was lying down with him. And that was a problem for - William's parents, because they wanted to sleep by themselves, in their own bed.

Not all problems with sleep associations involve a parent's actions. Alexa was a sixteen-month-old girl who slept in bed with her parents. They liked having her there, but the situation presented some difficulties. Alexa went to sleep at 8.00 p.m, but only if her mother was in bed with her (her mother had to be there, but she - didn't have to do anything). Usually her mother could slip away once Alexa was asleep, but she would have to hurry back if Alexa wakened before her parents had come to bed for the night. Since they all shared one bed, that particular problem didn't come up when Alexa woke later in the night. But Alexa also liked to fall asleep lying across the bed with her head resting on her mother and her feet against her father. Her mother found that position physically uncomfortable, and it usually kept her awake much of the night. If she tried to move Alexa, or if they tried to get Alexa to rest her head on her father instead, Alexa would cry. Alexa's father, who also found this arrangement uncomfortable and was annoyed at being physically separated from his wife, often ended up sleeping in another room.

Still, Alexa's parents liked keeping Alexa in their bed and didn't want to move her to a separate room. Fortunately, Alexa's disruptive patterns could be corrected without giving up co-sleeping. She just needed to learn to fall asleep lying in a normal position instead of across the bed, with her head on the mattress rather than on her mother, and without depending on either parent to be there with her.

Sam, aged two, was another child who had always had trouble going to sleep and staying asleep. His parents took the path of least resistance, letting him fall asleep on the couch in the living room while they watched television. When they followed this routine, the bedtime struggles seemed to disappear. Sam could then be moved into his bed at his parents' convenience, usually without waking him. However, he would wake up several hours later, call out and point towards the living room. If his parents lay down with him or took him into their bed, he stayed awake, insistently repeating, 'TV, TV!' He did not seem to be afraid, but he was demanding. Most nights his parents gave in, taking him back to the living room, placing him on the sofa and putting on a DVD. He hardly seemed to care whether or not they stayed with him. Soon he would fall back asleep on the couch, where he would sleep through until morning.

Sam had certainly developed poor associations with falling asleep, even though they did not include any special need to be close to his parents. Furthermore, although he needed the lights and television on to go to sleep, the constant light, and the frequent speech and music changes, also stimulated him and tended to keep him awake. He would be better off learning to associate falling asleep with a dark, quiet environment.

Even children who always fall asleep under nonstimulating conditions – perhaps alone in their own beds in a dark, quiet room –

can form associations that interfere with falling asleep. Jacob, for example, was an eight-month-old who always fell asleep with a dummy in his mouth. He would get drowsy, start to fall asleep and stop sucking. But when the sucking motions stopped, he would wake – just as Betsy did when her parents stopped rocking her too soon – and start sucking again. Usually that pattern repeated until he fell asleep deeply enough not to notice when he had stopped. But occasionally his dummy would fall out of his mouth before he was completely asleep, and he would wake fully and cry until one of his parents replaced it. Whether he fell asleep quickly at bedtime or not, he would still wake three or four times later in the night, find his dummy missing and cry until it was replaced.

(Actually, Jacob's parents learned to race into his room and replace the dummy at the first sign that he was waking, because when they didn't, he often got so upset that he couldn't go back to sleep for a while even after the dummy had been replaced. At one point, at a friend's suggestion, they tried what I refer to as the 'sprinkle technique': they sprinkled ten dummies around the cot in hopes that Jacob would randomly find one of them whenever he started to wake. This approach, although creative, almost never works. By the time Jacob was awake enough to find and retrieve one of the dummies, it was too late for him to slip quickly and easily back into the next sleep cycle.)

Kaitlyn was very similar to Jacob: at eighteen months of age she still fell asleep at bedtime sucking on a bottle. She, too, woke several times each night, but she always went back to sleep after she was given another bottle. Since her parents could simply hand her a bottle and leave the room, the problem was not an expectation that her parents be in the room or holding her. That she didn't need to be held during the feedings made it clear that her association was only with the bottle. That she drank only an ounce or two each time made it clear that her middle-of-the-night association with the bottle was only as a dummy, not as a source of food. She certainly was not being fed excessively, as discussed in Chapter 6.

What Jacob and Kaitlyn had in common was that, although they both fell asleep alone in their own beds, they were still dependent on conditions that they could not re-establish by themselves (unlike a child who depends only on sucking his thumb, say). Someone else had to get up, come in and replace the dummy or bottle.

How to Solve the Problem: The Progressive-Waiting Approach

The goal of this approach is to help your child learn a new and more appropriate set of associations with falling asleep so that when he wakes in the middle of the night he will find himself still in the same conditions that were present at bedtime, conditions that he already is used to falling asleep under. But, to do this, you must first identify the pattern of associations that is currently interfering with his sleep (and yours) and which he must unlearn. Almost anything can become associated with falling asleep. Feeding, sucking on something and being rocked to sleep or given a back rub are common examples; others include being patted, walked or driven around in a car (or even just being in a car seat); lullabies; DVDs; music; and fans or white-noise generators. Even simple tuck-ins and good-night kisses can become a poblem if they need to be carried out repeatedly at bedtime and again during the night. Fortunately, it doesn't take most children very long to learn to give up old habits and take on new and better ones.

If you have a child like Betsy who is still in a cot, treatment of improper sleep associations is fairly simple and the improvement will be quite rapid. However, the problems can be solved regardless of the sleep setting. Programmes for treatment are described below. Variations for children no longer in a cot will also be explained.

As you help your child to learn a new set of sleep associations, you will need to be understanding, patient and consistent until he adapts. Since you will be changing some familiar patterns, at first you will not always be doing what your child wants. Anytime you have to say no to a child, there will probably be protests and there may be some crying, but you can keep them to a minimum. A young child's sleep will show marked improvement, usually within a few days to a week.

Think again about having to sleep without your pillow. If you had to start sleeping without it regularly, for health reasons perhaps, you would probably find it difficult at first. You would be uncomfortable at bedtime; you'd thrash about, searching for a satisfactory position. You might be angry at your doctor, even if you understood why it was important to make the change. Even after you finally fell asleep, you would still find it hard to return to sleep after night-time arousals for a while. The only way you could learn to fall asleep easily without your pillow would be by actually doing it – over and over. If you kept going to sleep with the pillow and had someone sneak it out from under you after you were asleep, you would never get used to the change. But if you persisted in trying to get to sleep without the pillow, each time it would be easier, until at last it would begin to feel normal and familiar. At this point your night-time wakings would also cease to be a problem. So it is with the children I treat.

The programme I used with Betsy and her family usually works well. Together we first identified the troublesome sleep associations that Betsy needed to unlearn – namely, being rocked by her parents at bedtime and after night-time wakings. Then we decided upon the new associations that Betsy's parents felt she needed to learn to replace them – namely, being alone and in her own cot; that is, Betsy had to learn to fall asleep at bedtime under the same conditions that would be present when she woke spontaneously during the night.

I used a 'progressive-waiting' approach, which is very effective and which I will explain in detail here. The chart on page 74 (Figure 4) will help you to understand this method.

Once Betsy's parents understood her problem, we were ready to begin treatment. Each night, at bedtime and after night-time wakings, Betsy's parents were to make sure that she fell asleep alone, without them in her room. They would allow her to cry for gradually longer periods before briefly returning to her, but they would always leave while she was still awake. They would repeat this process until she finally fell asleep. Each night they would begin with a longer waiting period than they'd started with the night before.

FIGURE 4. HELPING YOUR CHILD LEARN
TO FALL ASLEEP WITH THE PROPER ASSOCIATIONS:
THE PROGRESSIVE-WAITING APPROACH

NUMBER OF MINUTES TO WAIT BEFORE
RESPONDING TO YOUR CHILD

		If Your Child Is Still Crying or Calling Out		
Day	At First Wait	Second Wait	Third Wait	Subsequent Waits
1	3	5	10	10
2	5	10	12	12
3	10	12	15	15
4	12	15	17	17
5	15	17	20	20
6	17	20	25	25
7	20	25	30	30

For simplicity, most of the following instructions assume your child sleeps in a cot or bed in his own room. However, variations of the same programme are also described in case your child sleeps in your bed, or in his own bed or cot in your room (see below).

1. Pick a starting bedtime no earlier than the time your child usually falls asleep, even if that is later than his usual bedtime. In fact, you may find that making bedtime even thirty to sixty minutes later than usual for the first several nights will help him fall asleep more quickly and speed up the learning process. However, his morning waking should not be moved later, and his naps should be kept to their normal length.

2. Put your child into the cot or bed awake, in the place you want him to be sleeping for the night. Let him fall asleep under the same circumstances that will be present when he wakes normally during the night (in his cot or bed, not being held or rocked). Let him fall back asleep the same way after night-time wakings.

3. If he cries or calls for you at bedtime or upon waking at night, check him briefly at increasing intervals. This chart suggests the number of minutes to wait before going in to him. (Most families find the waiting intervals shown on the chart to be workable. If the intervals seem too long for you, start with

intervals you feel you can manage – for instance, one, three and five minutes the first day. Any schedule will work, as long as the waiting periods increase progressively, and as long as you continue the process long enough for your child to get practice falling asleep under the desired conditions.)

4. When you reach the maximum number of minutes to wait for a particular night, continue to leave the room for the same interval – no longer – until your child finally falls asleep while you are out of the room.

5. By the third or fourth day, your child will most likely be sleeping very well. If further work is still necessary after that, continue following the chart down to day 7; if at that point the problem is improving but is still not fully re- solved, continue to add a few minutes to each interval on successive days. But if things are not improving or are getting worse, you may have to re-think your approach (see 'If Things Are Not Getting Better' later in this chapter).

6. Each time you go to your child, spend no more than one or two minutes with him. Remember, your job is to reassure him (and yourself), not necessarily to help him stop crying, and certainly not to help him fall asleep: the goal is for him to learn to fall asleep on his own. (Even if he does start to calm down when you are in the room, the crying will probably intensify when you leave again.) You may replace a fallen or lost blanket or doll, but if he throws them out of the cot or bed, you should not replace them again until the next time you come in.

7. If your child wakes during the night, re-start the schedule with the minimum waiting time for that night and work up to the maximum again from there.

8. Continue this routine after each waking until a time in the morning (usually 5.00 a.m. to 6.00 a.m.) after which it is unlikely that your child will fall back asleep, even if it is earlier than he has usually been waking. If he wakes at that time or later, or if he is still awake then after waking earlier, get him up and begin the morning routine. Do not let him go right back to sleep in another room – the entire night's sleep should be in one place. If he is still asleep at his usual waking time in the morning, wake him up then even if he was awake part of the night.

9. If your child sleeps in a bed in his own room but will not stay there, put a gate on his doorway (effectively making his entire room a cot) and return to the gate at the increasing intervals, as above. It is not a problem if he falls asleep on the floor for a few nights. If a single gate is not sufficient, you may need to use two gates or temporarily close the door as described for limit- setting problems in Chapter 5.

10. If your child sleeps in a cot in your room, you should put him into the cot at bedtime and then either speak to him briefly at the scheduled intervals from your bed, or – if your presence in the room is too stimulating, or if you prefer it – leave the room and come back in to check him at those intervals, as you would if he were in his own bedroom. (If he learns to fall asleep with you out of the room, you will have more freedom in the evening. You can accomplish the same thing even if you stay in the room as long as he doesn't know you're there – for example, if he can't see you from his cot, or if it is fairly dark and you are quiet.) When he wakes at night, do the same.

11. If your child sleeps in his own bed in your room, use the same approach unless he refuses to stay in his bed and either follows you out of the room or tries to get into your bed. In either of these cases you will need a gate at your doorway (as described in Chapter 5). Leave the room and close the gate behind you for progressively longer intervals until he stays in his own bed.

12. If your child sleeps in your bed, you may be able to lie still and withhold your responses to him for the appropriate intervals. If that isn't possible, you may have to get out of bed and check from a chair in the room. You may even have to leave and check from outside the room, and as above, a gate may be helpful in that case.

13. Use the same waiting schedule for naps, but if your child has not fallen asleep after half an hour, or if he is awake again and calling or crying vigorously after even a short period of sleep, end that nap time. He may fall asleep on his own later in another room, which is fine, at least initially, as long as he does it by himself, without the associations you are trying to break. However, the amount of time he spends napping should not be allowed to increase – that is, he should not be making up in the daytime any sleep he lost the night before. Also, don't allow naps to run so late (past 4.00 p.m., perhaps) that they will interfere with falling asleep at night.

14. Be sure to follow your schedule carefully, and chart your child's sleep patterns daily (See Figure 5 on page 77) so you can monitor his progress accurately.

15. Additional information on enforcing desired sleep habits when your child sleeps in your room is discussed overleaf ('Co-sleeping and Related Considerations') and in Chapter 5 ('Setting Limits When Your Child Shares Your Bedroom').

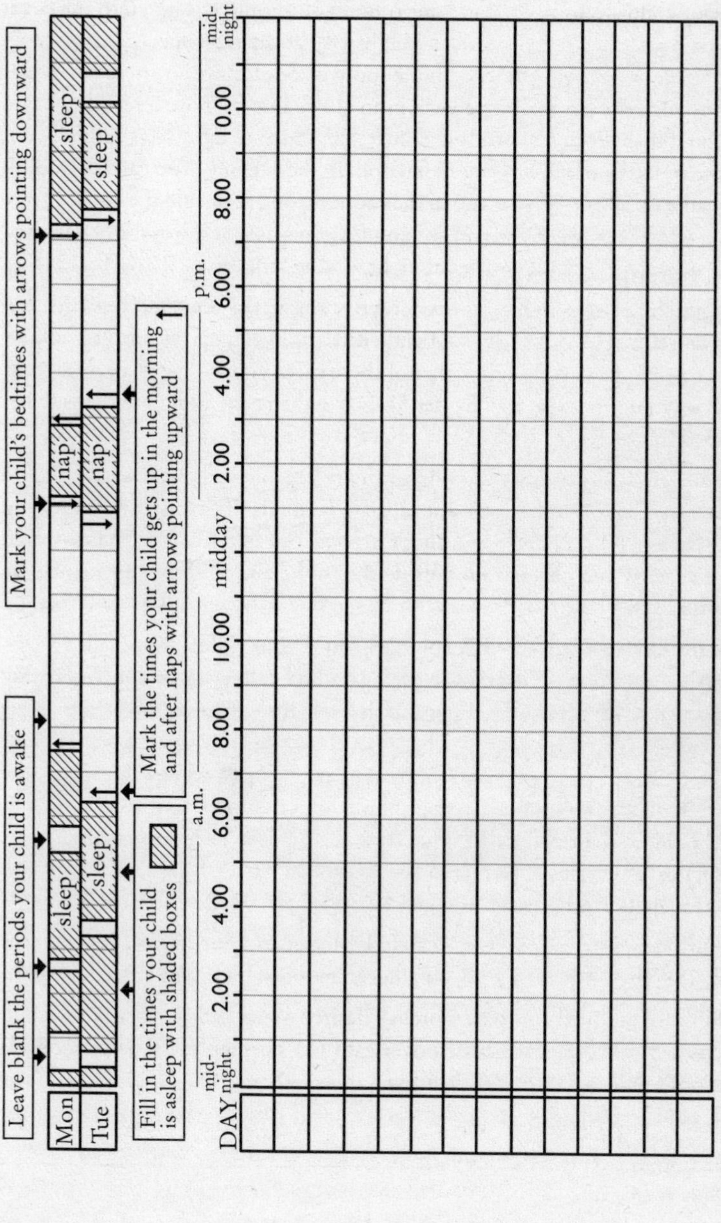
Leave blank the periods your child is awake
Mark your child's bedtimes with arrows pointing downward
Mon
Tue
sleep
nap
sleep
sleep
nap
sleep
Fill in the times your child is asleep with shaded boxes
Mark the times your child gets up in the morning and after naps with arrows pointing upward
DAY
mid-night
2.00
4.00
6.00
a.m.
8.00
10.00
midday
2.00
4.00
6.00
p.m.
8.00
10.00
mid-night

FIGURE 5. SLEEP CHART FOR PARENTS TO USE

I asked them how long they felt they could listen to Betsy cry before feeling they had to do something. Although they thought they could probably tolerate up to fifteen minutes of crying, we decided to begin with three. I find that three to five minutes is usually a good starting point, but, as noted in Figure 4, if that seems too long you can even start with one minute.

On the first night of the treatment programme, we agreed, Betsy's parents would get her ready for bed half an hour later than usual, play quietly and talk with her for a little while, then put her in her cot awake, without rocking her or rubbing her back. Then they would leave the room, returning after three minutes if she was still crying vigorously, to reassure her that they were still there to care for her (and also to reassure themselves that Betsy was all right despite the crying). They would stay in the room for one or two minutes, but they would not pick her up or begin rocking her: they were *not* there to help her fall asleep. It was crucial that she fall asleep by herself, in the cot with her parents out of the room. Her parents agreed that they would speak to her briefly and replace her blanket if necessary, but then they would leave again, whether or not she was still crying and even if she cried harder when they left.

If Betsy continued to cry for five more minutes, her parents would return to reassure her briefly in the same way. If she was still crying ten minutes after that, they would return again. Ten minutes was the maximum wait for the first night: after that point they would return to Betsy every ten minutes as long as she continued crying, until she finally fell asleep while they were out of her room. At any point, if she stopped crying or subsided to mild whimpering between checks, they were *not* to go back in: the one thing they did not want to do was to interrupt Betsy as she was starting to learn how to fall asleep on her own.

If later in the night Betsy woke up and began crying hard again, they would re-start the same pattern as at bedtime, waiting for three minutes, then five minutes, and working back up to ten minutes. They would continue this programme over the rest of the night until an hour before her usual waking time: since Betsy usually woke at 7.00 a.m., that meant that if Betsy woke after 6.00 a.m., they were to get her up for the morning (by that time she was unlikely to get any more sleep no matter what). If Betsy was still asleep at 7.00 a.m., they would get her up no matter how much she'd been awake during the night.

At nap times, Betsy's parents would use the same routine. But if after half an hour Betsy had either cried the whole time or had fallen asleep and wakened again, they would end that nap period. If she fell asleep later on the floor or in the playpen, that would be all right. The important thing was that she was falling asleep alone, without being rocked. As long as she had to spend time in her cot every day, she would eventually start to nap there once she had begun to associate that environment with falling asleep.

On the second day of the programme, Betsy's parents were to start with a five-minute wait and work up to a maximum wait of twelve minutes. Each night after that the waiting times would become a little longer, as shown in Figure 4 (page 74).

I told them to expect the first night or two to be difficult – though only rarely will a child cry for several hours – but by the third or fourth night things should be going fairly well. I also told them that if things were not improving markedly over the first few days, or at any time that they decided that the amount of crying was more than they were willing or able to accept, that we would consider shifting to an even more gradual multi-step approach (as described in the next section).

Her parents braced themselves for the worst and found that things went much better than they had expected. The first night was difficult, but Betsy did fall asleep during the third ten-minute episode of crying. She woke three times during the night, but each time she went back to sleep more rapidly. On the second night, Betsy fell asleep at bedtime after only one visit, and when she woke during the night she fell back asleep on her own so quickly that no checking was needed. On the third night, Betsy fell asleep on her own before even the first visit, and again she went back to sleep quickly on her own when she woke during the night. By the end of the first week, hardly any night-time wakings were still apparent. Over the months that followed, her sleep remained excellent. Her naps improved just as quickly: there were difficulties the first two days – during her first nap time on the first day, she did not sleep at all – but by the third day she was doing fine (see Figure 6, page 81).

Betsy's response was typical. Her parents also reported that as Betsy found it easier to fall asleep on her own at bedtime, they heard shorter and shorter episodes of whimpering when she woke during the night before returning to sleep on her own. Within a week she did not cry at all during these wakings. Of course, she continued to wake periodically during the night, as all people do, but she returned to sleep so rapidly and uneventfully that to be aware of these wakings one would have had to observe her closely all night.

For Jacob and Kaitlyn, who needed a dummy or a bottle used as a dummy to fall asleep, we used a routine similar to the one we used with Betsy: the parents would check on them at gradually increasing intervals, without giving Kaitlyn a bottle or replacing Jacob's dummy. In each case, I recommended that the parents not stay with their child while he or she learned to fall asleep without the bottle or dummy, since that would only produce new associations that would then have to be broken, too. Like most children who already know how to fall asleep in bed alone, Jacob and Kaitlyn needed only a few opportunities to practice falling asleep without the bottle or dummy.

Because the parents were permitted to go in to see their children while they were crying or calling, rather than leaving them alone all night, they could see that although they were unhappy they were otherwise fine. This gradual approach is better for your child, and easier on you, than going 'cold turkey'. Such a drastic approach – putting your child in the cot at bedtime, shutting the door, letting him cry and not returning until morning – would probably work eventually if you never gave in, but it is far from ideal. It would be unnecessarily painful for you and difficult for your child, and you would surely be tempted to quit. If, like Betsy, your child has always fallen asleep in your arms, and if you have always gone to him quickly when he wakes, then to stop this behaviour all at once would mean going directly from one extreme to the other. Such an abrupt change would be very confusing to your child. He has learned to

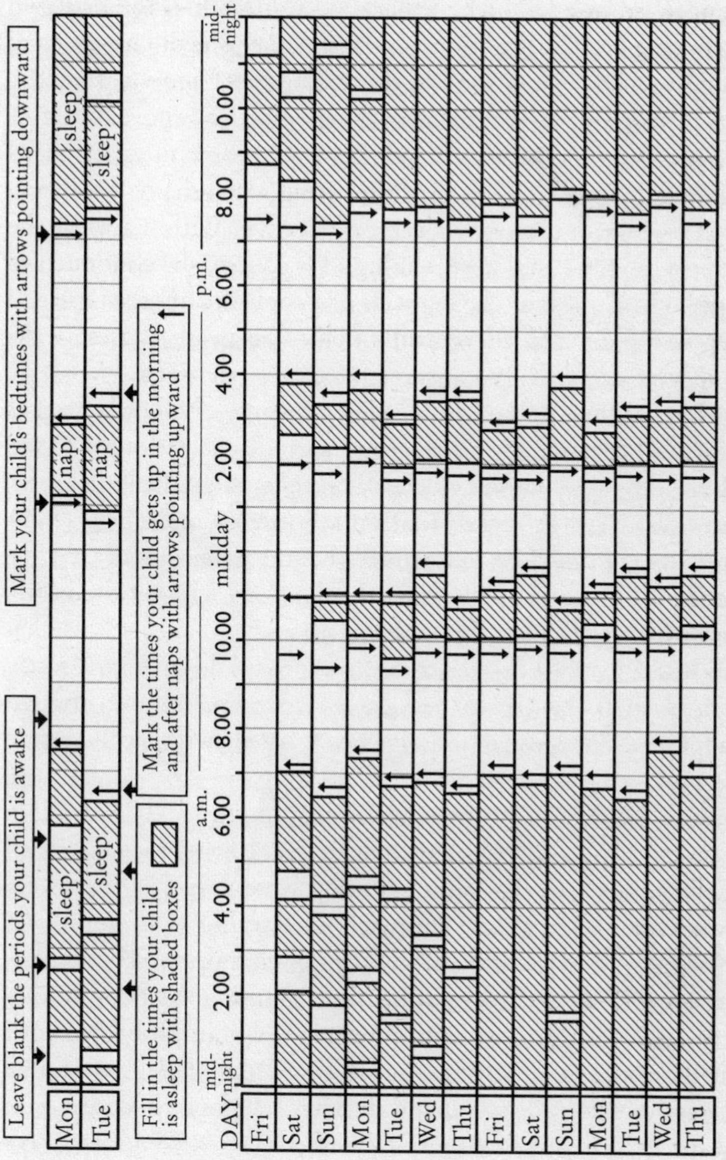

FIGURE 6. BETSY'S SLEEP CHART

expect your prompt appearance when he cries. What is he to think if you don't come in? Where are you? Will you ever come back?

When parents say to me, 'If you're going to suggest I let my baby cry, forget it; we already tried that and it didn't work', often what they really tried is this cold-turkey approach. If you've tried that technique, you likely found – quite understandably – that you couldn't stand to listen to your child cry alone in a room for an hour or more night after night without being able to check on him. Although a child under one year old can sometimes make the transition under these conditions with only a little crying, even on the first night, an older child is more likely to cry constantly or intermittently for hours for a night or two. The longer your child cries, the more likely you are to give up and go in to console him, reinforcing the very habits you are trying to break. It is easier to maintain your resolve, and easier for your child, if you can periodically look in and check on him. Remember, as I told Betsy's parents, if even that proves to be too much for you or your child, you can switch to a more gradual approach (see below).

You may also have misunderstood the thinking behind a cold-turkey approach. Parents are sometimes told that they're 'spoiling' their child by not letting him cry, implying that the crying itself should lead to better sleep. That is untrue: better sleep comes only when your child learns to fall asleep and return to sleep without your intervention, and that happens only when he gets practice at it. Crying does not help children to develop appropriate sleep associations; for that reason, as well as out of compassion, we should try to keep crying to a minimum. When parents tell me they have tried helping their child by 'letting him cry for several nights', usually that's exactly what they did: they let him cry, but *they did not let him fall asleep on his own.* They may have let him cry for a few minutes or for an hour or more, at bedtime or night-time wakings or both, but in the end they always went in eventually to do whatever was necessary to help him go to sleep. In effect, then, all that crying was for nothing; their child only learned that he must cry longer to get what he wants. It is not practice in crying but practice in falling asleep under new conditions that a child needs to learn. If you are going to rock your baby to sleep in the end, you would do better to rock him at once and skip the crying altogether.

The gradual approach accomplishes the same goal in a much more compassionate way. Your child has to learn some new rules, but he will not understand them at first. He should know that you are still nearby and taking care of him, and he can learn that only through experience. If you abruptly began staying out of his room all night, he would still learn that you always come back eventually and that you aren't abandoning him, but the lesson would be unnecessarily harsh. By waiting only a short time before going in to check him, you put him through much less uncertainty. He will begin to see after only a few wakings that you are still around and responsive to him. He may be *angry* that you are not rocking him, but since you keep returning, he will not be *frightened* by your apparent disappearance. As you increase the waiting times, he'll learn to anticipate that as well. Eventually he will simply find it preferable to go back to sleep than to cry for fifteen or twenty minutes knowing he won't be rewarded with rocking, holding or nursing. At the same time, he is learning to fall asleep, and feel comfortable, alone in the cot or bed.

MAKING THE CHANGES IN ONE STEP OR SEVERAL

Habits associated with falling asleep can be changed all at once (as we did with Betsy, Jacob and Kaitlyn) or little by little. Several different associations, such as back-rubbing and dummy use, can be changed at the same time or consecutively. Even a single habit, such as being rocked, can be broken into components, and then the components can be addressed one at a time – first eliminating the actual rocking motions, then being held, then having the parent in the room at all, for instance. Similarly, night-time feedings can be tapered gradually rather than stopped suddenly (see Chapter 6).

Most families choose to correct their children's sleep associations in a single step. However, you can choose to teach your child new associations in two steps or even more if you think it will be better or easier for you or for him. But bear in mind that at each stage you will have to start the learning process over again. How long that takes depends on how many steps are involved. It might sound easier for your child to learn new sleep habits in a few small steps rather than in one big one, but that is only occasionally the case.

Children are very quick learners. A child who has always fallen asleep one way can learn to fall asleep a new way after just a few nights' practice. (It's their slower-learning parents who may take a month or more to master new sleep habits.) That is both good news and bad news: sleep problems can develop over just a few days, but they can be solved just as quickly. Even if your nine-month-old has been sleeping fine on his own for months, if he gets an ear infection that keeps you up with him for a few nights, afterwards he may suddenly have trouble getting to sleep, or back to sleep, without being held. (Events like this probably account for the increase in night-time difficulties that many children experience in their second six months of life.) On the other hand, even if you have been rocking your nine-month-old to sleep all his life, he can learn to fall asleep without rocking in the same few days.

Because children learn so quickly, it often doesn't matter how many changes they have to master at once, so it can be better to go through the process just once and be finished with it as quickly as possible. However, in certain situations it makes more sense to solve the problem one step at a time. Thus, for a child who always gets very anxious when apart from his parents, or a child first learning to sleep in a room by himself, you might chose to work on certain of your child's habits first, such as dependence on a dummy or being rocked or sleeping in a new bed or room, and leave the separation problem for last. (Techniques for managing the anxious child are further discussed in Chapter 7.) However, if your child is *not* reassured by your presence in the room – for instance, if he only gets angry at you for being there but refusing to pick him up – then leaving the room from the start may actually make the change in sleep habits easier. If you are unsure whether to try a one-step or multi-step approach, you can start with either one and, if it isn't working well, switch to the other.

Similarly, while spacing out night-time feedings in an effort to reduce or eliminate them, as discussed in Chapter 6, many parents initially prefer to respond to their child whenever he calls and in whatever way will comfort him (other than feedings). In one or two weeks, after the night-time feedings have been phased out, the parents can change the child's other associations as a second step.

Finally, children with special needs may require changes to be made in very small steps with very gradual changes, sometimes for the parents' sake as much as the child's. It is very hard to refrain from responding to a child who is blind or has cancer, and a child with major neurological abnormalities may simply be unable to master the changes except in small steps, with long learning periods at each step. In some cases all the desired changes may not be possible.

ASSOCIATIONS TO THE BREAST, BOTTLE OR DUMMY

It is not necessary to wean your child in order to break the association of nursing with falling asleep. Nor, probably, will you have to give up the bedtime feeding, which is usually the last feeding to be phased out, anyway. You may try to eliminate nursing during the night (as described in Chapter 6) while still allowing your child to feed at bedtime, even if he falls asleep at the breast or with a bottle. If you are trying that approach, continue the bedtime feeding as usual, completing the feeding and then moving the baby to the cot. You don't have to wait until he is deeply asleep to move him; in fact, it's better if he knows he is being moved so there will be no surprises when he wakes up. If he is still awake or wakes during the transfer, respond to his cries at progressively longer intervals, as usual, until he does fall asleep. Since you have already fed him, you should not bring him back to the breast then or try to re-start bottle-feeding.

But if you find that your child has trouble giving up feedings during the night as long as he continues to fall asleep while feeding at bedtime, then you should consider separating the last feeding of the day from bedtime. Move the feeding a little earlier in the evening; if your child starts to fall asleep, stop the feeding, wake the child enough that he will be aware he's being moved, and put him in his cot or bed to continue falling asleep. You may need to do the same at nap times. Many parents choose to take this step even before they know whether it will be necessary, since it makes the bedtime process go more quickly and easily and frees a nursing mother from being the only one who can put the child to bed.

If your child is consuming large amounts of liquid at night, his sleep may be disturbed for reasons other than sleep associations (such as hunger signals, altered body rhythms and increased wetting, as discussed in Chapter 6). But a sudden end to nursing at night would be hard on both you and your child; it's better to gradually reduce the number and frequency of feedings. (How to solve problems caused by these excessive feedings is also discussed in Chapter 6.)

If your child uses a dummy only when going to sleep, then once he has learned how to fall asleep without it, he will no longer use it at all. But if he has a dummy in his mouth most of the day, it will be harder to stop its use at night. In that case, I suggest that you first work to cut down on his use of the dummy during the day. Decide on certain periods in the morning and afternoon when you will not let him use the dummy; then increase the length of those periods gradually day by day. During those times, give him extra attention and divert him so that he will have an easier time getting used to the dummy's absence. You may have to listen to some protests as he learns to feel comfortable without the dummy during the day, just as you may when he learns to give it up at night. Once he is using the dummy mainly at sleeping and resting times, you can eliminate it and begin a progressive programme like the one we used for Jacob. By now he will be quite used to being without the dummy and will only have to learn to fall asleep without it.

Stopping the dummy at night is easier than most people realise, particularly for a child between four months and twelve months old. It isn't that hard to stop later, either, but the older the child, the harder it seems to be (because he can protest more verbally and stay awake longer). There is no good way to eliminate night-time use of the dummy gradually; limiting the minutes it can be used during the night is too frustrating and confusing to work. This part you must do 'cold turkey'. But even if your child has the dummy with him all night, he probably doesn't suck on it more than ten or twenty minutes total, since most sucking takes place in short intervals as he is going to sleep. Often, falling asleep just once or twice without the dummy is enough for a child to master sleeping without it. If he is very sleepy at bedtime, the learning will be even easier, so starting with a later-than-usual bedtime the first two nights will help. Sleeping without the dummy should certainly be routine after one or two days.

The 2005 recommendation of the American Academy of Pediatrics to let babies fall asleep with a dummy in their mouth to decrease the risk of SIDS and related conditions – possibly by disrupting sleep and causing more wakings – was discussed in Chapter 3. Still, if this guideline is strictly followed, and dropped dummies are never replaced to aid return to sleep later in the night, the child likely will learn to sleep both ways (especially if dummy use during the day is limited). If the baby continues to have difficulty falling back asleep without it at five to six months – when the likelihood of SIDS has become small – then stopping the dummy even at times of falling asleep would pose little risk, even if these recommendations prove to be well grounded.

CO-SLEEPING AND RELATED CONSIDERATIONS

Proponents of co-sleeping often suggest that you can avoid the problems discussed in this chapter simply by having your child sleep in bed with you. It is true that sleeping together does avoid some problems. Parent-child separation is not an issue, at least if you are prepared to be in the bedroom as soon as your child goes to bed. If it is physical closeness with you that he wants and expects, then being in bed with you should make him happy and able to sleep. But inappropriate or undesirable habits and associations can develop wherever the child is sleeping. That he is in your bed does not mean that he won't expect to have his back rubbed or be fed or nursed repeatedly; he may still need a dummy replaced, or you may still have to rock him each time he wakes. If he just needs a few pats on his back during the night it may not be difficult for you, but if he needs long periods of patting at bedtime and again several times during the night, you have a problem. If you have to move to the rocking chair to get him back to sleep every time he wakes up, he may just as well be in his own room, except that you don't have to walk as far. Finally, if your child uses you as a soothing object, instead of an appropriate transitional object for that purpose (as discussed in Chapter 3), the situation may be even worse. If you are a nursing mother, he might use your breast as a pacifier every time he stirs, easily ten times or more during the night. Or, like Alexa, he may insist on falling asleep in a way that he likes but that is uncomfortable for you, such as on top of you or sideways in the bed, or he may demand to stroke your face while he sucks his fingers or nurses.

If your child sleeps in a cot in your room, the basic situation is mostly the same as if the cot were in his own room. However, the reassurance of simply being able to see you immediately whenever he wakes may not be enough to let him fall back to sleep quickly. Instead, seeing you may be a temptation that is difficult to ignore and that may actually make it harder for him to get back to sleep without your help (in the same way that a child may have a harder time being with a babysitter when he can hear his mother's voice in the next room than once she's left completely). Bringing him into your bed at these times will allow you to get back to sleep as fast as possible, and that's fine if you're happy with those sleeping arrangements; but if you're not, then you may still need to make changes.

Even if your child sleeps in your room or bed, his sleep association problems can be solved. If he is in a cot in your bedroom, treat the sleep problems exactly as if the cot were elsewhere: put him down at bedtime, leave the room and return for brief visits at increasing intervals. He will learn to fall asleep in the room alone and without rocking or patting, allowing you more freedom in the evening. If he wakes at night, you can try lying quietly in bed, responding to him at timed intervals as before. (You can do the same at bedtime if you don't mind always having to be in the room when he falls asleep.) But if your presence is too stimulating, you may have to leave and make your visits from outside the room. Once he gets used to falling asleep without your intervention, you should be able to stay in the room. Some parents prefer to sleep in another room for a few nights, until the child has mastered the new patterns. You may also be able to make a 'room within a room' with a concertina-style room divider or by hanging a sheet or blanket from the ceiling – if your child cannot see you in bed, you can limit your responses to him without having to leave the room yourself. The inside of the divider could be decorated for him.

If your child sleeps in your bed, or if you stay in his while he falls asleep, undesirable habits can still be dealt with as discussed below and in Chapters 5 and 6. If your child sleeps in your bed, then it is easiest if there are two parents working together to solve the problems, although a single parent can do it all if necessary. There is no need to let your child use your body in a way you find unpleasant, and there is no need to rock, pat or walk him during the night, either. You must simply refuse to go along with these demands and let him fall asleep anyway. If he uses you but not the other parent as an object for soothing himself, turn away or move to a chair until he returns to sleep. If he is big enough to pull at you or follow you out of the bed, you may have to leave the room and temporarily close the door or gate. (You can even sleep in another room for up to a week until the problem is resolved. The other parent can usually stay in the room.) Come back at increasing intervals, and each time you return, get back in bed and stay as long as your child does not make the objectionable demands. If he does, leave again for a longer time. The choice you present to your child should be 'me on my terms or nothing', where the terms are those you have decided are best for his – and your – sleep. Your child should find this an easy decision.

Alexa's parents used this method to deal with her preference for sleeping positions that interfered with their own sleep. Her mother left the bed every time Alexa tried to lie on her; each time she left for a longer period, while Alexa and her father stayed in bed. Whenever Alexa tried to turn sideways and force her parents apart, her parents placed her on a blanket on the floor, again for a longer period each time. The positions she favoured were no longer associated with anything pleasant. Soon both behaviours stopped.

Even if your child does not co-sleep with you in your bedroom, he still may be used to having you come into his room, at bedtime and after night-time wakings, and lie with him until he falls asleep. You can break that association as well. If your child is old enough to understand, explain to him that you can no longer lie down with him while he falls asleep. Make sure you have an appropriate and pleasant bedtime ritual (see Chapter 3). When you finish your story, game or quiet talk, tuck your child in and leave the room, but leave the door open. Some children will call out or cry; others will get out of bed. If your child only calls out, he can be handled in the usual manner by progressively increasing the interval between your responses. You can go back into the room when it's time to respond, but do *not* lie down with him, and always make sure you are out of the room when he falls asleep.

But if your child will not stay in his room when you leave, then you need to use a boundary of some sort, such as a gate or the door, as discussed earlier and in Chapter 5. If he is old enough, usually three or three and a half, you may want to try a reward system to help speed the initial phase of re-learning. If the rewards are especially successful, you may not even need a boundary. Otherwise, you can still use them along with a boundary and appropriate limit-setting. You can set up a chart like the one described in Chapters 5 and 7, letting him earn stars or stickers and occasional small prizes for going to sleep without getting out of bed. The chart will help to motivate him to try to fall asleep without having you there, and he will feel that you are working together to solve the problem. When the novelty of the rewards wears off, he may begin to make more demands at bedtime again. If that happens, be especially careful not to give in, or the old problems may re-appear. Since he has already learned to fall asleep on his own, it is no longer a matter of teaching him how to do it, but simply of enforcing the rules. Be firm, and use a boundary at the doorway if necessary: the good sleep patterns will return quickly.

Because William, the three-year-old who needed his parents in bed with him, and Sam, the two-year-old who fell asleep on the sofa with the television on, were old enough to get out of bed on their own, the progressive-waiting approach had to be applied using the option of a boundary. William's parents put up a gate to help keep him safely in his room. He put up major struggles over the first few days. His parents got little sleep and began to wonder if the plan would work. But they persevered, and by the middle of the first week William was beginning to sleep much better. By the end of the week, he was protesting only mildly when his parents left the room, and before long he was sleeping continuously through the night.

Although Sam did not need his parents present when he fell asleep (he only needed the television), the need to learn to fall asleep alone in his bedroom was similar to William's – and so was the treatment. Unfortunately for Sam, however, his existing associations with falling asleep did not even include his own bedroom. He had no formal bedtime ritual at all, and when he awakened in the night, he could re-create the conditions he associated with falling asleep only by going to the living room and playing while the television was on.

His parents instituted a pleasant bedtime ritual ending with a fifteen-minute period of story-reading that Sam enjoyed. Still, at first, he did not like being told to stay in his room, and he tried to come out until his parents, too, put up a gate. Like William, Sam struggled valiantly over the first few days to maintain the status quo, but by the start of the second week he, too, was sleeping normally.

A consistent, progressive programme for learning new routines can be difficult to enforce initially, but it works remarkably well in a variety of situations. If your child's problem is similar to those of the children described in this chapter, your approach to solving it can be very similar as well. Younger children are usually easier to deal with but, at least after the first three months of life, children of all ages with these problems will respond well to the programme *if* their parents are willing to stick to it.

IF THINGS ARE NOT GETTING BETTER

The programme of progressive waiting is designed to treat only one specific sleep problem: the situation where your child has come to inappropriately associate something you do, or allow him to do, with the process of falling asleep. If this is indeed your child's problem, and it is the *only* problem, you should have no more than a few difficult nights as he adapts to the new patterns. By the third or fourth night, certainly within a week, everything should be much better. If it isn't, you should be looking for a reason.

If a week or so has gone by without improvement – or, even worse, if your child's periods of crying have grown longer and more intense – then don't continue the programme. Stop and review the situation. There are a number of possibilities to consider before you decide what to do next. You may have made the wrong diagnosis; you may have made the right diagnosis but be treating only one part of a complex problem; or you may somehow be treating the problem inappropriately.

Procedural Considerations

Something you are doing, or not doing, could be interfering with your progress. Some parents have trouble following the programme strictly and consistently. Common errors include letting your child fall asleep on his own at bedtime, but then rocking him during the night; staying with him until he falls asleep at bedtime but insisting that he fall back asleep alone later in the night; letting him fall asleep alone at bedtime and early in the night, but moving him into your bed when he wakes near morning; handling his pleas or crying differently from night to night or responding differently when you think he is making enough noise to wake his siblings; and, in two-parent families, having each parent enforce the programme in his or her own way. If you do any of these things, matters may not improve.

If you stay out of your child's room for a certain length of time as planned but then, after checking him, you end up staying in his room until he falls asleep, you will not make much progress: remember, it is having him finally fall asleep the new way that matters, not the waiting. If you start with short waiting intervals and don't increase their length, your child may come to expect several visits from you before he goes back to sleep. The reason for increasing the times is to reach a point where he is alone long enough to fuss for a while and then settle himself before you have had to go in even once. The best thing you can do for your child at night is to give him a clear and definite understanding of what is to happen. Enforcing routines inconsistently will only make problems worse.

Similarly, if you can't enforce consistent, clear rules, you may not see progress (see Chapter 5). Perhaps you insist that your child start falling asleep alone, but you still have to put him back into his room over and over after he runs out. (For him, it may be a game.) Or you may be unable to insist that he stay in bed all night because he quietly sneaks into your bedroom without waking you. Or you may have stopped allowing him to watch television at bedtime, but he still watches in the middle of the night because there is a television in his room or because he can sneak into the den. In setting new routines, you will succeed only if you enforce them completely and throughout the entire night.

Schedule Considerations

The treatment can be undermined if the plan does not take into account your child's daily schedule and biological rhythms (see Chapters 9 through 12). The progressive-waiting programme assumes that your child is sleepy and capable of sleep at the times when you are using it. If he isn't sleepy, no programme – regardless of how strictly and consistently it is applied – can help him to fall asleep. If your child has been falling asleep at 9.00 p.m. and you set his bedtime at 7.00 p.m., he will have about two hours to complain before he even begins to get sleepy. That is why I suggest you start with a bedtime no earlier, and probably a little later, than the usual time he falls asleep. If you are not sure what time to start with, remember that it is better to err on the late side at first than to put your child to bed when he is still wide awake. You can always move his bedtime earlier again after a few days.

Similarly, if your child is usually awake for an hour or two in the middle of the night, but he is happy as long as you are there playing with him, then you may simply be keeping him in bed longer than he can sleep. In that case he will have an hour or two to fill in the middle of every night before he is capable of falling back asleep. As will be explained in Chapter 11, you will need to cut back the length of time he spends in bed accordingly before you try to teach him a new pattern of associations.

If your child loses sleep while you are teaching him new patterns because he is up crying during the night, don't let him sleep later than usual or take more naps or longer ones the next day. If you let him make up in the day the sleep lost at night, you will only succeed in shifting some of his sleep from the night-time to the daytime, ensuring that he will be awake and crying more the next night. If he ends up short on sleep one night, that's okay: it will actually work to your advantage the next night.

If you are not sure when your child is even capable of sleeping, perhaps because his schedule and hours of sleep vary so much from day to day, work on developing a consistent schedule that works for him. You should find a schedule in which he falls asleep quickly at bedtime (even if he needs help to do so) and falls back to sleep quickly after waking during the night (again, even if he needs help) before you start enforcing a programme of changes.

Anxiety

Your child may be frightened. If he shows signs of separation anxiety in the daytime, he may not be able to tolerate separation at night. Leaving him alone in his room for longer and longer periods will not help – in fact, it may make matters worse. If that seems to be happening, then choose a multi-step approach: as described earlier and in Chapter 7, you should work on all other associations first and deal with the separation problems later. You may need to sleep in the same room as him all night, but even then you can still insist on sleeping on a separate bed or mattress, refuse to hold or rock him or eliminate a dummy. If he keeps pulling at you or getting into your bed, you can still leave the room for increasing periods of time, except that when you return you should agree to stay as long as the undesirable behaviour does not resume.

Confusional versus Habitual Wakings

When you think your child is awake at night, is he really awake? When you go to him, does he respond appropriately, calm down quickly and let you know what he wants, or does he push you away and keep thrashing and kicking? Children experiencing a *confusional arousal* or *sleep terror* are not awake enough even to realise that you are there, much less to learn new patterns of associations. How to recognise and treat these partial arousals is discussed in Chapter 13.

Medical Considerations

It is quite uncommon for pain to be the cause of frequent or nightly wakings in children, but you may need to rule out the possibility. A child who is in pain at night can usually be distinguished from one who is simply unhappy. The child who wakes because of pain may be somewhat comforted by being held, but the pain will not go away: he will still show signs of being in pain, and he will not return to sleep quickly. He will probably experience similar periods of pain in the daytime as well. On the other hand, if your child is happy if you hold him, give him his dummy, or allow him to play, or if he sleeps well when you let him sleep in your bed, then you can be sure that he is not in pain. Pain and other medical situations are discussed further in Chapter 8.

GENERAL OBSERVATIONS

There are some general points that are useful to keep in mind as you try to determine the cause of your child's sleep problem and try to correct it.

1. *Changes you need to make to correct a problem of inappropriate sleep associations are not being made solely for your own benefit – more important is that they are also to benefit your child.* Being able to fall asleep easily, and trusting that things won't change once he does, is a better way for your child to go through the night.

2. *Ideally, the conditions associated with falling asleep should not be stimulating, like television, and they should not involve continuous activities such as sucking on a bottle or dummy.* It's best for children to learn to fall asleep in a cot or bed in a room that is fairly dark and quiet (no lullaby CDs, television or sound machines). After their first few months, children should not need to be held, rocked or patted, or need to be soothed with a bottle or dummy or at the breast, just to fall asleep. (Bedtime feedings are fine even after the early months as long as the child doesn't come to depend on them to fall asleep throughout the night.)

3. *When children wake during the night, they should be where they were when they fell asleep, with the same people there (or not there): they should be able to trust that no changes were made after they fell asleep.* They should not have any jobs to do – checking, calling, sucking, eating, watching, listening, pleading or demanding – before falling back to sleep. All they should need is to find a comfortable position and continue quickly into the next sleep cycle.

4. *If your child wakes crying at night but quiets rapidly and returns to sleep promptly once you re-establish the conditions that were present at bedtime – such as rocking him in your arms – then you can be certain that he has merely learned to associate the wrong conditions with falling asleep.* There is no inherent abnormality in his ability to sleep. The physiological systems that control sleep in a child cannot prevent him sleeping well only when he is not being held or rocked. If these systems were not working properly, your child would not sleep well under *any* conditions. So you can be sure that the cause of his sleep disturbance is not a neurological abnormality, a dietary imbalance or food sensitivity, or significant discomfort.

5. *Don't start too young.* Parents frequently ask at what age they should start a progressive-waiting approach. It is difficult to give a

precise answer to this question, but there are some guidelines. Most children start to sleep through the night on their own within three or four months after birth. (Note that all figures here are based on the due date, so they will be later for children born prematurely.) Newborns do not sleep through the night, and you should not try to make them. Sleep (particularly REM sleep) in the newborn is broken by many wakings. At these times, and during the periods of change from one sleep state to another, an infant's sleep patterns are particularly vulnerable to disruption. Your newborn should not have to negotiate these periods without comforting and help. At any rate, a full night is too long for a newborn to go between feedings.

By the time a child is around three months old, significant developmental changes have taken place. Now most sleep should be occurring at night, and the pattern of sleep stage cycling should be fairly mature (see Chapter 2). A baby's sleep patterns often improve markedly around this time, so unless you are having unusually severe problems, it is a good idea to wait until your child is three or four months old before you institute major changes. If at that point you only need to get up briefly once or twice a night to settle your child, you might want to wait a few weeks and see what happens; often, such sleep patterns continue to improve on their own.

But even a two-month-old should not be up more than two or three times during the night. If your baby is up more than that and always goes right back to sleep when you help, you might see if he starts to do better if you do not always respond immediately. (Remember, the methods in this chapter are designed to help you treat *habits*, not other sleep problems.) If his sleep does not improve over a few days, you should probably give him the benefit of the doubt and wait a few weeks before trying again. (Similarly, as discussed in Chapter 6, you should not have to feed a healthy two-month-old hourly across the night, and it is fine to start spacing out the feedings then, but it is too early to aim at eliminating them altogether.)

If a marked problem persists at three or four months, you can then consider a real effort to make changes. By the time the baby is five months old, you can consider making changes even if his sleep problems are relatively minor.

6. Your child's sleep associations at one time (say, bedtime) may not always affect what happens at other times (such as later in the night or at nap times). Rocking your child to sleep or patting his back is not *necessarily* wrong, or even certain to cause trouble. If your child falls asleep rapidly, is easy to move to his cot or bed and sleeps through the night (i.e., puts himself back to sleep quickly after normal wakings), and if you are happy with this routine, then there is no problem at all. For example, even if you rock your child for five minutes at bedtime or nurse him to sleep over ten minutes, you may be able to transfer him easily into his cot or off you onto the mattress, and he may re-settle himself quickly and then sleep through the night. You would have reason to change the routine only if problems emerged – if, for instance, the bedtime routine becomes prolonged, as it was with Betsy, or if your child begins waking most nights and requires your presence each time.

To take another example, your child may fall asleep alone at bedtime and nap time but need to be rocked after night-time wakings. Or perhaps he falls asleep easily at day care, even though his sleep associations there differ completely from those he has at home. Children with sleep patterns like these have learned to associate different conditions with falling asleep at different times or in different places. This is no more or less normal than needing the same conditions each time one falls asleep.

7. If your child falls asleep by himself at nap time but needs you at night, then you can expect the re-learning to go very quickly. He already knows how to fall asleep on his own; he simply has to learn to associate that behaviour with the night-time as well as with nap times.

8. The amount of help a child needs to settle during the night may vary depending upon the time. A child who wakes frequently at night may sleep well for several hours before his first night-time waking and after his last one. For example, he may sleep soundly from 7.00 to 10.00 p.m. and from 4.00 to 7.00 a.m. but be restless, waking frequently, between 10.00 p.m. and 4.00 a.m. This variation is only a reflection of his normal pattern of sleep state cycling. As you learned in Chapter 2, children spend the first few hours of the night in deep sleep and often return to that same state near morning. During the period of lighter sleep in between, they are more subject to wakings.

9. *If you have been going in to your child during the night to help him to fall back asleep, you may have been told that you were 'spoiling' him.* That is not true. Spoiling a child means giving in to his demands regardless of what is best for him. If you are comforting him at night, it is probably because you feel that it is the right thing to do for him, not because you cannot say no or are incapable of discipline.

Repeatedly going in to comfort him, however, is often not the best thing to do. By doing so, you may only be strengthening a habit, not responding to a real need. In the daytime, you may find it easier to distinguish your child's wants from his needs, and you can deny him any inappropriate requests without difficulty, even if he cries. But if he wakes and cries at night and only settles when he is nursed or rocked, you may mistakenly believe that he is hungry and needs to be fed or that he is in pain. You could also jump to the conclusion that he has some inherent problem that makes it impossible for him to go back to sleep without gentle rocking. You know that a colicky baby of two months might need to be walked; you might imagine that by the same token it is appropriate to walk a sleepless, crying child of six, eighteen or thirty-six months. The real problem here is not that you are spoiling him, but that you do not yet know enough about sleep and sleep associations to distinguish his wants from his needs. Once you understand that what he needs is to learn a new way to fall asleep – whether or not it is what he wants – you will find it easier to see that this need is met.

10. *The process of learning new sleep associations will not hurt your child.* Parents want their children to feel safe and cared for. When they realise they will have to let a child do some crying, they often fear that the experience will be traumatic, causing permanent psychological harm. While this concern is understandable, long experience has shown that there is nothing to worry about. Allowing some crying while you help your child learn to improve his sleep will never cause psychological damage. It will probably be harder on

you than on your baby. Even the most worried parents I have worked with have told me afterwards that their concerns about the re-learning process proved groundless and that, if anything, once the child's sleep improved, both they and the child were happier.

A young child cannot yet understand what is best for him, and he may cry if he does not get what he wants. As his parents, you have to be the judge of what he can and cannot have or do. You want to do what is best for him, and that should include helping him form good sleep patterns. If he wanted to play with a sharp knife, you would not give it to him no matter how hard he cried, and you would not feel guilty or worry about psychological consequences. Poor sleep patterns are also harmful for your child and it is your job to correct them. Doing so is a sign of caring, not of selfishness.

Of course, if your child does not get enough love and attention overall, then he may well develop psychological problems. But if you consistently show your love and provide warmth and care, then a little extra crying for a week or so – no matter how upset or angry it sounds – will not hurt him in the least. Even when children become more 'clingy' for a day or two, as sometimes happens, the parents are invariably convinced by the rapidity with which this behaviour resolves and the child's sleep improves that they have done the right thing. In fact, with respect to possible psychological effects, your family situation can only improve when your child sleeps better at night. He will feel better and be less irritable during the day. If there are no changes or surprises during the night, he will be more trusting. Because of these changes, and because you yourself will be more rested and have less to be angry about, you will enjoy your child's company more, and your interactions with him will improve as well.

11. Since it is important that you follow through on your programme consistently, wait for a convenient time to begin. Don't start at a time when you cannot afford to lose sleep yourself, such as before an important meeting or a job interview, or when someone is coming to visit. You may want to wait until a Friday night to begin, so that you have the weekend to catch up on any missed sleep.

12. In most cases, once you decide on a waiting schedule, follow it closely (or at least don't go in too soon). Know ahead of time how long you are supposed to wait and keep track of the time. Ten minutes can seem like an hour in the middle of the night. Sometimes, too, it may be better *not* to go in to your crying child even when the time is up. If you can tell that he is beginning to calm down, you may only interrupt the calming process and make things worse if you go in and leave again. If you sense that waiting a bit longer will actually be easier on him, then wait and see if he continues to calm down on his own. Remember, you can always go in if he becomes more upset.

13. In two-parent households, parents should share the responsibilities, if possible, so that the same adult does not have to handle all bedtime and waking interactions during the re-learning period. Your child should feel comfortable with either parent at bedtime and after wakings, so it is better if both parents participate. You do not have to alternate strictly; just pick a schedule that suits you. One parent may find it easier to get up in the first half of the night and the other parent may prefer the second. Or work demands may call for one parent to do more on weekends and the other on weekdays. If one parent has handled all the bedtimes and wakings until now, the other parent may have better luck breaking the old associations.

When a child cries and one of the parents responds, it is probably best if that parent continues to be the one who responds until the child falls asleep, so that the child won't sense that he can control who comes in by crying enough. For similar reasons, it is good advice not to let your child insist 'I want Mummy' or 'I want Daddy'. Decide who will handle each night's bedtime routines, and stick to it. You will do more to convince your child of your love by staying than by giving in to his demands for the other parent. Once he learns that you really mean that you want to be the one to care for him at that time, he will look forward to it (if it is part of the usual bedtime ritual), and he will be more reassured. The same applies to your responses at night-time wakings.

14. Occasionally, as parents increase the time they wait before responding, their child cries so hard that he vomits. If that happens, go in even though the time isn't up yet. Clean your child up and change the sheets and pyjamas as needed. But do so quickly and matter-of-factly, and then leave again. If you reward him by giving him too much attention, he will only learn that vomiting is a good way for him to get what he wants. Occasional vomiting will not hurt your child, so don't feel guilty that it happened. Like the crying, it will soon stop.

15. *If you have other children, especially young children, you may be concerned that they will be kept awake by the noise of crying during the re-learning period.* You probably don't need to worry too much. If the other children wake, tend to them as necessary, but don't let your fear of their being wakened interfere with your ability to stick to the programme. Remember, even if their sleep is disturbed for a few nights, it will return to normal quickly. They will probably sleep through most of the fuss anyway. If a child who shares a room with the one doing the re-learning complains about the noise, or if it seems to be disturbing him greatly, let him sleep in another room for a few nights. Generally the child with the sleep problem wants his brother or sister back, and that provides further motivation for him to co-operate. If the child you are helping sleeps in a cot, you can instead move the cot (rather than the sibling) to another room for the few days necessary.

16. *When you are considering a programme that involves some crying or screaming at night, it may seem that it would only be practical if your family lived alone on a deserted island.* If you live in an apartment building, you may have to contend with neighbours and your landlord. Explain to your neighbours what you are doing and tell them the problem should only last a few nights. Start the programme at the weekend if they prefer. If they are not willing to go along, perhaps you can wait until they will be away for a few days. Or you may have to use a very gradual approach in which you stay in the room initially to keep crying to a minimum.

17. *During the re-learning process, it is better not to use a babysitter.* But if it becomes necessary for a night or two, let the babysitter put your child to bed in whatever way is easiest. It is not fair to ask a babysitter (especially a grandparent) to follow your

programme, and letting a babysitter put your child to bed differently will not really affect what he is coming to expect from you. Nothing will be lost; just be sure to re-start the programme the next day. Once the new routines are well established, however, you might ask your babysitter to try them.

If your child is left with a babysitter most days, the babysitter will know your child well and he or she can participate in the re-learning programme for nap times. When a babysitter or day care provider handles nap times differently from the way you handle bedtimes, there are usually fewer problems than there would be if you handled both yourself but did so inconsistently. If it is not possible to involve the babysitter, or if it seems inadvisable (because the babysitter is very young, perhaps), then you may have to institute the programme only at night. It will still work.

18. *Once your child has learned to fall asleep by himself with the proper associations, he will probably continue to sleep well, but there may be occasional disruptions.* If you are visiting friends or relatives, your child may have to share your room, and you may want to respond to his whimpering quickly so that it doesn't disturb your hosts. Or your child may be ill, perhaps in pain, so you sit with him or take him into your bed. When you get home or the illness passes, he may want to continue going to sleep under these 'new' conditions. If you give in, the temporary change may well develop into an ongoing sleep disturbance. This is a common problem, especially during the second six months of life. Making changes on a holiday or during an illness is necessary and reasonable. But if these changes lead to new associations that cause your child's sleep to remain disrupted after he is back home or recovered, then all you need to do is go back to the progressive programme described in this chapter for several days to re-establish the proper patterns.

Since it is not difficult to re-establish good sleep habits, you should not hesitate to take care of your child in any way he needs if he is ill or frightened or while travelling. In fact, it is important to show him you are available when he truly needs you. That trust makes it easier for him to handle other times by himself. It's best, however, to make as few temporary changes as possible. If you have to spend some extra time in his room, you may not have to stay all night. He may want a glass of water, but you probably won't have to re-start feedings or bottles. Do only what is necessary, so he will have less to re-learn later.

CHAPTER 5

The Problem of Limit-Setting

'I want a glass of water'. 'One more story'. 'Another kiss'. Requests like these, benign though they may seem, can ruin your evening and disrupt your night as well if they are endlessly repeated. The youngster making these demands *could* fall asleep, if only he would stay in bed and stop calling out. This is a problem of limit-setting. As you will see, the appearance, causes and treatments of this problem overlap considerably with those discussed in the chapters on associations, feedings, schedules and anxieties, and elements of any or all of these can appear in the same child. The problem of limit-setting, however, tends to occur more in the toddler and older child than in the infant, and the interactions involved often take place before a child goes to sleep rather than during the actual transition to sleep itself.

Often this problem appears suddenly when a child learns how to climb out of a cot or is moved to a bed. Until then, the bars of the cot represent the parents' authority: the child can call out, but he can do little else to get his demands met. Once this control is gone, parents perhaps just assume that their child will continue to stay in bed at night on his own. But for a two-, three- or four-year-old, or even for an older child, the impulse to get up can be too strong to resist. There might be something he wants to do or someone he wants to be with. He may hear people talking and laughing; or he may hear nothing and wonder where everyone is. The temptation for your child to be part of whatever is happening outside his room can be overwhelming. He starts to make demands, trying to get you to come back in with whatever else he wants. If you don't respond, he may come out of the room after you, or he may find another way to get you to come in, perhaps by making enough noise to wake a baby brother or sister. Some children only have to threaten to wake their siblings to get the desired response.

WHO'S IN CHARGE?

Children are smart. They do what works and they don't do what doesn't. They may run through a litany of requests, but they will settle on the ones that get the most predictable responses. Most children settle on similar 'curtain calls', like the typical ones for more water, stories or kisses, as mentioned at the opening of this chapter, or perhaps:

> 'Rub my back some more.'
> 'I need to go to the bathroom (again).'
> 'Please tuck me in (again).'
> 'Sing me another song.'
> 'I want to say good night to Daddy.'
> 'I need to tell you something.'

If a child has difficulty with self-control, then it is best if that difficulty can be done away with at bedtime and during the night. Controlling the child is the parents' job – or should be. Ask yourselves, 'Who is in charge?' Frequently, when parents describe to me what happens at night in their household, it is clear that they are not. They tell me that they know they shouldn't give their child a second full bottle each night at bedtime, then add: 'But she *demands* another bottle.' Or they agree that their child should be away from the television and in bed by 9.00 p.m., then say, 'But she *insists* on watching another programme.' Or, after telling me that his wife has to handle all his daughter's bedtime routines, a father may explain that he tries, 'but she won't accept me.'

If you find yourself explaining away bedtime difficulties with words like 'demand', 'insist' or 'won't accept', then you are not the one running the show at night. Young children simply should not be allowed to demand or insist on anything that is not necessary, certainly not at bedtime or during the night. If they are given this power, they will use it; the situation goes downhill from there, and rapidly.

For example, Megan, a sweet and generally well-behaved four-year-old girl, turns her bedroom into Mission Control at night. She calls out for a glass of water, but when her father brings it in she sends him out, saying 'I want Mommy.' When her mother returns with the water, she, too, is sent out because 'it's in the wrong glass', and then again because 'it's not full enough'. Soon her parents are running upstairs and downstairs, trying to meet all her demands. The wrong person is in control, and no one is sleeping.

Learning to set limits appropriately is an important part of becoming a parent. All parents do set limits; they just don't all set them for the same reasons or with the same level of consistency. No parents would willingly let their two-year-old play with matches or run into a busy street, no matter how long he protested. They might not like listening to him cry when he is told no, but they are unlikely to feel guilty about it, either. And since these rules are firm and absolute, he will eventually stop trying. He would not think better of his parents if they let him do what he thought he wanted and he was then injured as a result. What lesson would he have learned, then?

Setting limits is relatively easy (at least emotionally) when the consequences are life and death. You don't feel you are depriving your child when you stop him playing with the electrical socket, although you might when the consequences are not so dire – for instance, when you refuse to get him an extra glass of water. But to the young child, these situations are indistinguishable: both cases are a matter of 'I want this; can I have it?' If you set a limit for a good reason, you have no cause to feel guilty or fear that you are hurting your child or losing his love, whether that reason is to protect him from harm or merely to keep his bedtime habits under control.

Of course, it is also important that you do not set limits capriciously based on how you feel on a given day, and also that two parents do not set limits differently (which can become an unintended game of 'good cop, bad cop'). Being overly strict is as bad as being overly lax. You should try to find a proper level of firmness, and that level should not change day to day or parent to parent, from daytime to bedtime, or from bedtime to the middle of the night.

Nurturance and proper limit-setting are not opposites: they are different ways of showing your child how much you care. If limits are set properly, a child will learn that they are in his best interest and that they are a sign of your love and concern. Think of the best teachers you had in school. In all likelihood, these teachers were strict enough to keep your class controlled, but they were also able to communicate their love and care for each student. If a teacher turns over control to the students, chaos ensues – no attention, no learning. That may be fun for a day, but not for much longer.

DIFFICULTY SETTING LIMITS

Some parents are always able to set limits well. Others set them effectively only during the daytime, weakening at night as they try to avoid battles and get to sleep themselves. Still others set limits poorly and inconsistently at all times.

If you are having trouble setting limits, there may be a variety of reasons. You may never have considered how important limits are for your child, and you may never have learned how to go about enforcing them. Aspects of your child's sleep schedule may be undermining your attempts to control his night-time behaviour. You may have feelings of guilt that make it hard for you to be firm. Your child's resistance at bedtime may have indirect benefits for you ('secondary gain'), which can in turn make you reluctant to follow through consistently, if at all. Finally, there may be underlying problems at home that interfere with your ability to control your anger and set and enforce proper limits while remaining nurturing and supportive.

Let's consider each of these issues in turn:

Knowing why limits are important and how to set them. If you think it's tolerable that your four-year-old son comes into your bed each night, against your will, and kicks you or your partner until one of you has to move to another room, then you may not understand the importance of setting and enforcing rules. The same could be said if you see nothing wrong with letting your child determine when and where he will eat, what television shows he will watch and when he goes to bed, or if you believe you should always buy him anything he wants (to keep him from throwing tantrums in public, perhaps). If you know these scenarios are wrong but you - don't know how to change them – if you can't keep your two-year-old in his room after you say good night, or can't even avoid going back to tuck him in repeatedly – then you need to learn some specific techniques. Later in this chapter, I will describe some techniques you can use at night; although, if you are having trouble controlling your child all day long, you may want to seek some general help in behaviour management. First, however, you should be aware of the important considerations of schedule, guilt and psychosocial factors as well as feedings, fears and associations.

Schedule. If limit-setting at night is the only problem, then when you start to set limits properly, your child will begin falling asleep quickly and easily. But if his bedtime is set too early, before he is sleepy, then he will not be able to fall asleep no matter how strict you are. In fact, at a too-early bedtime he may be more wakeful than at any other time of the day (see below, and 'The Circadian System and the Forbidden Zone for Sleep' in Chapter 9). It makes no sense to force your child to stay in bed and try to fall asleep when he feels wide awake and his mind is active.

Guilt. Setting limits at bedtime is often difficult even under the best of circumstances, and it can be far harder if your child has an underlying medical or emotional problem, or if you are unable to spend as much time with him as you'd like. You want to show your love clearly, and you worry about how your child feels when you seem to ignore his crying and pleading. And if your child is deaf, has had heart surgery or is on chemotherapy, or if you work two jobs or travel a great deal, just how tough do you want to be? There is usually no easy answer. In such situations, setting necessary limits all at once may be too wrenching, and you might find it easier to follow a programme that helps you to regain control in a series of small steps: for example, at one- or two-week intervals, you could first eliminate extra television, then extra drinks and so on with back-rubbing, sitting on his bed and sitting in his room.

Secondary gain. If failing to enforce appropriate limits at bedtime, or giving in to your child's demands at night-time wakings, has some positive consequence for you, this so-called secondary gain can make you hesitate to change things. For example, you may enjoy cuddling with your daughter on the sofa while she falls asleep at bedtime – you just don't like having to cuddle repeatedly throughout the night. Secondary gain can also involve more complicated scenarios. In some families, the child's wakefulness at night keeps the parents from fighting, and his presence sometimes even serves to keep the two of them physically apart all night, which one or both of them may find desirable. One might say that their child is doing them a favour, at least at some level, but even if this is so, family therapy is not a job any child should have to take on.

Problems at home. If limits are to be set properly at night, the child must be given proper support and nurturance during the day. The two go hand in hand. But it can be difficult to provide nurturance in a family experiencing marital difficulties, or if a parent is depressed, abuses alcohol or other drugs or is otherwise ill. A child who does not get enough proper attention during the day may be willing to accept punishment just to get *some* sort of attention at night. In this context, setting limits may be difficult, if it's possible at all. If major problems like these are making it hard for you, or if you are unsure even what limits should be set given the difficulties at home, I urge you to seek help. What is best in these situations varies considerably from home to home and cannot be decided without skilful counselling.

LIMITS, ASSOCIATIONS, FEEDINGS, SCHEDULES AND FEARS

As I mentioned at the beginning of this chapter, several overlapping syndromes can complicate limit-setting. If there is a component of associations (see Chapter 4) in addition to the limit-setting problem, the treatment required is basically unchanged. Different approaches are called for, however, if you have a frightened child (see Chapter 7) or if your child's sleep schedule is inappropriate (see Chapters 9 through 12).

If a child who is clearly not frightened or anxious requests a series of tuck-ins at night, and then goes to sleep alone and sleeps through the night, or perhaps requires at most one or two more tuck-ins during the night, the behaviours in question are part of the pre-sleep routine but not part of the process of actually falling asleep. Unlike the situations where sleep associations become a problem, he falls asleep and wakes under the same set of circumstances. The tuck-ins have become a possibly unwelcome habit, though, and the habit persists (and is reinforced) because limits are not being set.

Another child may request that you sit in the room or on his bed while he falls asleep. He may even hold on to you so that without even opening his eyes he can be sure you haven't left. You may have to return and repeat the process during the night when he wakes. If that happens frequently enough, you may well end up sleeping in his room part of the night. Now we have an association problem as well as a habit, because you are there when he falls asleep but may be gone when he wakes. Both problems are treated the same way.

Habits and associations may also both be present if a child sleeps with his parents all night and insists that he sleep between them while they move to the very edge of the bed. If the child also demands and receives access to the breast or bottle at each night-time waking, there is probably an additional element of excessive feedings, which may have to be dealt with (as described in Chapter 6) before the rest of the problem can be addressed. If your child stalls with an hour of repeated requests every night at bedtime but then sleeps through the night, his bedtime may be too early or his time of waking too late. A schedule adjustment may be called for rather than limit-setting, or in addition to it (see Chapters 10 through 12).

But if your child wants you in his room because he is truly frightened (not the 'pseudo-anxiety' discussed in Chapter 7, where 'I had a bad dream' is just one more item on the litany of 'curtain calls'), then setting firm limits and refusing him access to you at night could make matters worse. In that situation, you must deal with the fears first. As described in Chapter 7, that may require you to sleep in his room temporarily while the fears are addressed. Taking care of his fears is the main thing that matters at first. You can still limit extra drinks, stories and even the amount of time you spend lying in bed with him, but you should not insist that your frightened child be in his room alone.

Setting Limits at Night

Whether or not you find setting limits difficult to do, if you have come to understand that limits are important, and that a lack of limits is contributing significantly to your child's sleep problems, the suggestions in this and following sections should be useful.

You will notice that the treatments of limit-setting problems may be similar or identical to those previously described for inappropriate sleep associations. That is because there may be considerable overlap between the two types of problem. If your child keeps demanding you return to do something he wants *until* he is ready to go to sleep – such as repeatedly tucking him in – that part is a limit-setting problem; but if you always end up interacting with him *while* he falls asleep – perhaps rocking him – that part becomes a problem of sleep associations. The same activity may be both: for example, if your child insists you sit in his room singing to him before and while he falls asleep. The differences between these two problems may be slight, and both problems often resolve with similar if not identical treatments.

Your job is, first, to decide which of your child's behaviours and demands you would like to end and in what ways you give in unnecessarily or inappropriately at night, and then to develop a plan that will enable you to stop these behaviours. Whichever demands and responses cause protracted bedtimes and night-time wakings are the ones you must stop.

Your child should have an appropriate bedtime routine, like those described in Chapter 3. It should take place in the room where your child sleeps, and its length should be reasonable and determined by you, not by your child. For young children, five to fifteen minutes is usually adequate, but you may want to allow somewhat longer times if your child is of school age. Don't let the routine in the bedroom last so long that your child is not sure when it will end. Provide a warning ('Last story', for instance) and stick to your rules: if you give in to requests for extra stories only some of the time, those requests will still likely be repeated every night. If you want to allow a small drink before saying good night, include it in the formal routine; do not make your child ask for it. You may decide to end with a kiss and a tuck-in, and then leave. If you want to lie down with him briefly – for one minute, perhaps – then, again, it should be a formal part of the ritual, not something your child demands, and you must be prepared to leave when the time is up. If you are sloppy about enforcement, your child will learn that there is always a possibility that further demands will be rewarded.

If your child is still in a cot that he cannot climb out of and he makes demands from the cot, you need only respond briefly at progressively longer intervals, as in the treatment for association problems described in Chapter 4. The process is exactly the same. If he sleeps in your bed but cannot yet leave the room on his own, then you may have to leave the bed yourself for progressively longer intervals (you can move to a chair, for example, or even leave the room temporarily, as discussed below).

If he is able to leave his room (or follow you out of your shared room), the problem becomes a little harder. No matter how much he yells, how strong he is or how well he can climb, you *must* be stronger than he is. If he ends up in control instead of you, the only lesson he will learn is that he can always get his way. Thus, if he starts coming out of his room when you refuse to keep going in, you may have to put up a gate. (You may have to do that even if he sleeps in your bed, if he follows you out of the room.) If he can kick down the gate, you may have to screw it into the door frame. If he can climb over it, you may have to put up a double gate – two gates, one above the other – until he agrees to stop climbing. If he can get over a double gate, you may have to start closing the door. Do whatever it takes to enforce the rule, just as you would if he tried to play with matches. You must win because it will actually be scary for him if you do not. Only when you have successfully settled the issue will he see that you are really in charge; only then can he stop trying to find ways to outsmart you; only then can he stop worrying about whether you will respond supportively or angrily; and only then can he see that you are really taking care of him. Finally, then, he can relax, with no job to do except to go to sleep, and the matter is solved.

You should only set limits that are necessary. Some children never come out of their room at night, whether the door is open or not, and they rarely will challenge your control. Children like that do not need a gate, and they are easy to set limits for. Other children will find a way to get out through six inches of open space between the top of the gate and the ceiling, and if they cannot get out, they will set about systematically destroying their room. These children desperately need to have limits imposed. Take from the discussion that follows just those techniques your child needs.

The Barrier or Boundary: General Considerations

The cornerstone of setting limits at night is ensuring that your child stays in the room where he should be sleeping. If he doesn't stay in the room, you can't enforce any night-time rules at all; to enforce them, you must be prepared to use a barrier. Taking him back to his room over and over is not effective – in fact, he will probably perceive it as a game, especially if he has to be chased about the place, or if he can sneak out of the room when you're not watching. Threats and punishments are counterproductive: a young child should not be punished for a lack of self-control at night, when self-control is hardest. Do not insist that your child take on a job that he cannot yet handle; you must take it over for him.

If you dislike the idea of having a barrier, remember that in any case your young child cannot be allowed to wander freely about the house while you sleep. He may usually go to your room, true, but he could just as easily go somewhere more hazardous, such as the kitchen. He may also be confused in the middle of the night, half-awake and unsure of where he is going and why, and that will put him at additional risk. (Some children consciously and intentionally head away from their parents at night so they can do things that they are not normally allowed to do.) A strategically placed gate at the top of the stairs or in the corridor will keep your child in a restricted part of your home and probably safe. But you are still better off requiring him to stay in the room where he sleeps and putting the gate at the doorway of that room to enforce the rule. One of the worst things you can do is to leave his door open and lock your own: now he is kept away from you but 'confined' to the rest of the home, while you're locked in. Who's in control now?

Remember, problems such as those discussed here often start when parental controls, symbolically and physically enforced by the bars on the cot, are lost. When that happens, it is entirely reasonable to replace those controls and make his entire room a 'cot'. The gate accomplishes that. Your child is free to wander about his room, just as he was free to move about his cot, but he cannot go anywhere else. And the gate ensures only that he stay in his room, nothing more. You cannot keep him in bed, and you shouldn't try. If at first he falls asleep on the floor by the gate, don't worry; you can always move him to his bed once he is deeply asleep, and in any case, sleeping on the floor by the gate usually stops on its own before long, unless he can see you from the gate. (If he can, you are providing a temptation for him to stay by the gate instead of returning to bed. It is even worse if he can see you doing something he would like to be doing himself, such as watching television. You will find it easiest to set limits when temptations like these are gone.

You would not put sweets on the dinner table if you didn't want your child to eat them for dinner. The gate takes away the temptation for your child to leave the room, since he can't. Closing the door to your bedroom, or the living room or wherever you are, far enough that he won't be able to see you takes away the temptation for him to stand there and watch.)

Usually a single or double gate will suffice for a child under four. If your child is a climber, avoid concertina gates with large diamond-shaped holes that he can use as finger holds and toeholds. A nylon mesh gate like a window screen or one with vertical bars will be hardest to climb.

A gate is far preferable to a closed door, for several reasons. Most children like to sleep with their own door open, because an open door helps them to feel connected to the rest of the home. That is also why children often prefer that their parents' door not be completely closed, either. For the same reason, being able to hear the sounds of people moving about the home is often more reassuring than disruptive. If your child's door is completely closed, he can only imagine where you are and what is happening on the other side, and that can be scary, which is not the goal. Locking the door all night is rarely a good idea – probably never, for an otherwise normal child. You may have to close the door for increasingly long periods to help a child who is too big for a gate (see below), but the eventual goal here is to have the door open, and that approach presumes he can develop enough self-control to master staying in his room.

The gate should be presented as what it is: a tool to help your child stay in his room at night and keep him safe. (The word *help* here is more than a euphemism: many children do want to stay in the room and make their parents happy, but they just cannot overcome the temptation to leave.) Closing the gate should be part of your bedtime routine. When you go into your child's room to start your stories or songs, close the gate behind you, and begin with an activity he looks forward to; if you close the gate only when you leave or when you are angry, that's what he will learn to associate with it. When you have finished your bedtime routine, quickly step over the gate (or open it and quickly close it again behind you) and leave. Remember to then stay out of his line of sight. (It is usually a good idea to remain on the same floor as his bedroom, at least until problems have been resolved.)

From this point on, handle the situation just as you would if your child were in a cot and you were helping him to break a pattern of inappropriate associations (see Chapter 4). Follow the chart for the Progressive-Waiting Approach in Figure 4 on page 74. If he keeps calling, yelling or crying, come back to the gate at the increasing intervals listed in the chart to reassure him briefly, and then leave again. Usually it is best not to actually enter his room, just as you would not climb into his cot, unless something truly needs attention. (If he throws his teddy bear or other special object out of his bed, don't go in to replace it unless he can't find it; if he loses it again, don't go in to replace it until your next scheduled trip back.) There are two reasons not to go into his bedroom. First, you do not want to reward him for calling. Second, if you do go in he may grab you, and then you will have to pull him off and race him to the gate, which is unpleasant for everyone. Check on him until he falls asleep, and repeat the checks during the night as needed.

The Barrier or Boundary: Using a Gate

To properly enforce the boundary, you must first make sure the barrier is effective. If you are using a gate, remove any chairs and stools that your child could use to climb over it. Second, you must behave consistently for this plan to work. You cannot give in on occasion just because your child's crying is intense or prolonged, and you must not handle wakings in the middle of the night differently than at bedtime, or respond differently from night to night. Inconsistency is unfair to your child. It will be easiest for him to learn if your actions and responses are always consistent and predictable.

Just like the inside of a younger child's cot, the room must be made safe – windows locked or protected, sockets covered, no sharp-edged furniture. If your child's behaviour escalates to the point of wildness, you may have to go further. For this child, even more than for others, it is critical that you get control back. If he topples dressers, knocks over lamps and throws toys, remove them from the room. Once something comes out, it does not go back until the nights have quietened down. In extreme cases – which, fortunately, are rare – it is necessary to start with the room empty except for a mattress.

If setting limits is new to you, some of the techniques suggested here may seem harsh. But an out-of-control child is not a happy child. A gate will allow you to remain calm and supportive, since you can set limits without physically restraining your child. If you are fighting with him, controlling yourself is very hard, and if you get angry and lose control, he gets the wrong message. It is much easier to continue talking to your child in a warm, reassuring and controlled way when you are on opposite sides of a gate than when you are carrying him back to his room kicking and hitting you.

To some extent, the bigger your problems are at the start, the easier you may find setting limits to be – after all, things cannot get much worse. It can be more emotionally difficult to set limits when a child's requests are almost trivial, like asking you to pull up the covers twice a night. Meeting those requests may take no more than ten seconds each time. But if you cannot get right back to sleep yourself after these nightly requests, your own sleep could be badly disrupted. You might have to do something about these demands for your own sake; but in this case there is a lot of room for things to get worse before they get better, if your child reacts strongly to new limits. In such situations you have to decide whether the problem is important enough to fix and whether the time is right to fix it. On the other hand, when the problem is relatively mild, positive reinforcement, even without firm limit-setting, may be all that is necessary (see below), and the cure may prove to be as mild as the problem.

Rarely do normal children actually hurt themselves in reaction to the establishment of clear, firm and appropriate limits. Occasionally a child will engage in self-destructive actions, such as biting his arm, banging his head into the floor or wall, scratching (if he has eczema) or wheezing (if he has asthma). Obviously, you cannot let truly harmful behaviour go on. The goal is to stop such behaviour without at the same time rewarding it. If your child reacts in this way, you may need some help in designing an individualised and gradual programme; fortunately, however, these situations are uncommon.

Once you have regained control and your child has stopped challenging you, peace returns to the night. The hours before bedtime are free of tension. Your child stops running away when you go to put him in his pyjamas. Both you and your child start to look forward to bedtime as the special time it should be. Children find that they can relax, and they are happy that they are no longer displeasing you. All of this happens because you took back control. The gate often becomes a symbol of this change, and the same child who fought the gate initially may now remind you to close it every night. It not only keeps him in his room but it also keeps his emotions in check. The gate is an extension of you, doing what a parent is supposed to be doing: taking care of your child.

If after some days or weeks your child asks that the gate be left open, try it. Some children will now be able to stay put on their own. For others, despite the best of intentions, the open doorway remains too great a temptation. Take care of each child according to his individual needs.

The Barrier or Boundary: Using the Door

For a child who is too big for a gate, probably between the ages of four and six, you may have to close the door. (Doing so with an older child is also possible, but the older and bigger they are, the more difficult it becomes to enforce limits with this approach.) Each time your child leaves his room, take him back and close the door, keeping it closed a little longer than the time before. Because this technique requires the child to be shut behind a closed door, and the goal is to develop control, not fear, we usually start with short times like fifteen seconds, as shown in the chart in Figure 7 on page 121, and slowly work up from there. If you feel that you and your child can tolerate longer times, you can start on line 3 of the chart or lower.

Close the door only if your child leaves his room, and close it only for the specified time. He should learn that his leaving his room triggers a definite response which *increases each time* and over which *he has no further control.* Don't agree to open the door as soon as he gets back in bed, since as soon as you have opened the door he may get out of bed again, knowing full well that he can get the door opened any time he wants.

Similarly, closing the door does nothing if he can open it. Stay on the other side of the door and hold it closed as needed. If you have to, you can put a hook and eye on your side of the door so it will stay closed – but just for the designated time. Do *not* lock the door and leave; stay by the door, where you are only a few inches from your child if he is right on the other side. You can say something through the door periodically to let him know you are there, but do not let him draw you into conversation. Do not answer any questions: he will be trying to take back control, which you cannot allow.

Open the door at the end of the allotted time, whether he is in bed or kicking at the door from the other side. You are using the closed door only to keep him in his room, not to control the rest of his behaviour. Keep following the chart. He must learn that he is not allowed out and that nothing good happens when he tries to come out, only longer periods with the door closed. If he does not like the door closed, he will stop leaving his room. (Remember that even if he stays in the room, you should refuse to respond to any of his habitual requests or demands if you want them to stop.)

What if your child needs to go to the toilet? Usually, if he went at bedtime, he won't need to go again until the middle of the night, if at all. If he always uses the toilet (appropriately) at that time, of course you must continue to allow him to go, without it triggering any door-closing. (A younger child, for whom you are using a gate to set limits, eventually may be able to go by himself once the gate is no longer needed, although most toilet-trained two- and three-year-olds still need help at night.) But if his request to use the toilet is only a stalling tactic, if he goes into the toilet but little or nothing happens, you can refuse.

FIGURE 7. HELPING YOUR CHILD LEARN TO STAY IN HIS ROOM

NUMBER OF MINUTES TO CLOSE THE DOOR IF YOUR CHILD WILL NOT STAY IN HIS ROOM

If Your Child Continues to Come Out of His Room

Day	First Closing	Second Closing	Third Closing	Fourth Closing	Fifth and Subsequent Closings
1	¼	½	1	2	3
2	½	1	2	3	5
3	1	2	3	5	7
4	2	3	5	7	10
5	3	5	7	10	12
6	5	7	10	12	15
7	7	10	12	15	20

1. This chart shows the number of minutes for which you should close your child's door if he will not stay in his room at bedtime or after night-time wakings (if he is too big for a gate). (The times listed are ones that most families find workable. You may change the schedule as you think best, as long as the times increase progressively.)

2. Keep the door closed for the number of minutes listed, even if your child goes back to bed sooner. You may speak to him through the door occasionally so he knows you are there, but do not let him draw you into conversation.

3. When it's time to open the door, speak to him briefly, offer encouragement and leave. If he leaves his room again, put him back inside (no need to tuck him in) and shut the door for the next amount of time listed.

4. Once you have reached the maximum number of minutes for the current night, continue keeping the door closed for that amount of time until he finally stays in his room.

5. If your child wakes during the night and will not stay in his room, begin the door-closing schedule at the minimum time for that night and again work up to the maximum.

6. Continue this routine as necessary after each waking, until a time in the morning (usually 5.00 or 6.00 a.m.) after which you feel further sleep is

unlikely. Then begin the day. (If the time of morning waking remains too early for you, it can be adjusted later as described in Chapter 10)

7. If your child wakes and calls or cries but does not get out of bed, switch to the progressive-waiting routine described in Figure 4 on page 74.

8. Be sure to follow your schedule carefully and chart your child's sleep patterns daily (see Figure 5 on page 77) so you can monitor his progress accurately.

9. Remember, your goal with this technique is to help your child learn to fall asleep without you being there. You are using the door to enforce this behaviour in a controlled way, not to scare or punish him. Reassure him by talking through the door; do not make threats or raise your voice. Because you are progressively increasing the length of time during which the door is closed, your child is spared the anxiety of having no idea when it will be opened. He will learn that he can keep the door open all night just by staying in his room.

10. For this programme to be successful, you must return your child to his room as soon as he leaves it, even in the middle of the night. If you wake in the morning to find him on the floor in your room or outside your door, you will not be solving the problem. If that happens, put a bell or some tin cans on your door, or place a chair in front of the door, to make noise and warn you when he is coming in. If you prefer, or if he tends to go other places than your room, you can put the bell or cans on his door instead so you will know when he is leaving his own room. Or you can put up a gate on his doorway; even if he can open it, you can make it impossible for him to open it quietly.

11. By day three or four your child will most likely be staying in his room, but if further work is necessary after day seven, just continue to add a few minutes to each door closing on successive days.

12. You can try the same routine at nap time. (Bear in mind, though, that most children too big for a gate will no longer be napping, or can stay awake through a nap if they want.) If your child has not fallen asleep after half an hour, or if he is awake again and out of bed after getting some sleep, end the nap period for that day. But if you fail to make progress at nap time, especially in an older toddler, it may be best to focus your efforts at night and work only on having a regular quiet time in the middle of the day, not necessarily in his room. If he still needs a nap, it will come back eventually.

13. The first few nights can be difficult, but with a later-than-usual bedtime, clear resolve on your part and perhaps support from a sticker chart (as outlined later in the chapter), they can also be surprisingly easy. Children vary in their

willingness to struggle. Some will learn quickly that they prefer staying in their room to having the door closed on them even briefly. Other children are willing to accept longer closed-door periods before giving in. Either way, if you persevere, the situation should improve substantially within one week, two weeks at most, provided that you follow the schedule consistently: your child must learn exactly what to expect. If you are lenient at some times and firm at others, your child will always have reason to believe that *this* time you may give in.

If your child stays in his room and calls for you, switch to the chart in Figure 4 on page 74, returning to the doorway (but not inside the room) for reassurance at increasing intervals. Go back to the chart in Figure 7 (above) if he comes out of the room again.

Setting Limits When Your Child Shares Your Bedroom

Even if your child sleeps in your room and you want him to be there, he can stall, make unnecessary demands and otherwise behave inappropriately. He may keep asking for extra stories, additional television or more drinks. He may demand that you stay and your partner leave; he may insist that both of you stay; or he may give orders about where on the bed each of you is to sleep. He may insist on twirling your hair, stroking your cheek or lying on top of you.

Although in this situation the child cannot be confined to his own room while you sleep elsewhere, you still have to remove certain temptations and enforce limits. You may have to make changes, such as unplugging the television or moving it out of the room for a few nights. If your child tries to leave your room at night, you may have to set up a gate or be prepared to close or even lock your door (acceptable in this case because you'd be in the room with him). If he keeps disturbing you at night by trying to get something from you or do something to you, move to a chair for increasingly long periods. (Use chart in Figure 4, page 74, as a guide for times.) If your child is old enough to follow you there, or if for any other reason you find it difficult to refuse his demands while you are in the same room, you may have to leave the room for the designated periods with the barrier in place until the demands cease.

If there is only one parent and no partner who can remain in the room to be sure your young child is safe, or if a child beyond the toddler stage is too destructive to leave alone in your room even for short periods, you will have to find another place for him and at least one parent to sleep, somewhere you can enforce limits safely and effectively, until he accepts the new rules and you can all move back to your bed.

Sticker and Point Charts: Positive Reinforcement

When your child is unable to control his behaviour by himself, you have to set limits for him and enforce them. But sometimes a child capable of controlling his behaviour has simply got into the habit of making demands. Such a child frequently can be coaxed into giving up those demands by providing him with motivation in the form of rewards for the desired behaviour. For some children, rewards alone are all that is necessary. For others, limits and rewards can be used together: once the child stops testing limits, he starts earning his rewards.

Enforcing limits with barriers and other responses that your child perceives as negative may be necessary, but it is certainly not fun. Working out a reward system with your child, on the other hand, can be fun, and reward-conditioning is entirely positive. When I use rewards to help a child I see in the office, I enjoy it; and children who succeed in following a reward-based programme are as happy as they come.

Start your reward programme by negotiating with your child, at least if he is three or older. (Using a reward system with younger children is difficult: their language skills are limited, and although they like getting the rewards, they usually won't make the connection when they are protesting at night.) For example, ask your child if he would like to be allowed to stay up later (see sections above and below and Chapter 9). He will doubtless say yes. Then ask him if, given the (temporarily) later bedtime, he would be able to stay in his room and stop calling or making other demands. You could also ask him if it would help if you stayed on the same level of the house, or in the next room of your flat, while he went to sleep.

Next, discuss a sticker chart with him. Set up different award levels for different levels of achievement, so he can be successful even when he cannot do everything you hoped for. For example, offer two stickers for quietly staying in the room at bedtime, one if he calls out but doesn't leave the room. Offer another three for the rest of the night, depending on how well he does: three if he stays in bed all night and doesn't call you, two if he calls during the night but stays in his room, one if he comes out only once and no stickers if he leaves his room more than once. (Later in the learning process, you might reduce the middle-of-the-night awards to only one sticker if he calls and none if he leaves his room even once.) If the problem behaviour occurs mostly at bedtime, you can focus the rewards there. For example, you might give him three stickers if there are no bedtime problems, two stickers if you have to come back once, one sticker if two trips are required and none if you must return more than twice. Another one or two stickers could be earned for good behaviour later in the night.

For three-year-olds, the stickers are their own reward. Youngsters a little older may be better motivated if you let them earn a small present each week by doing well and accumulating stickers. School-aged children may also like the idea of earning presents but find stickers babyish; they are often happy to negotiate a system based on points. If presents are to be earned, they should be small, costing perhaps a couple of dollars. The rewards are meant to be symbolic, not out-and-out bribery, and small presents can be given weekly. Remember that if young children have to wait too long to earn anything, they will lose interest. (Older children may be able to postpone the weekly rewards in favour of a bigger one, perhaps earned over several weeks.)

If necessary, begin by rewarding your child for meeting relatively modest goals. There is no point in offering rewards for tasks the child cannot yet do or can do only occasionally, and a child who feels he cannot earn his rewards will stop trying. Besides, success breeds success. Err on the lenient side at first in giving out stickers or points. If you're using small presents, award them as long as your child is trying hard and having some success. Don't be so strict that he can fail by falling one sticker short.

Set up a chart with your child and have him participate in designing it, as well as in applying stickers or recording points; he may want to decorate it and show it to others. Be creative – the possible ways to set up a sticker chart with a child are endless. Make your system fit your child. Make a big deal of the chart and of your child's success; it should be fun for everyone. If he is working with you and trying to succeed at night, rather than fighting against your attempts to regain control, you are way ahead of the game.

If stickers alone are not enough to get your child to stop calling or stay in his room, be prepared to set limits anyway, including the use of a gate or a closed door. If he takes to the rewards at all, the limit-setting will be easier. Once he is quietly staying in his room, he will begin getting stickers, earning rewards and feeling proud of his success. If the reward approach works well, continue it as long as your child's interest lasts. Usually problems won't re-surface after his interest fades, but if they do, be prepared to set or reset whatever limits are needed.

Late Bedtime

It is crucial that your child be sleepy and ready to fall asleep when you start this programme. If his bedtime is too early, what looks like a limit-setting problem may really be related to his schedule (see Chapters 9 through 12). Remember, a child gets more alert late in the day before he gets sleepy at night. If he keeps leaving his room at night saying that he is not sleepy, chances are that he really isn't sleepy enough to fall asleep. Even if you sit or lie down with him, he will probably be unable to fall asleep until a later hour.

When you start any programme of limits or rewards, your child's bedtime should be set no earlier than the time he has recently been falling asleep most nights; in fact, it is often helpful to begin thirty to sixty minutes later than that time, even if it means a bed-time between 10.00 p.m. and midnight. If he falls asleep at different times on different nights, start at the later end of the range – better to start with too late a bedtime than with one too early. Leave his wake-up time and nap times unchanged, unless they have been in-consistent or otherwise inappropriate – such as waking too late in the morning or napping too long or too late in the day.

Controlling his schedule in this way guarantees that he will be very sleepy at bedtime. That in turn helps to keep the amount of protesting to a minimum and gets the learning process started with as little difficulty as possible. Once he gets into his sleep phase (the period that runs from when he is first ready to fall asleep at night to when he is ready to wake for the day in the morning – see Chapter 10), he gets sleepier and sleepier until it becomes difficult for him to stay awake. Use this powerful drive to your advantage. If, on the new schedule, you always have to wake him up in the morning – a sign that he needs more sleep than he is getting – you should have no trouble gradually moving his bedtime earlier again.

You may be pleasantly surprised to find that with a later bedtime all of your child's bedtime problems disappear. And if that happens, night-time problems are likely to resolve as well. As we've seen in the context of other problems, when a child wakes during the night, he tends to resume whatever he was doing when he went to sleep. If he started the night with an hour of calling and leaving his room, he will likely start up again at his first waking; but if he starts the night by going right to sleep, he is more likely to go right back to sleep after waking later in the night.

Even if problems remain despite the later bedtime, there should at least be some improvement: your child will find it much easier to stick to a reward programme if he is very sleepy, and his struggles over limit-setting won't go on for so long.

Allowing your child to stay up later than usual does not mean you should allow unsupervised or inappropriate activity. The televi-sion and computer should be turned off at a reasonable hour. You may also have to be more available to your child during these extra hours for play, stories or conversation, depending upon his age. Once the limit-setting problem is solved, you can re-adjust his schedule as needed.

Siblings

It can be difficult to use a closed gate or door to set limits for a child who shares a bedroom with a sibling, younger or older. If the sibling who does not need limit-setting is old enough, he can open the gate or door as needed (for example, to use the toilet). But if he is too young to do this himself, you can ask him to call you, when he needs to use the toilet or is done sleeping for the night, until the other child has learned enough self-control to stay in the room without the boundary.

Siblings often sleep through any noise their brother or sister might make, whether they sleep in a separate bedroom or share the same one. But if a child protesting new limits at night is able to make enough noise to disturb his sibling, the sibling may need extra attention from you during the night until things quieten down; you may also have to let him sleep elsewhere (such as in another bedroom, on the sofa or on your floor) for a few days to a week, until the protests stop. The noisy child will see that his behaviour caused him to be left alone in the bedroom, and that may provide him with an extra motivation to settle down. It's always better to deal with a sibling's disturbed sleep for a few nights than to give up on a plan of limit-setting for the other child (which will only teach him that screaming gets him what he wants).

Sometimes a sibling undermines the parents' efforts at control; for example, an older sister may unlock her brother's gate, let him into her bed or move into his bed. It is not the role of a sibling to play parent, and you should not allow it to happen. Talk to the sibling: explain what you are doing and why, and make it clear that he or she can help her brother or sister most by not interfering. Usually this discussion is all that is needed to ensure siblings' co-operation. If their interfering behaviour persists, however, it means they, too, need limits set, and you must be prepared to stop them. It may be enough for you to move them temporarily to another room, even yours, or for a parent to stay with them in their own room, for the few nights it takes for the other child to start sleeping well.

Limit-Setting Problems: Some Examples

Isabella was a five-year-old girl whose behaviour had never been a big problem. Her 8.00 p.m. bedtime went fairly easily, except that she never went right to sleep. She would call for her parents every ten minutes or so, and when they returned she would ask to be covered again and to get another kiss. Her parents always complied, although when she sometimes asked them to stay with her, they usually refused. If they did not respond when she called from her bed, she would come out of her room and call again. If they still did not respond, she would go and find them. This pattern would repeat itself about five times until she finally fell asleep at 9.00 p.m. Some nights she would become upset, especially when her parents were slow to respond, and then she might not fall asleep until 9.30 or even 10.00. When she woke at night she would call for another tuck-in and another kiss. If her parents were asleep and did not hear her, she would walk quietly to their room and stand by their bed until one of them woke up and walked her back. After her parents finally gave in, she usually went right back to sleep, but it was happening three times a night and her parents were getting tired and frustrated.

Since Isabella never fell asleep before 9.00 p.m., it seemed likely that she was being put to bed too early: she didn't wake until 7.00 a.m., and she was getting ten hours of sleep. It was hard for her to lie in bed for an hour waiting to fall asleep (see Chapters 9, 10 and 11).

The difficulty of falling asleep at 8.00 had led to the repeated calls for tuck-ins, and now the calls had become a habit to be repeated at each waking. Isabella never resisted when her parents left her room, and she would leave the room only when they didn't answer her calls. She was clearly not frightened.

Helping Isabella and her family was easy: we moved her bedtime to 9.00 p.m. She was happy to have the later bedtime, and in exchange she said she could stop calling and leaving her room. (Note that she was getting no less sleep than before, perhaps even a bit more once the wakeful periods during the night were eliminated.) We supported the change further with a sticker chart. Isabella did very well from the first night on. When I saw her next she was gleefully waving her chart for me to see. No stronger measures were ever necessary.

Michael, a two-and-a-half-year-old boy, had an 8.30 p.m. bedtime, which he was comfortable with. Since moving from a cot to a bed four months earlier, he had developed night-time habits that were making his mother very unhappy. He liked having a bedtime story, but he never wanted his mother to stop and leave the room. When she tried, he would run after her. So she got in the habit of sitting on his bed and making up stories until he fell asleep. If he did not fall asleep quickly, it soon became hard work. Sometimes she would stop, thinking Michael was asleep, but he would open his eyes and say 'More story!'

Often, tired out after forty-five minutes, she would leave despite his protests. Michael would call from his bed for a few minutes, but then he would get up, find her and ask her to come back and continue the stories. Sometimes she would give in; sometimes she would let him stay up until she had finished her work, and then she would take him back to bed. Sometimes, if it got late enough, she would fall asleep in Michael's bed. If she fell asleep before he did, he would wake her and tell her to keep talking. Sometimes he would let her rub his back instead. Either way, he could close his eyes and still be sure she was in the room. When he woke at night he would call, and she would return quickly (if she had been able to leave in the first place). She would lie down with him, and usually she could get him back to sleep by rubbing his back. At this point, she would stay with him until morning.

Michael's difficulties at night came from a combination of association and limit problems, and there were sleep schedule considerations as well: although his bedtime was 8.30 p.m., he usually did not fall asleep until 9.30, and he generally didn't wake until late in the morning, between 7.30 and 8.00 a.m. His mother wanted to sleep in her own bed without him. She should have been able to, since Michael was not an anxious child; he separated easily during the day and was fine with babysitters. In fact, when he had a babysitter he went to sleep late but alone and with no trouble.

Getting Michael to sleep well without ruining his mother's sleep required consistent limit-setting. We temporarily made his bedtime 9.30 p.m., an hour later than usual but matching the time when he usually fell asleep; his morning waking was to be a little earlier than usual, namely 7.00 a.m., so that eventually we would be able to move his bedtime earlier as well. His mother set up a gate and established a routine for Michael's bedtimes, during which the gate was kept closed. She would read him one story and make up one short one; then she would tell him she was leaving and go, closing the gate again behind her. Michael called at first, and even came to the gate. His mother responded briefly at intervals, following the chart in Figure 4 on page 74. The first night, Michael fell asleep on the floor and she moved him back to bed. By the third night the calling had stopped and he was sleeping through the night. The next week, his bedtime was moved back to 9.00 p.m., and by the week after that it was once again close to 8.30.

Kyle was a four-year-old boy whose bedtime was a horror. On a typical night, tensions started to rise after dinner; although Kyle was playing, he also kept checking nervously to see if bedtime was near. At 8.00 p.m., when he saw that his parents were about to get him into his pyjamas and clean his teeth, he tried to run away. His parents, already upset, had to bring him screaming and fighting to his room. Sometimes he hit them or kicked them. Putting on his pyjamas, a major task, usually required both parents. Whatever parts of his pyjamas they got him into, he took off again. Often he managed to squirm away from them and run back to the living room, and they would have to chase him down and start over. He had his own bed, but they could not even get him to stay there for a story. If they tried, he would bolt again. Sometimes they sat and held him struggling in bed, but they always grew tired before he did, and eventually they would give up and let him go. Kyle would then play in the living room for another half hour, at which point his parents would try again to get him into bed, to no avail.

This exhausting process went on for hours every night. Kyle would finally fall asleep in the living room with the television on between 10.00 p.m. and midnight, usually by 11.00. His parents found that they needed to wait another half hour before they could be sure he wouldn't wake when they moved him to his bed. Now they could go to sleep themselves, but they would usually wake around two o'clock in the morning to hear him back in the living room. The television would be on, and the room was often a mess. Putting him back to sleep was no easier than at bedtime. Kyle could be up another hour or two, and he usually fell asleep in the living room again. This time one of his parents would stay there with him. He usually slept until morning, waking between 6.00 and 9.00 a.m., depending upon how much he had been up the night before. During the day his parents could not make him take formal naps, but he did usually fall asleep on his own for an hour, sometimes early in the afternoon and sometimes late. At day care, which he attended three days a week, he took a regular nap on a mat like everyone else, without a struggle.

Kyle was clearly out of control. Although his parents had been trying hard to make bedtime work, they just did not know how. Part of the problem was that Kyle's schedule was so varied and inconsistent that it was impossible to be sure where his sleep phase fell – that is, when he was physiologically ready to fall asleep and when he was ready to wake (see Chapter 10). The inconsistency in the times of morning waking led to inconsistent nap times, which in turn led to wide variations in the times he would fall asleep at night and in the lengths of his night-time wakings. It was important to get Kyle settled down, but I knew it would not be easy. I also knew from my interactions with Kyle and from reports of his behaviour at day care that he was a normal youngster who responded well when appropriate limits were set and enforced.

To set limits correctly at night, we needed to know when Kyle would be ready and able to sleep. We started with a schedule that allowed him too little sleep, ensuring that he would be sleepy both at bedtime and also during the periods at night when he used to be awake. Bedtime was set at 11.00 p.m., and he was to be wakened by 6.30 every morning. He was to be allowed no more than ninety minutes of nap time, none of which was to take place after 3.30 p.m., and he was not to be allowed to sleep at other times. As soon as things started to improve, we could gradually move his bedtime back to a more reasonable hour.

Within the structure of this schedule, we could begin setting limits. A double gate went up in Kyle's doorway, and a chair and a toy box were removed from his room so he couldn't use them to climb. His pyjamas were to go on at 8.00 p.m. in a setting that had nothing to do with going to bed, and once he was in them, he would be allowed to watch a DVD he liked. The quicker he got into his pyjamas, the more time he had for the DVD. Once he got the idea, he stopped resisting, and getting him ready for bed became easy. From 8.00 to 11.00 p.m. there was no longer a reason for fighting or chasing, and the parents kept themselves available to play with him or read to him during that time. He could also watch appropriate DVDs, but only until 9.00.

At 11.00, his parents were to take him into his room, close the gates behind them and offer to read him a story. If he accepted, they would read him *one* story and then leave. If he started fighting, they would leave immediately. This time the lesson was, if he wanted the story, there could be no fighting; if there was any fighting, there would be no story. Once out of the room, his parents were to respond to his yelling by returning to the gates, without entering his room, at increasing intervals until he fell asleep, and they were to repeat this pattern of responses as often as necessary during the night. They no longer had to struggle to hold him on the mattress: now the gates took care of keeping him in his room. They could stay calm, and threats were unnecessary.

The first two nights were a challenge – Kyle was accustomed to getting his way at night. Escalation had always worked for him before, and now he had to learn that even yelling louder got him nowhere. But by the third night matters had improved considerably.

By the end of the first week, he was accepting a bedtime story and was not even fighting when his parents left. In fact, it was actually becoming difficult to keep him awake until 11.00, so we gradually moved his bedtime earlier. By the end of the second week Kyle was going to sleep at 9.00 p.m. and waking at 6.30 a.m.

Because Kyle was already four years old, we were uncertain whether he would continue napping after his sleep at night improved. Therefore, we planned only to offer a nap, not to insist on one. He started to nap regularly at 1.00 p.m. on the sofa, and since that was working well, we made no effort to change it. When I next saw the family, it was clear that more than Kyle's sleep had improved. His parents reported that he was much happier than he'd seemed before, that he wasn't angry at them and seemed to enjoy being with them more, and that his behaviour throughout the day had improved as well.

Ashley was a two-year-old who slept in bed with her parents. They liked having her there and had no desire to move her to her own room yet. However, nights were difficult, at least for her mother. As Ashley went to sleep, she liked to climb up on top of her mother and stroke her hair or face, sometimes even scratching her, while she sucked her own thumb. Once she was asleep her mother could usually ease her back onto the mattress, but over the course of the night Ashley would wake several more times, climb back up and begin stroking again. Her mother found the behaviour very unpleasant, and the loss of sleep made her tired and grumpy during the day. Nevertheless, she felt it was her job to do whatever Ashley wanted during the night. Night-time was a time for closeness and support, she felt, not withdrawal and frustration. Sometimes Ashley's father tried to help to get Ashley back to sleep, but that never worked, at least not if her mother was still nearby; Ashley wanted her mother, her mother's face and her mother's hair. However, on the occasional night when Ashley's mother was out late, her father had little trouble getting her to sleep.

Like Michael, Ashley was suffering from a mixture of association problems and limit problems. It was fine for her to sleep with her parents, but there was no need for them to put up with her annoying habits. They could be close and supportive without letting her do everything she wanted. Besides, letting Ashley learn that she would be allowed to annoy someone else at will was teaching her a bad lesson.

So her mother told her that from now on she had to sleep next to her, not on top of her, and without stroking her face or hair. When Ashley fought this new rule, her mother got up and left the room, while her father stayed behind; if she called, her mother came back in periodically to reassure her that she was nearby, but she did not get back into bed until Ashley was asleep. If, later during the night, Ashley tried to re-start the unacceptable behaviour, her mother again stopped her and left again until she went back to sleep. For a few nights Ashley's mother had to spend part of the night on the sofa while her father remained with Ashley in the bed. But on each of these nights Ashley was learning to fall asleep on the mattress instead of on a person, and without stroking or annoying anyone. A few nights were all it took. After that, Ashley's mother had only to threaten to leave to make her stop, and a few nights after that she stopped trying to sleep on top of her altogether.

CHAPTER 6

Feedings During the Night:
Another Major Cause of Trouble

Perhaps surprisingly, night-time feedings are a frequent, if easy to miss, cause of major sleep disturbances. Once your baby is about three months old, she should not require more than one feeding during the night (in addition to a feeding at bedtime), and that last night-time feeding will probably be given up at some point over the next month or two. You certainly should not have to continue getting up repeatedly during the night to feed her. If you do, the sleep disturbance associated with these excessive night-time feedings can be dramatic, and if you allow the night feedings to continue, the problem may go on for a very long time – years, even. On the other hand, when you begin to eliminate the extra feedings, the improvement in sleep is usually very rapid.

You may find that having your child fall asleep as you feed her in your arms is rewarding for you and satisfying for her. There is nothing wrong with continuing to nurse your child to sleep during her first year, as long as you enjoy it, as long as you can easily transfer her to her cot or bed as soon as she is done, and as long as she begins to sleep through the night. But if it's difficult to put her down after feedings, or if she wakes repeatedly and has to be fed each time before she can go back to sleep, then she is developing a sleep problem, and the feedings are almost certainly the cause.

A baby with this problem has learned to associate nursing with falling asleep, as described in Chapter 4. In addition, if your child drinks large amounts of milk or juice at night, her sleep may be disturbed for other reasons as well: for instance, if her nappy is soaked, the discomfort can certainly wake her. Furthermore, extra nutrients ingested at night will stimulate your child's digestive system, which should ordinarily be relatively inactive during the night. The process of metabolising those nutrients will alter patterns of functioning in other body systems; it will trigger or inhibit the release of many different hormones and it will raise the body temperature, which is normally low at night. The overall result is that many important biological rhythms that are closely tied to the ability to sleep are disrupted.

Even the timing of a child's feelings of hunger can be affected. We all get hungry at the times of the day or night when we are *accustomed* to eating. This timing is learned – it is not simply determined by the number of hours since our last meal. If, for example, you change your dinner-time from 5.00 to 7.00 p.m., then – after a period of gradual adaptation – you will find that you don't get hungry in the evening until two hours later than you used to, even if your breakfast time and lunchtime remain unchanged. Similarly, if your child is used to being fed often during the night, she is likely to wake up hungry. She will eagerly nurse or take her bottle, but she has simply *learned* to eat on this schedule and does not actually need food at these times. This learned hunger then becomes a trigger for extra wakings. Her sleep at night won't consolidate into long periods, but – like the sleep that occurs in the daytime – it will remain as mere naps between wakings and feedings.

Sleep disruptions caused by too much feeding at night occur most often in children under two years old who are still breastfeeding or using a bottle. Kayla, for example, was eight months old when I first saw her. Her parents told me that she fell asleep easily at bedtime while nursing at the breast, and once asleep, she could be moved into the cot without difficulty. She would sleep for two and a half hours, but then wake crying. Her father was unable to comfort her; only her mother seemed to be able to put her back to sleep. When she picked Kayla up and nursed her again, Kayla would stop crying and go back to sleep within ten minutes. But she would continue to wake up every hour or two, and each time the same process had to be repeated. On most nights Kayla woke five or six times for feedings, and her soaked nappies had to be changed at least once. Since Kayla's mother was always the one to take care of Kayla at night, she was exhausted and frustrated. Occasionally she was so tired that she wanted to let Kayla cry, but her husband insisted that she respond. That made her angry with him as well as with Kayla, and there was a great deal of tension in the family.

You will probably recognise by now that Kayla associated falling asleep with being held and nursed. That was true, but it was not the whole story. When such associations are the only problem, there will usually be only a few apparent night-time wakings, times when the child wakes fully and needs help returning to sleep. Kayla's wakings, however, occurred too frequently – up to once an hour – to be explained by sleep associations alone. Something was either waking her more frequently or causing her to wake fully almost every time she stirred.

Allison, another child I saw with this problem, was two years old and had never once slept through the night. She was no longer held or rocked to sleep, but her parents handed her a bottle when she was placed in her cot. She always finished all 235 millilitres – sometimes 350 – then she turned over and fell asleep. After about three hours, she would wake crying and wouldn't stop until she was given another bottle, after which she would fall asleep quickly again. She woke four to six times a night, and each time she needed another bottle to go back to sleep.

Often, when Allison woke, she was soaking wet even though she was in double or triple nappies. At each waking her mother or father would go in, change her if necessary, hand her another bottle and leave. When Allison's parents went to bed they would prepare four or five bottles and leave them in the refrigerator or on Allison's windowsill. The entire burden did not fall on Allison's mother as it had on Kayla's, and since Allison did not need to be held, her parents could go right back to sleep themselves. Still, after two years, they too were tired and frustrated, and they usually went to bed early in the evening just to be sure they could get enough sleep.

Allison, like Kayla, had associations that interfered with falling asleep – in this case, sucking on a bottle. However, she did not need the bottle to actually fall asleep; that was evident because she usually finished the bottle, tossed it aside, rolled over and then went to sleep without having the bottle in her mouth. Her sleep disturbances evidently had to do with the large amount of milk she drank during the night.

Both Kayla's and Allison's wakings had probably begun as the normal arousals of an infant who is just beginning to develop good sleep habits. But when their parents tried to 'treat' these wakings with extra feedings, the wakings became excessive. The 'cure' for normal wakings had become the cause of abnormal ones.

IS YOUR CHILD'S SLEEP PROBLEM CAUSED BY NIGHT-TIME FEEDINGS?

Although your baby may give up regular night-time feedings on her own by the end of her first three months, it is not reasonable to expect or insist that such a young infant give them up altogether. But if your child is at least three months old, still nurses or requires a bottle at bedtime and needs to eat again several more times during the night, then the extra feedings may well be causing the extra wakings. If that is the case, you may be able to help her to sleep better by decreasing the number of these feedings.

If your child nurses only for a minute or so at the night-time wakings, or takes just a few sips from the bottle, she is not taking in much food. Rather, she is behaving like a child who is dependent on a dummy: it is the breast or bottle itself that she needs before she can go to sleep, not the food. This pattern can be stopped immediately, as discussed in Chapter 4. On the other hand, if she takes in a substantial amount of food – from extended feedings at the breast, or from bottles adding up to more than 235 millilitres over the course of the night – then she has learned that certain times of night are mealtimes. To eliminate these feedings suddenly would be neither wise nor kind.

Frequent nappy changes are another clue that your child's feedings at night may be excessive. Most babies three months or older do not need to be changed at night at all. If your baby's nappies are often soaked when she wakes during the night, then it is likely that she is drinking too much. She certainly cannot be thirsty or getting too little to drink if she is wetting that much. Medical causes such as diabetes are extremely unlikely, certainly if the same problems (of excessive feeding and wetting) do not occur in the daytime. If you are at all concerned, consult your GP. But in all likelihood your child probably simply has a habit of taking in too much fluid at night.

The amount of milk or juice your child drinks during the night may be considerable. If she finishes four full 235-millilitre bottles, she is drinking an entire litre! That is a large amount for even an adult to consume overnight, and an adult who drinks that much at night will not sleep well, if only because it will mean extra trips to the toilet. It should not be so surprising to find that your child, like Allison or Kayla, does not sleep well, either.

HOW TO SOLVE THE PROBLEM

If you have concluded that excessive and unnecessary feedings at night are disrupting your child's sleep, you will be relieved to learn that although such feedings can produce especially severe sleep disturbances, this problem is also one of the easiest to treat. There are two tasks you need to carry out. One is to reduce or eliminate the night-time feedings, thus avoiding their various sleep-disrupting effects and also helping your child learn to get hungry only at reasonable times during the day. The other task is to teach your child new sleep associations so that she can fall asleep without being held, without eating and without sucking on the breast, bottle or dummy. You can take these jobs on simultaneously or one at a time.

To address the problems caused by the feedings, begin by gradually decreasing the number of night-time feedings or their size, or both (see below for more about these options). Don't stop the feedings suddenly: although your child would not suffer from lack of nourishment, she has become accustomed to being fed during the night and she will probably be hungry. A programme designed to allow new patterns to develop gradually will be easier for her, and also for you.

Your goal is to gradually move your child's feelings of hunger out of the night-time and into the daytime by eliminating the feedings at night – or, if you have a young infant, at least to move some of the feedings to the daytime by spacing them farther apart at night. If your child feeds substantially at only one or two of the feedings, then the other 'feedings' are not a response to hunger and can be eliminated immediately, like a dummy. The real feedings can then be reduced gradually. Once there is only a single remaining night-time feeding left, you can choose to stop that feeding straight away (instead of gradually) if you prefer, since the total amount ingested during the night is now fairly small.

It is not always necessary to eliminate night-time feedings altogether; in fact, for a young infant that would be inappropriate. Still, it is unpleasant and usually unnecessary to nurse or feed a baby hourly throughout the night; if your child is an infant, you may simply want to decrease the number of feedings. It's entirely reasonable to cut back to two night-time feedings by the time your child is two or three months of age, one feeding by three or four months and none at all at five months. Many children give up night-time feedings altogether around the age of three or four months; basically no normal, healthy, full-term babies still *require* a night-time feeding when they are five months old, and you can certainly insist on stopping them altogether at that point if you want to.

(There is nothing wrong with continuing a single night-time feeding for some months beyond that point, if you enjoy it, but be aware that this is a choice, not a response to your baby's biological needs. However, if you have to feed her several times during the night, it may not be so nice for your child, even if *you* don't mind.

Instead of allowing her an uninterrupted night's sleep, you're making it necessary for her to wake up repeatedly, call for you or go and find you and perhaps wait for you to get up and prepare a bottle, before she can go back to sleep. After all, if she weren't hungry at these times, she could just stir and go right back to sleep. Furthermore, if she relies on the breast or bottle to go back to sleep, she has another problem as well: if she happens to wake too soon after a feeding and is not yet hungry, or has completed a feeding but is still awake, then what is she to do? She is accustomed to nurse to go back to sleep, but now she doesn't want to feed, or cannot, because she is not hungry. This is unpleasant for her, and it should be unnecessary.)

Use the chart in Figure 8 on page 143 as a guide. Whether you are nursing or feeding by bottle, the key is to increase the minimum time between feedings. Note how close together your child's night-time feedings are currently, and use that interval as the point from which to begin adjusting the feeding schedule. (If there is a range – perhaps one to three hours – start with the shortest interval.) For example, if you are starting with an interval of two hours on the first night, don't allow your child to feed until at least two hours have passed since the previous feeding. If your child wakes before two hours have passed, she will have to wait for her next feeding; if she wakes later, she can be fed immediately. Increase the minimum time between feedings by thirty minutes each night.

If you are bottle-feeding, you may find it helpful to decrease the amount offered at each feeding as well. Note how many millilitres your child drinks at each waking. (If there is a range, start with the largest amount she takes most nights.) Each night, in addition to spacing out the feedings, decrease the amount in each bottle by 30 millilitres. If you're aiming to eliminate night-time feedings altogether, keep this up until you reach 30 millilitres per bottle. Because you also have been spacing out the feedings, there should now be only one or two night-time feedings left, totalling 30 to 60 millilitres for the entire night. On the next night, eliminate night-time feedings completely.

(Many parents find that the night-time wakings decrease markedly

FIGURE 8. ELIMINATING EXTRA FEEDINGS AT SLEEP TIMES

Day	Minimum Hours Between Feedings (Nursing or Bottle)	Millilites in Each Bottle (if Bottle-Feeding)
1	2.0	210
2	2.5	180
3	3.0	150
4	3.5	120
5	4.0	90
6	4.5	60
7	5.0	30
8	Night-time feedings may be stopped (see below)	

The millilitres and times in this chart are general guidelines. You can alter them to fit your own desires and your child's current feeding schedule.

1. If your child takes less than 235 millilitres in each bottle, start with 30 millilitres less than she usually takes and continue reducing from there.

2. If the minimum time between your child's night-time feedings is already more than two hours, then begin with the line in the chart one half hour longer than the current minimum and continue increasing the times from there.

3. If you are breast-feeding, just increase the minimum time between feedings according to the first two columns on the chart. Don't worry about the exact amounts consumed at each feeding.

4. By day seven, you will probably be feeding only once during the night, five hours or more after your child first falls asleep. If your child is young and you want to continue one feeding at night, you can stop here. Otherwise you can stop all night-time feedings the next night. If you are nursing, and the remaining feeding seems to be a substantial one, or if you are bottle-feeding and have not made the feedings smaller, you can also choose to continue moving that last feeding further away from bedtime, an extra thirty minutes each night, until it moves out of the night-time altogether.

5. If you prefer, you can decrease the size and number of feedings every other day instead of every day. It will just take a little longer.

even before the feedings are completely eliminated, and that the remaining very small feedings – 30 to 90 millilitres – sometimes seem more upsetting to a child than comforting. For this reason, parents sometimes decide to stop the feedings a day or two earlier than originally planned.)

If you are trying to reduce the number of night-time feedings to one or two, rather than eliminating them altogether, then you may not need to decrease their size at all, unless any are more than 235 millilitres. (Most night-time feedings should be in the range of 120 to 235 millilites. Giving more than 235 millilitres is unnecessary, if the goal of the feeding is only to satisfy hunger, and feedings of less than 120 millilitres usually reflect a habit of sucking more than they do true sensations of hunger.) Apart from that, all you need to do is to progressively increase the time between feedings (perhaps to somewhere between three and six hours, depending upon your child's age and your goal) until you are down to the number of night-time feedings you want.

If you are working on sleep associations and hunger patterns simultaneously, put your child in bed as soon as each feeding is over, even if she wakes and begins to cry. If you nurse her and she sleeps next to you, move her off of you when the feeding is done so that she can learn to fall asleep without using your breast as a dummy. You've just fed her, so she is not hungry; now you are only changing her expectation of what happens while she falls asleep. (Remember, if she is asleep or almost asleep in your arms and never knows that she is being moved away from you, then when she wakes during the night she may be surprised to find she is no longer where she was when she went to sleep.) If she protests, follow the progressive-waiting programme described in Chapter 4, responding to her briefly at increasing intervals until either she goes back to sleep or it's time for her next feeding. Within a week, if all goes well, you will have finished cutting down on or eliminating the night-time feedings. After that, continue applying the technique of progressive waiting at any wakings at night (except for feeding times) until the wakings stop. It should not take more than another few days.

If you hand your child a bottle in the cot and she takes it by herself without being held, then you don't need to work on her sleep associations directly. Since she already falls asleep by herself without being held, she does not have that association. As you eliminate feedings from the night-time, the association of falling asleep with sucking will also disappear (as long as you do not introduce a dummy to replace the bottle).

But if you are keeping some of the night-time feedings, it is particularly important to dissociate feeding from the act of falling asleep. Your goal in feeding her is to take away the hunger, not to get her to sleep. If she keeps falling asleep in your arms, or even just with the bottle in her mouth, it may be difficult to make the progress you would like.

If you are nursing and your nursing child sleeps in your bed, you may have to be firm when she tries to get at your breast before it is time to nurse. You may even have to get up temporarily and sit by the bed, or even leave the room (if there is another parent staying behind for safety), until your child goes back to sleep or it's time for the next feeding. Once the night-time feedings stop, that will no longer be necessary.

If you have chosen to work on the night-time hunger problem first and change sleep associations second, then don't change the bedtime ritual yet. Let your child fall asleep in your arms during or after feeding, if that is what she has been doing. If she wakes and cries before it's time for her next feeding, you can try to comfort her, if it helps. Do whatever seems to comfort her most: hold her, soothe her, rock her or talk to her. The purpose is only to calm her down and help her fall asleep while she learns not to expect a feeding. Sometimes it's best not even to try to help: if she sleeps in her own room, she may become more upset if you go in but refuse to feed her, and she may calm down more quickly without you there.

If you are a nursing mother, it may be difficult to hold your child without nursing her. You may have a let-down response, and your child will smell the milk and expect to nurse. In a two-parent family, it is often easier for the non-nursing parent to settle the child at times when she is not being fed. Your child may still seem a bit frustrated, but in this way she will learn not to expect you and to nurse so often during the night.

Once you have eliminated night-time feedings or cut them down to the number you want, and your child is falling asleep without nursing or taking a bottle (at least after night-time wakings), you have solved the problem of excessive fluids and broken the association of falling asleep with having the bottle or sucking at the breast. If she still needs you to hold her, rub her back or rock her before she can go to sleep, you can now begin to correct those associations, as described in Chapter 4. Once excessive feedings are no longer complicating the picture, the rest of the re-learning process usually happens quickly.

Even if you continue to nurse your child to sleep at bedtime and nap time, you may find that if you just eliminate the middle-of-the-night feedings, she will still be able to put herself back to sleep after waking during the night. That is fine, as long as it's working well. But if she isn't adjusting to this pattern – if it still takes a long time to transfer her from your arms to the cot or mattress, or if she wants to be nursed whenever she wakes during the night – then you must take more care to clearly separate the bedtime feeding from the act of falling asleep. Note carefully when she is getting close to falling asleep. Stop feeding her at that point, and put her to bed; wake her a little if necessary, so that she will be aware of being moved. Or move the final feeding a little earlier, so that she will definitely still be awake when you put her to bed.

A schedule with one or two night-time feedings is a little more unstable than one with no feedings, because it means that sometimes your child gets fed before she goes back to sleep during the night and sometimes she doesn't. If she has been waking once a night for a feeding, she may begin waking twice a night, and if you feed her at that second waking, she may begin waking three times a night. You can prevent this regression by sticking to a maximum number of feedings and a minimum time between feedings and, if necessary, by making certain that after she feeds she is always put to bed awake.

Some families find a slightly different approach helpful in cutting out unnecessary bottle feedings. Rather than spacing out the feedings and making them smaller, they progressively dilute the contents of each night-time bottle until their baby is just getting water. For instance, on the first night, instead of full-strength milk (or formula or juice), use a three-quarter-strength mixture – three parts milk (or formula or juice) to one part water. Dilute the bottle further every night or two, to half-strength, one-quarter-strength and then one-eighth-strength. Now, assuming your child is drinking the same number of millilitres of fluid as before, she is getting only an eighth of the amount of milk she started with. The next night, give her just water. Now she is not being fed at all during the night. Since she is taking only water, the *nutritional* effects are no longer important. She may still be wetting at night, but she probably won't feel hungry. Now the bottle is only being used as a pacifier, so you can stop using it the next night altogether. Help her learn to fall asleep without sucking, along with any other remaining inappropriate associations, by following the methods described above and in Chapter 4.

If you use this approach, stick to the concentration you offer each night, even if your child complains, and don't give in to demands for larger or more frequent feedings. Some children take the diluted milk without complaint; others complain considerably or refuse to take it at all. If she won't take the bottle, she probably isn't very hungry, and she will give up the extra feeding that much quicker. You can simply look in on her at increasing intervals; if she decides she wants the bottle after all, she can still have it. If you find this approach too difficult for your child, use the other approach of spacing out the feedings and making them smaller instead.

We used the methods described in this section with Kayla and Allison, and both girls soon started sleeping soundly through the night. Allison gave up the bottle within a week after the treatment began. Her mother followed the programme of progressively spacing out feedings and decreasing the amount of milk in each bottle, and she was surprised by how quickly Allison's night-time behaviour improved. Allison did cry a little when her night-time bottle was taken away altogether, but only for two nights and only for five minutes each time. Her parents can now enjoy their time together in the evenings, and they can sleep through the night again.

Kayla's mother continued to nurse her twice a day, but never at night. She occasionally nursed Kayla to sleep at nap time, because she found that it did not seem to affect the good night-time habits they had established, and because she still found it rewarding and pleasurable. Kayla's father came to understand that he had been wrong to insist that his wife get up to nurse throughout the night, and the tension between the parents eased.

OTHER POINTS TO KEEP IN MIND

Eliminating feedings at night may or may not lead to weaning. If your child always drinks from a cup except at bedtime, at nap time and during the night, you will be weaning her altogether if you discontinue all the sleep-time feedings. On the other hand, if she is not ready to be weaned, or if you do not want to wean her yet, you can still eliminate feedings during the night. Simply continue nursing or bottle-feeding her at other times as you always have.

Decreasing night-time feedings generally won't affect your child's daytime feedings much, unless she has been getting a significant part of her nourishment at night. In that case, you will probably notice that over several weeks she gradually feeds more during the day as her patterns of hunger and satiation change.

Feeding your child at appropriate intervals during the day will not interfere with her sleep at night or during naps. After about the age of two months, though, your baby's night-time sleep may be affected if she is given a bottle or put to the breast whenever she seems the least bit upset, fussy or demanding, even though it is clear to you at these times that she is not hungry and eats very little. Learning to associate the breast or bottle with a feeling of comfort is important, but it will become a problem if your child never learns to be comforted in any other way. If you find that you are using the breast or bottle as a pacifier too frequently during the day, consider offering them less often and less quickly. (Of course, you should not withhold feedings during the day when she actually is hungry, needs to be fed and takes more than 30 to 60 millilitres before being satisfied.) Your goal is to help your child learn other ways to calm herself, so that she will begin to associate the breast or bottle mainly with hunger and feedings. Once you have seen that your child can accept these changes without lasting frustration – on the contrary, she will probably be happier in the daytime – you should be able to work on the night-time changes more easily and with new confidence.

Feedings in relation to naps can be handled in any of several different ways. You can leave them unchanged, as long as your child falls asleep easily while feeding, can be transferred out of your arms easily and without waking and finishes her nap without needing to feed again. If you are trying to separate feeding from falling asleep, you can (if you choose) make the separation clear at nap times as well as at night. But if you put her to bed awake at nap time, it is reasonable to have a time limit: if she has not fallen asleep after thirty minutes of checking, pick her up and end the nap for that day. She may later fall asleep on her own in another room; that's fine as long as she does so without being fed. Alternatively, you can make the separation (between feeding and falling asleep) only at night to begin with, and once your child has learned how to fall asleep at night without feeding, you can start to do the same thing at nap time, asking her to do during the day what she has already learned to do at night.

MEDICAL CONSIDERATIONS

You should always avoid feeding your child when she is lying in her bed or cot, even if sleep disruptions aren't a problem. Simply handing a bottle to a child lying supine is a way to cause ear and dental problems. Because the *eustachian tube* (a small passageway to the throat that vents or drains the middle-ear cavity) is short and horizontal in young children, liquid – and bacteria – can easily pass from the throat to the middle-ear space if a child sucks on a bottle while lying on her back. The result can be a middle-ear infection, *otitis media*. Also, once your child's teeth erupt, she is at risk for tooth decay if she goes to sleep with milk or juice in her mouth, and this is just what happens when she falls asleep with a bottle in her mouth.

CHAPTER 7

Night-time Fears

Most children occasionally feel frightened at night, and fears can lead to sleep problems: frightened children do not like to be alone.

In this chapter, I will outline a number of considerations useful in assessing the severity of your child's night-time fears, and I will describe methods you can use to deal with them. Although professional help may be necessary for a very anxious child, you should be able to manage most anxiety-related sleep problems yourself by using such techniques as emotional support, desensitisation, rewards, schedule adjustments, negotiation, unlearning of automatic behaviour and limit-setting.

THE ANXIOUS CHILD

As your child grows, she will face many new challenges. She must learn to tolerate being apart from you during the day – alone in a room, with a babysitter or at day care or nursery school – and (at some point) each night when she goes to sleep. She must learn to control her behaviour, her bowels and her bladder; to hold feelings of anger, jealousy and aggression in check; and to master the give-and-take of interacting with her family and friends. She will learn, wonder and perhaps worry about death, God, heaven and hell. She will find pleasure in genital stimulation but may worry about masturbation. She will question her ability to perform on a par with her peers and wonder whether she can live up to your expectations of her.

Each stage of your child's development brings with it particular vulnerabilities to certain anxieties. For example, when she begins nursery school, her concerns about separation may increase for a while. She may be reluctant to leave your side during the daytime, and she may not want you to leave her at bedtime. If you get ill, she may feel guilty, imagining that her angry words or thoughts caused your illness and made you less available to her than usual.

Toilet-training presents other concerns. Your child may worry about her ability to control herself. She may even be tempted to soil. Yet at the same time, she wants to please you, and she may fear incurring your displeasure. For many toddlers these worries are heightened at night: how can they avoid soiling or wetting while they are asleep?

For a five- or six-year-old, a scary film can be particularly frightening. She may be very upset by scenes of kidnapping or those in which a child shows aggression towards a parent. Films can be very real to a child. All children have aggressive fantasies, and most feel a bit guilty about them, but seeing these thoughts acted out on the screen can become a source of great anxiety.

Although the ages from six to twelve are considered to be a period of relative psychological calm, children between the toddler years and adolescence face pressures in a number of areas: in school, on the sports field, at music class, in religious programmes, at home and even from their own thoughts. They struggle to make friendships and to find new role models apart from their parents; they are called upon to be increasingly independent and to become more sensitive to problems in the home; and they start to carve out their own identity. At these ages, previously unrecognised learning and psychological problems can become clearly evident.

Most children in this age range sleep alone. A child who is too frightened to do so may be embarrassed to have her friends find out. She may be unable to participate in events with her peers that require being away from home overnight, and she may find her self-confidence shaken and her self-image worsened.

Adolescents, too, wrestle with major worries as they undergo the rapid physical and emotional changes of puberty. They start to worry about the future – university, jobs, money. Teenagers' sexual feelings are very intense. Moral issues become more relevant, and adolescents face constant dilemmas as they struggle with new and important decisions. They must weigh personal desires against peer pressures and family standards in such areas as academic performance, sexual habits and drug and alcohol use. They may experiment with new value systems and abandon old ones. They may believe their parents no longer trust or support them, and they may reject their parents' help entirely.

Most adolescents with fears intense enough to affect their nightly sleep choose to suffer alone rather than to ask their parents for help. Such youngsters are in need of help, but they may be more likely to get this help through counselling than from the behavioural techniques described in this chapter.

BEDTIME FEARS

Anxiety is a common and important cause of bedtime struggles and night-time wakings. During the day it is relatively easy to keep worries under control. Most children have too much to do, and too many distractions, to sit and brood. But even a child who feels fairly confident in the daytime can feel insecure at night. Waiting for sleep to come, she may begin to worry. As she lies in bed in a dark, quiet room, there is little to distract her thinking, and her thoughts and imagination can run free. If she wakes during the night in a dark, quiet house with everyone else asleep, her anxiety can grow even worse. It's small wonder that even a child who has no difficulty going off to school may resist going to her room to sleep at night.

Because the ability to control one's thoughts and feelings diminishes as one gets sleepy, children often regress at night, and they begin to feel, and act, more childish. In this state, a five-year-old may need the same level of reassurance that a three-year-old needs during the day. It will not help to scold her or tell her she is being a baby. Better to try to understand why she is feeling insecure. At such times she may need you to be more involved in her care than you might be during the day.

Although certain anxieties are normal, or at least reflect internal struggles that are part of normal development, others are caused by external events. Any significant social stress over which the child has little control – illness; parental fighting, separation or divorce; alcoholism or other substance abuse; death – can lead to a great deal of worry, guilt, anxiety and fear at any age. At night, when a child must give up what little control she has over her world along with the ability to stay aware of what is going on outside her door, fantasies stimulated by these strong feelings are especially likely to emerge, and they can be quite frightening. Bedtime difficulties and fears are to be expected.

Tyler was a four-year-old boy who had never had many problems with sleep until, four months before I saw him, a loud thunderstorm frightened him in the middle of the night. From then on, Tyler was unable to sleep by himself. Each night one of his parents had to lie down with him from his 8.00 p.m. bedtime until he fell asleep an hour later. They kept reassuring him when he asked if there would be more thunder. If his parents needed to leave the room even briefly before he fell asleep, he would keep calling after them, and if he couldn't hear them, he would come out to see if they had gone downstairs and to get them to return. He insisted that two bright lights be left on in his room all night. Once he was asleep his parents could leave the room, but he always woke around midnight and began screaming. Usually one of his parents went in and lay down with him again. He would clutch them tightly until he returned to sleep. Often they would stay with him until morning to forestall any further screaming later in the night. If his parents did not respond to his screams quickly, he would run into their room.

They would let him into their bed, where he would sleep fine until morning.

During the daytime Tyler's fears seemed to disappear, although he stopped playing in his room alone; in fact, he spent little time there at all. He had no trouble at nursery school and on play-dates. Although he was a little apprehensive about being left with a babysitter, it was not a big problem (although the babysitter had to stay with him until he fell asleep or else he would stay up until his parents returned).

Tyler told me that he was too frightened at night to sleep alone, but when I asked what frightened him, he had no answers except thunder. I did not doubt that he found thunder frightening, but since I did not find him to be an unusually anxious child, I also felt that his night-time behaviour was based as much on habit as on fright, and his main anxieties now were actually secondary ones that had grown out of the initial fear. What started as a single scary night had become a series of nightly fears. Would his parents leave his room before he was asleep, or would he wake to find them gone? Could he get them to return quickly, or would he have to leave his bed and venture out to find them? Would he wake to find the lights turned off and the room dark? Would his parents become angry sharing his small bed or giving over part of their bed to him?

I also saw Rachel, a seven-year-old girl who was generally co-operative and well behaved. She was doing well in school. She had many friends and appeared busy and happy during the day. She seemed to get along well with her parents and her older brother, and there were no signs of any major problems in the family. During the day she did not appear at all fearful.

But her behaviour changed completely every night at bedtime. She begged to stay up. She was desperate to sleep in her parents' room and would do anything, even sleeping on the floor in a sleeping bag or accepting punishment, to be allowed to do so. If her parents tried to carry her to her own room she would hang on to their legs, sobbing. The struggle became so intense that her parents finally gave in and let her sleep on their floor most nights. Although that helped, Rachel still refused to go up to her bedroom ahead of her parents. Eventually she became reluctant to be on the second floor alone even during the day. She also disliked being left with a babysitter at night; when that was necessary, she always stayed awake until her parents returned.

As I spoke with Rachel and her family, it became clear that, despite her relatively untroubled daytime life, she did suffer from tremendous anxieties that became overwhelming at bedtime. In the quiet darkness of the night, while she lay in bed, disturbing fantasies which she could not control began to fill her mind. If she was alone, she would call or come out of the room in search of her parents. At Rachel's level of fearfulness, a firm response from her parents would only have intensified the problem. If they had tried to put her in her room and close the door, she would not have settled down or felt reassured: she would have become hysterical. Fortunately, they understood that Rachel needed sympathy and attention.

Rachel was helped by some of the methods described below – but only up to a point. She initially remained anxious and unable to sleep alone. Ultimately, Rachel's anxiety was brought under control through psychotherapy. As her general anxiety lessened, it became easy to help her and her family to re-establish normal routines at night.

Rachel required counselling as part of her treatment, but (as in Tyler's case, as you will see) psychotherapy is usually unnecessary; most night-time anxieties can be handled more easily. There are many things you can do by yourself to help, and these approaches alone are effective in most cases. If you are in doubt, discuss the matter with your paediatrician or consult a therapist to help you decide on a course of action.

EVALUATING YOUR CHILD'S FEARS

Not all complaints of being 'scared' at night mean the same thing. Some children complain of fears when they are really not anxious at all; others are truly terrified. Some children are only scared of insects; others seem to be frightened by everything. Some are only frightened at bedtime; others are just as scared throughout the day. For this reason, not all complaints of being scared at night should be handled in the same way. In deciding what kind of support your child needs, you may find it helpful to consider the following questions.

Is Your Child Really Frightened?

1. When she says she's scared, does she look and act frightened? When children wake their parents at night, they commonly explain themselves by saying 'I'm scared', or 'I had a bad dream'. But it is easy for children to say they are scared whether they are or not. Those words can be uttered by rote and without much real meaning. If your child reports her 'fear' in a matter-of-fact manner, and if she is calm and does not appear frightened, then in all likelihood she is not truly scared. Appearances are more reliable than words in this context. The complaint may be just one of many your child has tried; she may have abandoned requests for extra drinks or tuck-ins and started complaining about 'monsters' in her room because that complaint is the one that got the best results. As a parent, you do not want to respond to this 'pseudo-anxiety': your response will only encourage it. On the other hand, you do want to respond if the anxiety is sincere.

2. Is she really having bad dreams? All children have nightmares now and then, but if your child says she has a bad dream every night, remember that nightmares generally occur only occasionally and are not usually the cause of *frequent* night-time disturbances. Most children who complain of bad dreams *nightly* are unable to describe much about the dreams, usually because there haven't been any. After a truly scary dream a child will look and act frightened, and she will have a real dream story to report (in contrast to a vague reference to 'monsters' or 'bees' or 'robbers'). As always, judge your child's anxiety more by paying attention to how she appears and acts than by the particular words she uses.

(If she seems extremely frightened but cannot be comforted at all, make sure she is actually awake. What many families believe to be frequent nightmares are actually sleep terrors, confusional arousals or other similar partial wakings; see Chapter 13.)

When your child does wake truly frightened from a scary dream, she should not have to stay alone; yet you certainly want to avoid having to sit with her every night. You should help her to orientate herself and realise that she is not in any real danger. It may also help to discuss the dream with her matter-of-factly. You can do that briefly at the time, but longer talks are better done the next day (discussions in the middle of the night can easily become a bad habit). There are a number of good books for children about dreams and nightmares that may also be of use. Other aspects of dreams and nightmares are discussed in Chapter 14.

3. *Is she testing limits?* Distinguishing a child who is anxious at night from one who is only testing limits is important – the appropriate responses are quite different – but making this distinction is not always easy. An anxious child and one testing limits are both likely to resist going to sleep, make extra requests at bedtime, call out repeatedly and keep coming out of their rooms. Both may complain of fear (remember, a child testing limits will use whatever excuse seems to work). It is easiest to tell the difference in extreme cases: the anxious child appears very frightened, whereas the limit-tester may even be laughing. Furthermore, the firmer you get with the anxious child, the more terrified she becomes; a limit-testing child might become angry (not frightened), or her behaviour may simply improve.

Sometimes limit-testing problems and anxiety occur together, since poor limit-setting can cause a child to become fearful. Children need proper, predictable, consistent limits, and their absence can lead to increasing anxiety. If on some nights parents happily give in to extra requests while on other nights they respond with anger and threats, the child will not know what to expect. She might want to make one more request, but she will be understandably nervous about your response. Here is a case where setting night-time limits appropriately for an anxious child will help matters, whereas when the anxiety has a different cause, firm limits are likely to make it worse. If you are not sure that poor setting of limits is the key problem, err on the side of assuming that there is another cause to the anxiety. You can always set limits later.

4. Is she just not sleepy? If your child's problem is anxiety, then sleep should come fairly quickly on nights when you sleep together (if it is clear to her that you will be together all night). If it takes her just as long to fall asleep with you there, then she may be going to bed too early. As explained in Chapter 9, we all go through a period of extreme wakefulness in the hour or two before the time we usually fall asleep. Most children forced to go to bed too early act like children with limit-setting problems: they keep calling their parents and coming out of the bedroom with various excuses. Some very well-behaved children (perhaps too well-behaved for their own good) stay put, but without the option of reading or watching television, they may lie in bed, fantasise and eventually end up scaring themselves. Under such circumstances, these children do get a bit anxious even though they are not inherently anxious children. If the bedtime hour is adjusted, the anxiety disappears.

How Severe Is Your Child's Anxiety?

1. How intense are her fears at night? To help a child with anxiety-related sleep problems, you need to determine just how pronounced her anxieties are at night. Again, observe your child's behaviour – don't just listen to her words. It is usually obvious when a child is truly terrified at night. She will grow frightened, even panicked, as bedtime approaches. She will cling to you, cry and beg not to be alone. She may accept any punishment as long as she won't have to stay by herself. On waking at night she screams from under the covers, afraid to leave her bed or she races to your room. If, instead, she stops to gather up her blanket and teddy bear before calmly walking to your room and then patiently stands by your bed waiting for you to wake, she may be a little nervous, but it is unlikely that her fears are major. A fearful child may move into your room at night, but if the fears are very intense, she will not go back to sleep on your floor without waking you first. A child's fears cannot be very intense if she is able to go to sleep easily by herself on nights when you leave her with a babysitter. Similarly, the more fearful a child is, the less likely she will be to want (or be able) to sleep at a friend's house. Even during a sleepover at her own house, a very fearful child may risk embarrassment, leaving her friends in her room to join her parents in theirs.

2. *Is her anxiety present all day or just at night?* Anxiety that is present all day long is more worrisome than anxiety that only appears at night. You should be reassured if you find that your child has no difficulties during the day at home or in daytime programmes, and that she is social, enjoys being with others and is not easily panicked. If this is the case, night-time fears are likely to be isolated and easy to deal with. But if she seems anxious throughout the day, about many things and in various settings and activities, then it is less likely that the night-time anxiety can be solved simply and by itself; instead, more general psychological help may be indicated.

3. *Does she have trouble separating in the daytime?* Separation anxiety is common in young children but can occur at almost any age. It can start as early as about eight or nine months. Often a period of increased anxiety lasts several months and then gradually eases. A child having separation difficulties probably cannot be left easily with a babysitter, and she may still be up and awake when you get home; she appears panicky and cries each day when she is brought to day care or nursery school, and the panic does not disappear quickly when you leave; she resists going to school; and she refuses sleepovers with friends, or calls to ask to come home. She may refuse to leave your side when you are out of the house with her, and she may be reluctant to join in activities or play with others even if you are close by. At home, she may become upset if you leave the room, even for just a few minutes. If she has such difficulties with separation, expecting her to sleep in a room by herself may be unfair and unrealistic. In contrast, even if she is very 'clingy' at home, you should be reassured if you find that she does fine with

babysitters or at day care (at least once you've left), plays well with others and is not afraid to try new activities. If she handles separation well during the day, and particularly if she will go to sleep without a problem when left with a babysitter, you can be confident that she will be able to handle separation at night.

4. Is the anxiety of long standing or is it a recent development? A frightening DVD, something heard at school or a bad dream can cause short-term anxiety. Transient fears such as these afflict all children and do not imply a need for professional counselling. With support and understanding from parents at night as well as during the day, such anxieties generally resolve themselves within a few days or weeks. A child with occasional fears will find the extra compassion offered by parents during those fearful periods very helpful; just knowing that such help will be available when it is needed can reduce the severity of these fears and shorten their duration.

Long-standing fears, lasting several months or longer, are a cause for more concern. These fears can intrude into a child's day and affect her choice of activities. If severe, they increase the likelihood that the child will have difficulty coping with normal daytime activities. Such fears are not likely to disappear with support alone. Bear in mind that a scary film, seen once, generally won't produce major, lasting fears, but it can unmask anxieties that are already present. Therefore, even when long-standing anxieties seem traceable to a scary event, the real cause may be quite different from the initial trigger.

What Is Your Child Afraid Of?

1. Is there an identifiable external cause to her fear? Although single events like a scary film may expose existing anxieties, they can also trigger short-term worries and – if exposure is repetitive or ongoing – long-term fears. There may be a specific reason for your child's fear: last night's television porgramme, an illness in the family or a parent's absence due to a business trip. She may be afraid of a bully at school, an unsympathetic teacher or an upcoming exam.

Or the source of the fear could be trouble at home (perhaps parental fighting, drinking or depression). Depending on the nature of this cause, you may be able to provide enough help with understanding and support, or you may need to seek professional counselling.

2. *Does she seem to be frightened by many things, or is she just afraid of a few specific ones?* Some children are not frightened as a rule but do have significant fears of particular things, such as insects, spiders, snakes or fire. If, as with Tyler, the object of fear happens to be thunder, your child may have sleep problems only on stormy nights. On those nights, you need to make yourself especially available to her: if you refuse to comfort her at those times, she may become frightened every night, worrying that there will be a scary storm and she will have to get through it alone. To address fears of insects, spiders, snakes or fire, you can, for example, reassure your child by telling her about the precautions you've taken to avoid them (or, for snakes, that there are none where you live, if this is true), or gradually desensitise her through education (using books) and exposure (at zoos and museums). But, most importantly, you must assure her of your ability to protect her should there be any problem.

If, instead, your child is afraid about many things, day and night, she may have a more generalized form of anxiety. Unless these fears are minor and occur only occasionally, trying to deal with them with the behavioural techniques described below is unlikely to resolve them. Here, too, professional counselling will likely be needed.

3. *Is she afraid of 'monsters' and 'robbers'?* If your child develops feelings of anxiety that she does not understand, she is likely to use her imagination to come up with an explanation. She must find something she can believe to be a cause of her fears, something external and threatening over which she has no control: hence monsters and robbers. Such anxieties are especially common in young children. Often they relate to issues of control associated with toilet-training, hostility towards a new sibling or the need to keep aggressive impulses in check at day care or nursery school.

Remember, although the monsters or robbers are not real, your child's fear is genuine. It comes from real feelings, urges and worries. She does not understand that it is these feelings that are making her anxious. To resolve such fears, your child does not need protection from monsters: she needs a better understanding of her own feelings. She needs to know that nothing bad will happen if she soils, has a temper tantrum or gets angry at her brother or sister. At such times she can best be reassured by knowing that you are in control of yourself and – to the extent that she needs it – of her, and that you can and will protect her. If you can persuade her of these things, she will be better able to relax. Since these monsters represent your child's feelings, not things in the room, your calm, firm and loving assurance will do more to banish the goblins than will searches under the bed. Spending half an hour every night shining torches behind the furniture does little to reassure your child, and it might even reinforce her fears: why would you be looking so hard if monsters couldn't be there? The monsters are in your child's mind, and it is there you should focus your efforts. She certainly needs reassurance; whether she needs more than that depends upon just how frightened she is.

4. Is she afraid of the dark? Few children like to sleep in total darkness and there is no reason why they should. It is helpful if the bedroom is dimly lit by a night-light or by streetlights from outside, so that when your child wakes up at night, especially after a dream, she can see where she is, re-orientate herself within the room, re-establish a sense of reality and put the dream in its proper perspective.

If a child is afraid only of the dark, a night light (two to seven watts) usually suffices. But a nervous child may request additional lights: first a table lamp, then an overhead light. The room often ends up quite brightly lit: a total of 60 to 200 watts is common. Many parents turn the lights off after their child falls asleep, but when she wakes in the dark she gets scared and turns the lights back on, or a parent has to come in to do it for her. Other parents leave the lights on all night. But at night, even 60 watts is very bright (as we all know, our eyes adapt to the dark at night and become more sensitive to light; most school-aged children are able to understand this, too, if we explain it to them). Waking in that much light is a strong arousal stimulus not conducive to a rapid return to sleep.

Occasionally a child actually prefers darkness to the shadows created by a night-light. That is fine if it is really her preference and if, in fact, she does sleep well without any light. But for some children, the fear of 'shadows' is the same as the fear of monsters – that is, the fear does not originate in the shadows, but the child, having an anxiety she does not understand, tries to rationalise it by blaming it on something else. If the shadows are gone, she will find something else to be afraid of.

5. Is she afraid of having her door closed? Just as most children want some light in the room, so most want their doors at least ajar at night. This is particularly true of frightened children, although those whose fears take the form of robbers may actually feel safer with the door closed. In general, the open door allows a child to maintain a sense of connection (to what's outside), awareness (of where her parents are) and reality (where she is). Hearing her parents moving about or watching television nearby is reassuring because it reminds her that they are there. Once the door is closed and she can't hear what is really happening outside, she might use her imagination to decide, the same imagination that conjures up monsters. Don't worry that the usual noises of family activity will disrupt her sleep. If she is only scared at night when her door is closed, the remedy is easy.

6. Is there a self-reinforcing pattern to the fear? Most often, when an isolated event such as a scary film causes a child to become frightened at night, the fear lasts no more than a few weeks. Sometimes, however, the nightly memory of being frightened, and perhaps of her parents' inappropriate responses to the fear, leads to increasing anxiety that spirals out of control until the child reaches a state of near-panic. Each night the child remembers the fear of the night before, not the original trigger.

Suppose a child wakes one night from a truly frightening dream, wakes her parents and finds that they respond to being wakened with anger, threats and punishments. She is now as frightened of their response as she was by the dream. The next night she is afraid to go to bed, because she knows that if she has another frightening dream she will not be able to get help, and she also knows she may become so scared that she will *have to* wake her parents, which will only make them angrier. The fear of making them angry adds to her anxiety. If the next night goes badly, her anxieties may escalate until the night-time becomes a battle for her parents and a time of terror for her. What started as a single bad dream has become weeks or months of major disruption. At that point, the parents and even the child may have forgotten the original dream and have no idea what she is actually frightened about. No one is getting enough sleep, the parents are angry and the child is suffering terribly.

When I see a family at this juncture, I always consider the possibility that, even though everything seems out of control and the child is terribly frightened, the underlying problem may be less serious than it appears. With proper interventions, the spiralling process can be reversed and the escalated fears gradually brought back under control. It is of utmost importance that the child experiences falling asleep quickly and without fear, so the only bedtime memory the next night is a good one, and the spiral can become one of increasing confidence. Then, and only then, is it possible to decide whether a significant predisposing psychological problem exists.

How to Cope with Night-time Fears

If Your Child Isn't Really Frightened

Like most parents, you can probably tell if your child is really frightened. If you decide she does not look or act genuinely frightened, you must be firm. Stick with the bedtime routine and say good night. Do not return repeatedly. More guidelines for setting firm limits and getting your child to co-operate can be found in Chapter 5.

Be as sure as you can when you make this judgement. If a child is genuinely frightened at night, being firm in this way will not help. It may well make matters worse.

For Very Mild Fears

If your child begins to have difficulty going to sleep because she is worried or a bit fearful at bedtime, talk it over with her during the day. At night, be empathetic, reassuring and supportive. As long as her worries are relatively mild, you probably should not make any substantial changes in her bedtime and night-time routines. You might sit with her in her room a little longer than usual, but keep her on her normal schedule as much as possible (except, perhaps, for setting her bedtime later than usual for a while, as discussed below). Simply reassure her firmly and calmly that she is safe and that you will take care of her; then put her to bed with her usual story or quiet talk. Your child will be more reassured in the long run if you show her that you can take care of her than if you give in to her fears.

For More Substantial Fears

If your child is anxious at night, having more than just some mild worries, goal number one is to *do whatever you have to do to take away the anxiety.* Other issues can be resolved later. Therefore, all the suggestions below follow the same basic formula: *Start by doing whatever is necessary to help your child to feel safe and able to sleep well during the night* – but try not to do more than necessary. As things calm down, gradually reduce this extra support and boost your youngster's confidence at a rate she can tolerate.

For a child whose anxiety is mild, even very small steps can help. Keep in mind that the fear might be the outcome of a spiral that you need to reverse. The better each night is, the easier the next night will be. Try to keep to more or less the same schedule and routines as before, especially if the fears developed recently. Be sure to find time for your child during the day and evening. The bedtime routine should be pleasurable and unrushed: understanding and reassurance are important. Try to determine how much support your child needs to feel safe and secure, and offer it freely, at least initially. She must know that she can get help without angering or upsetting you. That knowledge alone makes the night less scary.

Every child is different, but for most children at least some of the techniques described below will be helpful. The techniques listed first may be enough to help a child with mild fears; those listed later may be needed for children with more severe anxieties.

Techniques to Help a Child To Feel Less Frightened and To Fall Asleep Quickly

1. Arrange for enjoyable time in her bedroom. If your child sleeps (or is supposed to sleep) in her own room or with siblings, but she doesn't spend much time there during the day, her associations with her bedroom may be only unpleasant ones. Spend time with her in her room during the day doing something enjoyable such as reading a story or playing a game. These visits should have nothing to do with bed or sleep. When bedtime comes, the final routines should take place in her room, they should be unhurried and they should include things she looks forward to, such as a story. If getting into pyjamas or cleaning teeth has become unpleasant, it should be done ahead of time.

2. Move her bedtime later. A (temporarily) later-than-usual bedtime can be very helpful for several reasons. The sleepier your child is and the faster she falls asleep, the less scary that night will seem, and the easier the next night will be. Make the new bedtime late enough that your child's mind is no longer active and she is having trouble staying awake. Take note of the time when she has actually been falling asleep, and start no earlier than that. The best idea is to set bedtime thirty to sixty minutes later than that time, for a while, to help to assure that she falls asleep as quickly as possible. Remember: better at first to put her to bed a little too late than too early.

It is critical that you get your child falling asleep quickly at bedtime. That will help not only with bedtime fears but also when she wakes during the night. When we wake at night, we all tend to pick up our thoughts where we left off before we last fell asleep. If you spend a long time worrying about something before falling asleep, you are likely to start worrying about it again as soon as you wake during the night, as if the intervening sleep hadn't even happened. Children are the same: if they fall asleep too quickly to worry or be scared at bedtime, then they are more likely to ignore their wakings during the night and fall back asleep without becoming frightened all over again.

3. Use stickers or other prizes as positive reinforcement. Rewards alone will never resolve significant anxiety, but they can help if a minor fear has spiralled out of control or if the complaint of fear has become more habitual than real. Nothing is better at helping a child feel less afraid than success at being unafraid – that is, the reversal of the spiral.

The reward system can work as described in the chapter on limit-setting. However, instead of backing up the rewards with limits, here you must leave your child the option of getting whatever she needs from you to feel unafraid. Where to start depends upon your child's current night-time behaviours, needs, and abilities. If she has problems only during the middle of the night, you can offer one sticker for going to bed without problems – she'd be certain to earn that one – and two if she has no problems during the night. Or you can offer three stickers for not waking anyone, two for just getting tucked back in, one if you have to walk her back to bed, and none if she needs more help than that. Again, success leads to more success. But your child must know that if she is very frightened, she can still count on you being there. If she believes that if she is too frightened to earn a sticker she will be left to cry alone at night, she will abandon the reward system altogether.

For school-age children, the attraction of stickers may be gone, but you can negotiate a similar system for points, with small, tangible rewards at the end of the week if things have gone well. Try to avoid large prizes – your child may work toward one, then quit trying once it is achieved – and never take back any prize your child has already earned. Don't set the reward too far in the future, or your child may lose motivation and interest. And don't be rigid about the number of stickers or points needed for a reward. If your child has been trying hard and making progress, reward her even if she's short a point or two. Make a big deal of success.

4. Teach your child to practise dealing with wakings and mild anxieties – alone. Some children automatically call out that they are frightened even before they actually are, sometimes even before they are fully awake. They may even start getting out of bed before they are alert enough to know why they are doing it. Getting children to interrupt this automatic behaviour can help, especially if it is supported with a reward system. I ask children to pause when they wake up and consider how they actually feel, instead of immediately calling for help. If they are not frightened, they should not call. Even if they are frightened or become a little nervous, I ask them to try to wait a bit longer. If they become very frightened, they can request whatever help we have agreed they might need and can have. The more nights without calling (whether they wake but control their calling, or don't wake at all) the more rewards they earn, and the more successful and competent they feel.

5. Talk to your child; ask her what she needs. Offer to help in ways such as those described below. I am always impressed by children's insight in assessing their own needs. If your child tells you that it is important for you to check on her but that you do not need to stay upstairs between checks, that is probably correct. Even if the initial requests are a bit more demanding than you wanted, start there. If you can get her falling asleep quickly and sleeping well, you are making progress. Support levels and rewards can be re-negotiated every week. A child who needed to be checked every five minutes at first might now just want you to make sure she falls asleep before you go to bed. A child who started out earning stickers just for staying in bed may now be able to earn them by not calling out or waking anyone.

6. *Set appropriate limits.* As described above, setting certain limits on an anxious child, such as requiring her to stay in her room alone, can have unwanted consequences: she may become more anxious, starting a spiral in the wrong direction. The *only* situation when this is not so is when the cause of the anxiety was the absence of appropriate and consistent limits in the first place. On the other hand, less drastic limits can still be set for an anxious child. For example, if you agree to sit with your child because she is scared, you can nevertheless refuse to read endless stories, to keep getting more drinks or to let her twist your hair. If she is scared, she needs you, not drinks and stories. As long as you are available, you can refuse most other requests and demands.

7. *Leave lights on and doors open.* Night lights can be very helpful, but bright lights (either used at bedtime or left on all night) should be turned down gradually at a pace the child can tolerate. The overhead light can be turned off in favour of the lamp; a 60-watt bulb can be replaced by a 30-watt bulb, then a 15-watt bulb and then the 7-watt bulb used in most night lights. If necessary, a dimmer control for the lamp or overhead light can easily be installed. If your child complains about the shadows, you can change the room's lighting pattern, but once you find a reasonable one, stick to it. Turning the lights on and off or moving them about the room every night will do little to allay your child's fear. Finally, leaving the child's door open is almost mandatory, unless she specifically requests that it be closed.

8. *Agree to check on your child periodically.* Children often call out repeatedly to keep tabs on their parents and to keep them from wandering too far away (in the child's judgement). Agreeing to check on your child until she falls asleep may fill this need. (Checking only means looking in on her to be sure she is all right and to let her see that you are near; it does not mean getting into extra night-time conversations or interactions.)

Explain that she does not have to call you and that you will keep checking on her until she is asleep. Make the initial intervals short, perhaps five minutes or even one minute if necessary, so that she can see you before she gets too worried. Most children are re-assured hearing you pottering around nearby as they fall asleep so they know you haven't gone very far. A later-than-usual bedtime will help assure that she falls asleep before you have had to look in on her many times. Once she becomes comfortable with this routine, you may be able to lengthen the intervals to ten or fifteen minutes. But trust is the key: she must know that you will do what you say. Don't wait longer than you agreed to just because she is quiet.

If she regularly wakes up during the night, you may have to agree to check on her then, too, but treat that as a short-term aid only: checking in the middle of the night is difficult since you must keep it up until she is back to sleep. Fortunately, once children find they can count on being checked during the night if they need it, their wakings at night often become very brief or disappear alto-gether.

Checking on a child once or twice at bedtime is not particularly difficult, but if it takes thirty minutes or more before she falls asleep, the checking process becomes burdensome. In this case, it may be that she is going to bed too early – this is especially likely if she is never frightened later during the night. (Children who are very frightened generally need to be checked by their parents, or to be with them, during the night as well as at bedtime.) On the other hand, if you need to check your child repeatedly *both* at bedtime and during the night, if the need does not diminish over a week or so of checking, if a later bedtime does not help and if each time you check her she seems truly frightened, then this approach may not be enough to help with her anxiety. You may need to stay with her all night (see overleaf), or her anxiety may be too severe to manage with behavioural techniques alone. But if she usually does not seem at all frightened even if she continues to call for checking, and espe-cially if only brief periods of checking are necessary before she goes back to sleep, it may be that the ritual has become a simple habit that you can change using techniques of negotiation, rewards and limit-setting as described above and in Chapters 4 and 5.

9. *Agree to stay upstairs until she is asleep.* Children often do not want to be the only one upstairs (or downstairs) while they are going to sleep. If that is the case, then agreeing to stay on the same level of the house as her bedroom, or in the next room if in a flat, until she is asleep, or until she says it is okay to go to another floor, may be all that is necessary. Keep your promise. If she does not have to keep checking to be sure you are still nearby, then she can relax and go to sleep.

10. *Agree to stay up later than she does.* Some children – especially those whose parents go to bed early – worry that they will be the last one left awake, and that in the middle of the night they will be the only one up. Racing to fall asleep before the parents do, they are certain to stay awake. Checking is helpful in this situation. You may not even have to check on your child at intervals, as long as you promise to be sure she is asleep before you go to sleep yourself. Also promise her that if she wakes in the middle of the night and needs your help, you will get up and stay up until she falls back to sleep. This is a burden if you have to do it frequently, but if you are willing to do it and make it clear to her that you are, the need usually disappears quickly.

11. *Sit in her room.* If checking even at short intervals is not enough to keep your child calm, you may have to stay in the room. That probably means sleeping there (see overleaf), but it may be enough to sit with her until she falls asleep. Sitting with her is fine if you don't have to stay long – another reason to start with a late bedtime – but it is very difficult to do repeatedly during the night. Your child may also fight sleep if she knows that you will leave as soon as she has fallen asleep. But if sitting with your child awhile is all that is necessary, it may get her sleep back on track. Then, as her anxiety eases, you can work your way back out of her room. By a process of *gradual desensitisation,* you can progressively move your chair farther from the bed, then out into the corridor; or you can work on leaving for brief but increasing intervals (see overleaf); or you can start a reward system. Do whatever works best.

12. Sleep in her room. For the child whose anxiety is severe, the suggestions above may not suffice. A child whose separation anxiety is such that she cannot allow you out of her sight even briefly during the day should not be expected to stay in a dark room alone for ten hours; nor should an older child with serious anxiety, regardless of its cause. If your child is sufficiently frightened, the only way to make her feel safe at night may be to be there yourself. Remember, your first goal – at first, your only goal – is to take away the fear and make the night-time pleasant again.

The fastest way to get things under better control is to offer to sleep in her room: preferably you will sleep in a separate bed or on a mattress on the floor, but if absolutely necessary, you may sleep in her bed at first and move to the floor as a second step. You could achieve the same effect by letting her sleep in your bed or in your room, but, assuming the long-range goal is to get her back to her own room, you will only be adding a step to the process, because to help her move back to her room you will probably still have to sleep in there with her initially.

Letting her move every night from her own room to a sleeping bag on your floor is also a poor technique. It forces her to get up and switch rooms in the middle of the night, which will hamper good sleep; it fosters an automatic habit of room-switching; and it forces her to sleep on the floor. Unless you take steps to change the sleeping bag routine, it may go on indefinitely (I have worked with families who have been stuck in this pattern for years), and your child may come to believe that she will never be able to sleep alone the way her friends do.

Start the night by lying down in your child's room while she goes to sleep. Don't leave before she falls asleep unless she says you can; wait until she is deeply asleep before going out and finishing your evening activities. Then, return to her room when you retire for the night. (If you hear her start to wake before that, you should return immediately.) The goal is for her to know and trust that you are there when she falls asleep and will still be there whenever she wakes. If you try to sneak back to your own room whenever she is asleep, you will undermine her trust and she will start trying to stay awake or re-awakening frequently to check on you.

Most children's night-time fears dissipate if a parent sleeps in their room with them. Your child should start sleeping well. And so should you (although in less than ideal circumstances). The idea here is to let things calm down, reverse the spiral, get back to normality and re-assess the situation.

If your child's night-time fears are only one part of a generalised problem with anxiety, then she will likely remain very anxious during the day even after things are going reasonably well at night. In this case, you may have to continue sleeping in her room until that anxiety is addressed directly. Consider seeking professional counselling, particularly if the anxiety is pronounced and long-standing.

If the day and night are going well, you may be able to start applying some of the approaches listed above as you would for a child with only mild anxiety. Once your child has gone a week or two without being very fearful at night, she may be able to release you at bedtime, as long as you stay upstairs and promise to come back if she is frightened.

Your child may now be sleeping well, no longer bothering to check that you are there during the night. In this case, if she can learn to fall asleep at bedtime without you in the room, the problem will be resolved. Your child may agree to this step, perhaps helped along with a reward system and some negotiation as described above. If she is not ready, you can gradually help to prepare her. Before she goes to sleep, you can leave her room briefly 'to get something'. How long you stay away depends upon your child's ability to tolerate your absence; it could be ten seconds or ten minutes. If she does not fall asleep immediately upon your return, you might go out again. Gradually, perhaps over a week or two, make the trips out longer and the trips back shorter until you're really just checking on her. Now your child is starting to get used to being in her room alone again – this is very important, because it means that simply finding herself in the room alone is no longer a cause for alarm. And she will start to fall asleep while you are out of the room – also very important, because if she wakes to find herself in the room alone, she will not find anything changed from the way it was when she went to sleep. Once she is comfortable falling asleep alone, you can plan on staying out of the room the rest of the night. If she starts waking again at night, use your judgement as to whether she is simply repeating old habits or is actually frightened. In the first case, set appropriate limits or respond briefly at increasing intervals as described in Chapters 4 and 5; in the latter, make yourself more available again.

Do Not Use Siblings (or Pets) to Do Your Job as Parents

Many siblings share rooms at night, and of course that is fine. But if a child is frightened at night, it is your job to deal with that fear, not her brother's or sister's. You should not make one child let her frightened sister climb into bed with her during the night, or force another child to go to sleep with his frightened brother, or move either of them into a frightened sibling's room or let the sibling move in with them. Nor should one child have to rely on another to feel safe at night. If two siblings have been asking to sleep in the same room, that may work out fine, but don't let one youngster's anxiety be the reason.

Buying a cat or dog (or using one you already own) to stay in your frightened child's room at night may or may not be fair to the pet, but either way it will usually not help your child. The bedroom door will have to be closed, to keep the pet from leaving the room, which might cause your child more anxiety. Even if a cat is there, your child may have trouble finding her; your child's sleep may be further disturbed by a dog trying to leave or by a cat patrolling the room throughout the night. In any case, the presence of a pet is not enough to allay significant anxieties in most children, and even when it is, the child only becomes dependent on the animal, and the cause of the underlying fears goes untreated.

How We Helped Tyler

Tyler benefited from a number of the techniques described in this chapter. I suggested to his parents that they spend time with him in his room each day for a game or a story. They were not to leave him there alone. Since Tyler rarely fell asleep before 9.00 p.m., his bed-time routine would not even start until that time. After a story, they would say good night around 9.30. Tyler would be very sleepy then: the late bedtime, along with an unchanged 7.00 a.m. wake-up time, guaranteed it. Tyler liked the later bedtime, and he thought he could stay in his room alone as long as his parents stayed upstairs and looked in on him frequently until he was asleep. Since they were to check him regularly even if he was quiet, he would not have to call. Tyler also agreed to let us turn off one of his lights at night, and over the next two weeks, his parents were to gradually replace the bulb in the remaining lamp with dimmer ones. These goals were further supported with a reward system that I negotiated with Tyler: he would be awarded stickers when there were no problems at bed-time, and more stickers when he handled the night-time by himself or with only a minimal intervention. The stickers could then be converted into small presents.

If Tyler woke up at night, he was to try to go back to sleep with-out calling or waking anyone. If he felt he needed help, he could call, and one of his parents would check in on him; if need be, they would check on him regularly until he was asleep again, as they did at bedtime. He was never to sleep in their bed, but if he was very scared on a given night, one of his parents would sleep that night in his room (on a separate mattress on the floor, so he could continue to practise sleeping in his bed alone) – but on those nights he would earn no stickers. Finally, any night there was thunder, a parent would sleep in his room and he would still get his stickers.

Most of the areas of concern were now covered. Tyler would be sleeping in his own bed every night. The long wait to fall asleep would be gone, making it easier to go back to sleep later in the night. He would start each night by falling asleep in his room alone, so that if he woke later in the room alone, nothing would be differ-ent. He would not have to keep track of his parents' whereabouts at his bedtime because they would always be nearby and checking on him, and he could always get more help later in the night if he needed it. Also, the bright lights would be gone. And he did not have to worry about the possibility of thunder because, if there were any, one of his parents would come right in. Furthermore, when he did well he got stickers and prizes.

In fact, things went very well. Tyler did call out a few times at bedtime the first night, but not often after that. He learned that his parents were close by and checking, as they had promised, and he started falling asleep too quickly to worry about checking anyway. He did need his parents to look in on him a few times during the night for a few nights, but once he saw that this help was always available, he stopped asking for that as well. All this time he was sleeping in his own bed alone all night, and each night was easier than the night before, as I had told him it would be. He was very proud of his stickers and the toy cars he got as rewards. Eventually the family was able to move his bedtime back to 8.30 p.m., and the lamp was replaced with a night-light. Soon he started wandering up to his room for toys during the day, and not long after that the fearful nights were only a memory.

FINAL CONSIDERATIONS

All the techniques mentioned previously should be considered guidelines. Try to design an approach that suits your child's needs, your own abilities and your particular living circumstances. Often trial and error will show you what works or what changes have to be made. Sometimes you will be able to move ahead faster than you expected; sometimes you'll have to go more slowly. But in the beginning, always give your frightened child the benefit of the doubt. Assume that her fear is real and remember that you must provide support before you begin making demands. If you aren't making progress, or if the progress stops, you may need professional help to decide how serious your child's anxiety is, whether your behavioural programme should continue and whether counselling is indicated.

CHAPTER 8

Colic and Other Medical Causes of Poor Sleep

Illnesses of various kinds can disrupt a child's sleep. Unless the illness is chronic, this disruption is usually temporary; a child in discomfort or running a fever might sleep fitfully at night and nap intermittently during the day until the illness resolves. Teething pain, for instance, can cause a young child to sleep poorly for several nights, but it will not interfere with his sleep for weeks on end, as parents sometimes suppose. In young children, even chronic medical conditions rarely cause sleep disturbances that continue for months or years. Still, if your child has consistently poor sleep and you have ruled out the more common causes – or, of course, if you know that your child has a significant medical problem – then you may have to consider a medical cause.

COLIC

In the early months, probably the most common cause of significant sleep disturbances is colic, a condition in which a baby has frequent spells of intense crying and is difficult to soothe. The episodes begin to appear in the first weeks after birth; they usually occur in the late afternoon or evening and can go on for several hours. If your baby is colicky, you may find you can help only by walking around with him for hours or by placing him over your legs while you rub his back. Often, nothing you do may seem to help.

A colicky baby often has a distended stomach; his legs will likely be pulled up toward his chest, and he may seem to feel relief when he passes gas or has a bowel movement. For these reasons, it is commonly assumed that colic is caused by intestinal pain. Whether that is true (or always true) remains uncertain, but in very severe cases of colic a paediatrician may prescribe medication to relax the bowels and ease the apparent discomfort. On the other hand, it's possible that the distention, the gas and at least some of the apparent discomfort may actually be caused by air swallowed during long periods of vigorous crying. The initial reason why the baby started crying, or cries so long and so hard, may be something else entirely.

Another possible contributing factor is sensory overstimulation. Colicky infants often seem to be unusually sensitive to events happening around them or to excessive handling and other stimulation, or at least they behave as if that is the case. Many professionals have concluded that these children see, hear and feel the world about them as an unpleasant and disorganised barrage of sensations. This chaotic input would be difficult for an infant to handle; the child could become upset and build up so much tension throughout the day that his coping abilities become overloaded. He would need to discharge this accumulated tension at the end of the day. Whether or not this explanation is true, colicky babies do act as if they have a need to cry and seem to do better when allowed to do so for a while.

If your baby seems to have colic, you should first try to comfort him; you might try rocking him gently, feeding him or giving him a dummy. If you find he cannot easily be comforted, allow him to cry for fifteen minutes while held calmly or alone in his cot. If he has not settled by then, try again to console him. Be calm and speak softly; try not to become frantic, and don't do anything too vigorous, such as bouncing him or running about the room with him. If he still isn't comforted, try again every fifteen minutes or so. Remember, since colicky babies seem to benefit from a period of crying, you are actually responding to his needs by letting him cry for a while. If you try too hard to stop the crying, you might just overstimulate him and make things worse. If he needed to be held, nursed or rocked, or just wanted to use a dummy, then those interventions would have calmed him down.

A child's colic often improves if he is allowed to cry undisturbed for just two or three consecutive colicky periods. His crying spells may get shorter and less intense in a day or two, and, if they do, he will probably sleep better as well. Babies hospitalised for severe colic often seem to be 'cured' just by being in hospital, probably because nurses are more likely than parents to allow an infant periods to cry by himself if he does not accept comforting.

Colic is discussed in all books on baby care, and if your baby suffers from it, you should also talk it over with your paediatrician. In almost all cases, the symptoms completely disappear by the time the child reaches three months of age. However, although colic is not in and of itself a sleep disorder, colicky infants often do develop long-standing sleep problems. These ongoing problems may look the same as those the baby suffered from during the colicky months, but they are not.

What happens is that the habits formed when your child was colicky can persist after the colic has disappeared. You may have spent a great deal of time walking, rocking and holding him, and otherwise trying to comfort him to help him get to sleep. Once the colic is gone, your child may still demand these rituals, not because he is in distress (despite his crying), but because he has come to expect them. If that happens, you will have to help him learn new, more appropriate associations with falling asleep, as discussed in Chapter 4.

The biggest difficulty here is deciding when the colic is gone. It goes away gradually, not overnight, so it may not be obvious to you when the time has come to change your responses. Keep in mind that colic is usually gone by the age of three months, and that it occurs during the day, not just during normal sleep hours. In fact, colic tends to be most severe in the evening, suggesting an interaction with underlying circadian rhythms, although it is not known which hormones or bodily functions may be involved. A colicky baby appears to be genuinely distressed, as if he is in pain and not merely hungry, frustrated or angry, and it is difficult to ease a colicky baby's suffering. So it is unlikely that colic is (still) the problem if your baby cries mainly at bedtime and during the night; if, despite the crying, he does not appear to be in pain; if the crying stops promptly when you pat his back, rock him, give him a dummy, or feed him; and if you can get him to return to sleep quickly when he does wake. Once you have realised that, you can go on to identify the real cause of the persisting sleep problem and take steps to correct it. If you don't, it may continue for months or even years.

CHRONIC ILLNESS

Chronic medical conditions can contribute to ongoing sleep disturbances in a variety of ways. A child's illness may cause pain or discomfort: skin irritation causes annoying itching; migraines cause night-time headaches and nausea; asthma makes breathing difficult. His sleep may be disrupted by the specific symptoms of his disease or disorder: perhaps he wakes feeling jittery or needing to urinate because of poorly controlled diabetes, or his sleep may be broken by epileptic seizures. The indirect consequences of a medical disorder can also cause trouble: for example, certain medications have side effects that interfere with sleep; an orthopaedic brace can cause discomfort or limit a child's ability to move; and even a child's anxieties about his condition can keep him awake.

If your child suffers from a chronic medical problem, you're probably well aware of it. The difficulty lies in sorting out which factors related to the illness – if any – are disrupting his sleep. Several factors may be contributing at once. This can be a very complex problem, possibly too difficult for you to solve alone. Ask your paediatrician or specialist for help.

Several conditions do merit special discussion here.

NOCTURNAL PAIN

When pain at night affects sleep, it is the pain, not the sleep itself, that must be treated. In most cases – for example, when a child is up at night after sustaining an injury or while teething – it is clear what is happening, and the solution is as simple as relieving the pain with medications or other treatments. Fortunately, most causes of pain are easy to recognise and resolve quickly. However, there are two especially common ones that often go unrecognised for long periods of time: middle-ear disease and gastro-oesophageal reflux.

Night-time pain from these or other causes often wakes children at unpredictable times during the night (not at a regular time, say, always an hour after the child falls asleep). If your child has awakened in pain, he will probably be crying and unhappy, and there will be no easy way to stop it. It makes little difference where he is. If he usually stops crying quickly and seems fine once you pick him up or allow him something he wants, then he's probably not in pain. Similarly, if he cries every night in his own bed but always sleeps soundly when you let him sleep in your bed, look for an explanation other than pain (he could not be suffering from reflux or middle-ear disease only when in his own bed, after all).

Middle-Ear Disease

Once identified, chronic middle-ear disease is usually easy to treat. In this condition, fluid collects in the middle-ear cavity behind the eardrum and does not drain satisfactorily. This fluid can become infected, but even if it doesn't, the fluid build-up alone can lead to a temporary loss of hearing, and if the fluid remains there long enough, it can permanently damage the bones of the middle ear.

When a child's middle ear is acutely infected, pressure in the middle-ear cavity increases, the eardrum bulges and the child likely experiences pain. When the fluid does not become infected, children usually don't complain of pain, but their sleep may nonetheless be disrupted – it is not clear how or why. It may be that when the child is lying down the middle ear drains less effectively than at other times, more fluid collects, pressure increases to a degree and the child feels enough discomfort to interrupt his sleep. Whatever the cause, children with persistent fluid behind the eardrum sometimes have significant sleep disturbances that cannot be explained any other way. It is striking that when these children are treated with proper medication, or, if necessary, by having drainage tubes inserted through the eardrums, not only are their middle-ear problems cured but often the sleep disturbances disappear as well.

Caroline was an eighteen-month-old girl who had a long history of frequent wakings at night despite the fact that she went to bed easily. On waking she usually cried. She calmed down somewhat if her parents picked her up, but she had a hard time getting back to sleep, no matter what her parents did. Even when they walked with her or rocked her, she usually whimpered for ten or fifteen minutes before finally going back to sleep. Nothing they tried seemed to help at all. Caroline's history did not suggest an obvious cause for her sleep disturbance, but her parents did report that Caroline had had three or four ear infections over the past year.

When I see a child with sleep problems like Caroline's – frequent unhappy night-time wakings, with difficulty returning to sleep regardless of anything the parents do – I always take a careful look at the child's eardrums before deciding on a diagnosis and plan of therapy. In Caroline's case, I found that she still had a build-up of fluid behind her eardrums. Not only were her ears better treated with drainage tubes, but her sleep problems went away, and we avoided a series of behavioural treatments that, in her case, would not have worked.

Gastro-oesophageal Reflux

Another cause of night-time pain is gastro-oesophageal reflux, what we commonly call heartburn. Ordinarily, food passes down from the mouth through the oesophagus and then through a valve that keeps food in the stomach and prevents it coming back up. This valve often functions imperfectly in early infancy (which is why spitting-up is so common). Other problems with the normal passage of food out of the stomach into the intestines can complicate the problem further.

Occasional spitting-up in itself is no more than an annoyance, and most reflux material is cleared fairly rapidly from the oesophagus by swallowing. But if stomach contents (which are very acidic) are repeatedly regurgitated into the oesophagus and remain there too long, they can burn and even scar it. Occasionally some acid even spills over into the trachea (windpipe) and possibly down into the lungs, causing coughing, gagging and occasionally pneumonia. Paediatricians and gastroenterologists have good techniques for evaluating these symptoms and many effective medicines to treat the problem. You should not hesitate to consult them.

When a young child is frequently up at night crying inconsolably, pain from reflux is one of the causes we must consider. Reflux occurs more often when a child is active than during sleep; most episodes of reflux at night are actually caused by movement and crying, not vice versa. Children with reflux generally also show symptoms during the day: they spit up frequently and perhaps gag and choke. If your child has no such symptoms during the day, then it is unlikely that he is experiencing much reflux at night.

When a child's symptoms suggest reflux as a possibility, further evaluation may be indicated, possibly including X-ray studies or direct monitoring of the level of acid in the oesophagus. Occasionally we simultaneously monitor a child's sleep and reflux patterns overnight in the sleep laboratory to see if reflux is actually causing discomfort and wakefulness. Treatment is generally by antacid or anti-reflux medication, sometimes started on a trial basis to help make the diagnosis. Surgery is only rarely indicated.

MEDICATION

Sleep medication is very frequently misused. In recent years doctors have begun to appreciate that sleeping pills have caused far more sleep disorders in adults than they have ever cured. That is equally true with youngsters. A child receiving sleep medication regularly may reach a point where without the medication he cannot sleep, yet his sleep on the medication is of poor quality. When a child is not sleeping well and nothing seems to help, the family feels frustrated and hopeless, and they often beg the doctor for help. Often the doctor will prescribe some sort of sleep medication. The ones most commonly used are the antihistamines, such as diphenhydramine (Benadryl); certain medicines for high blood pressure, such as clonidine (Catapres); and certain drugs used to treat depression, such as trazodone (Desyrel). All of these drugs cause sleepiness as a side effect. Major sedatives, such as chloral hydrate, and even major tranquillisers, such as those related to diazepam (Valium), are often tried as well.

Yet such medications rarely solve the sleep problems of a child who is otherwise normal and healthy. A child may even have a so-called paradoxical response to the medication, becoming 'hyper' and unable to sit still or sleep. In some conditions, such as sleep apnoea (see Chapter 17), certain medications can be very dangerous. Even if your child sleeps well on medication, he will be far better off if you can determine the cause of the disturbance and help him to learn to sleep well without drugs. Sometimes medication improves a child's sleep for several nights, even for a few weeks, but usually the old pattern returns. Besides, the stronger medications often affect a child's daytime mood and level of functioning: he may become overactive or clingy, cranky and babyish. Only occasionally will a short (one- to two-week) course of drug treatment break the cycle of a poor sleep pattern and allow a good one to emerge so that normal sleep persists after the medication is stopped. If this treatment succeeds, the medication probably did no harm, but proper behavioural approaches would probably also have been successful. If you are able to correct your child's sleep without medicine, you will avoid the nagging anxiety that he has an underlying medical or neurological problem that keeps him from sleeping well, and you will feel more confident in dealing with any problems that may emerge in the future without feeling that you have to head immediately for the medicine cabinet.

In my practice, I see far too many young children who have been given powerful medications in an attempt to relieve sleep disorders that could be corrected by other means. In many cases, whatever the child's problem, the medication only makes matters worse. Also, the child's daytime behaviour and his ability to concentrate and learn may well be compromised. This was the case with Joshua.

Joshua was a four-year-old boy described by his family as tense and irritable. His parents said he had great difficulty sleeping at night and wasn't very happy during the day. Because of the boy's repeated night-time wakings and his behavioural difficulties during the day (which were probably the result of his poor sleep), his parents had sought medical advice. Joshua ended up on three medications: a long-acting stimulant taken in the morning, a drug to induce sleep at bedtime and an even stronger sleeping pill to be taken if he didn't fall asleep quickly or woke again later in the night. He had been on these medications for ten months.

Joshua was so clearly an unhappy and irritable child that I was quite concerned. He interacted poorly with adults and peers, and I felt that a complete psychological evaluation would likely be needed. But first, to get a clearer picture of the situation and to establish a baseline for making further decisions, I had the family gradually stop Joshua's medications altogether. We also discussed changes to his sleep schedule and bedtime routines and ways for his parents to set limits. Joshua agreed to co-operate in exchange for stickers and prizes. When I saw the family several weeks later, - Joshua's parents were already vastly relieved. After a few difficult nights in the beginning, Joshua had begun going to bed easily and sleeping through the night for the first time in a year. In addition, he was much happier in the daytime and his parents had begun to enjoy his company again. When I saw him in my office, Joshua was smiling, obviously happy and good-natured in our conversation. In short, he was a delightfully normal four-year-old. His good sleep pattern and normal daytime behaviour have continued, and there has been no need for further intervention.

I almost never recommend medication for a child with difficulty falling or staying asleep, and when I begin to treat a child who has been taking medication just for his sleep, I usually try to arrange for a trial period off of the medication before doing anything else, as I did with Joshua. If your child is on medication just to help him sleep, you may want to speak with your doctor about doing the same.

Your child, of course, may have to take medications to treat other medical conditions. Phenobarbital and other drugs with sedative properties are often used in the treatment of epilepsy. Theophylline (Slo-Phyllin, Slo-Bid), aminophylline (Phyllocontin, Truphylline), metaproterenol (Alupent), albuterol (Ventolin, Proventil), terbutaline (Brethine, Bricanyl) and other similar medications with stimulant properties are used to treat asthma. Other stimulant drugs, such as the amphetamines (dexamphetamine, for example) or methylphenidate (Ritalin, Concerta XL), may be used to treat Attention Deficit Hyperactivity Disorder (ADHD). Some children need antibiotics on an ongoing basis as protection against recurrent infections. These and many other medications can interfere with proper sleep. Again, the various effects of the underlying medical disorder, the medication, and other causes of sleep problems have to be sorted out – not always an easy task. The dilemma can be further complicated if your child has had many hospitalisations and has become fearful at night, or if you (understandably) find it hard to set firm limits for your child because of his illness.

If it seems possible that medication may be causing the sleep problem, you should raise the issue with your doctor and discuss the several approaches that may be helpful. You may be able to change your child's dosage or the time of day when he takes the drugs, or your doctor may be able to suggest alternative drugs – even a temporary change will help you to determine whether the original medicine was causing the sleep problem. Asthma medications taken by mouth may also be available as an inhalant, with fewer side effects. Antibiotics themselves are unlikely to cause much of a sleep problem, but the additives in the liquid preparations may; switching to pills, or even to a different brand of liquid, may be helpful.

In any case, these changes will take time and require a certain amount of trial and error. But *do not make any changes before you talk to your child's specialist*. With his or her help, significant improvements may well be possible.

ABNORMAL BRAIN FUNCTION
AND A TRUE INABILITY TO SLEEP WELL

On occasion I see children who appear to sleep poorly because of some impairment in the brain mechanisms that control one aspect or another of sleep. Most of these children show general impairments significant enough to be obvious. Usually they are mentally retarded; they may suffer from spasticity and seizures; and they may be blind or deaf.

When such a neurological disorder is accompanied by a sleep disorder, we have to consider all the possibilities very carefully. For example, the child could have any of the sleep problems described in this book apart from his illness, and those problems can be solved in much the same way as for any other child. If your child has a neurological disorder or sensory impairment, it may be especially difficult for you to be firm at night – enforcing new patterns and setting new limits – but often the only way to solve his sleep problem is to accept that there will be some crying as, for example, you help him to learn new associations with falling asleep (see Chapter 4). Although it may seem harsh, it is in your child's best interest. You may just have to proceed more slowly than you would in the absence of the disorder. Instead of setting an initial goal of being out of the room while he falls asleep, say, you might simply work on helping him learn to fall asleep when you are out of his bed, even if initially you remain in the same room. Correcting an inappropriate sleep schedule is easier, and it is especially important for children with visual disabilities who have an impaired ability to rely on daylight to control their body rhythms (see Chapters 9 through 12). As described above, medications that your child is taking for his disorder could also be a source of his sleep problems. Finally, your child's neurological impairments could be directly responsible for his inability to sleep – that is, the brain systems that control sleep may not be working properly.

When I treat a child who is neurologically impaired, I first try to identify and treat factors apart from the brain damage, such as medication, inappropriate sleep associations or schedule problems. More often than not, this approach leads to a successful outcome, and the child's sleep problem is resolved in spite of the neurological disorder. Only after all other factors are eliminated do I conclude that the child is sleeping poorly as a direct result of the brain damage.

Sarah was a six-year-old girl with muscular dystrophy, which left her severely compromised. She was largely confined to bed, although she spent part of the day in a wheelchair. She took one medication, to help keep her muscles relaxed. Though she could not speak, she understood much of what went on around her. Her parents were devoted to her. They did not, however, like the fact that Sarah slept only about five hours each night, usually from midnight to 5.00 a.m. If she was put to bed early, she made noise until her parents came and stayed with her or brought her into the other room with them. Neither behavioural changes nor sleep-inducing medication seemed to help. The family had been told that the problem was part of Sarah's illness and that there was little that could be done.

However, when I met Sarah I discovered that, although she slept little at night, she usually slept about four hours during the day. She spent much of the daytime in bed, and when she was alone she often fell asleep for up to three hours at a time. This was due mainly to habit, not to the sedating effects of her muscle-relaxant medication (since her sleep pattern changed little when the medication was temporarily discontinued). It was clear to me that, despite her neurological illness, Sarah had a normal sleep requirement; the problem was that too much of her sleep took place in the daytime.

Even though Sarah had had this problem for years, it was fairly easy to fix. I simply asked her parents to keep her awake all day. They needed to get her out of bed more often, and at first someone had to be with her almost all the time to be sure she did not doze. I also changed the dosage and timing of her daily medication. Once Sarah was no longer allowed to sleep so much during the day, she started sleeping more at night. Within two weeks she was sleeping from 9.00 p.m. to 6.00 a.m. and never took more than a one-hour nap.

Although Sarah had a severe neurological illness, it was not the illness or even her medication that (directly) caused her sleep problem but her sleep schedule. The solution was an adjustment to her hours of sleep, not more medication.

Nicholas was a four-year-old boy who had moderate learning disabilites because of a birth injury. He had always been a poor sleeper and was now falling asleep no earlier than 10.00 p.m. (albeit fairly easily) and waking at about 4.00 a.m., after which he would stay awake for several hours or even the rest of the night. On waking he would call out, throw toys around the room and bang his head against the wall. During the day Nicholas sometimes napped for about thirty minutes, rarely longer. Nicholas's parents wanted very much to keep him at home instead of placing him in a residential treatment programme, but getting up with him every night was a tremendous strain, and some of Nicholas's behaviour posed dangers to him.

We began Nicholas's treatment by changing all of the possible behavioural factors we could identify, including how his parents handled his bedtime routines and responded to his night-time wakings, but he showed only slight improvement over a period of several months. Eventually, I had to conclude that behavioural intervention would not work and that he had a true inability to get the sleep he needed. The only other explanation, which seemed unlikely, was that he simply didn't need very much sleep (although even if that were the case, we had to do something since he could not continue to live at home if he slept so little).

In an extreme case like Nicholas's, when I know that brain function has been impaired and I'm convinced that the impairment is responsible for the sleep disturbance, I will consider the use of medication. Sedatives are sometimes effective. There have been a few reports suggesting that melatonin (a hormone, sold in health food shops, that is normally secreted during night-time sleep periods; see Chapters 9 and 10) can help children like Nicholas, and as far as we know at this writing it is probably a *relatively* benign drug (we do not yet know for sure what side effects it may have, especially when it is used for a long time); however, I have not found it particularly helpful. Usually we must resort to stronger medications. There is no single medication that is helpful to all children like Nicholas, and not all children respond best to the same drug. While I greatly prefer not to use such drugs, they do help children like Nicholas to go to sleep more easily and, more importantly, to sleep long enough for them and their families to get sufficient rest.

With the help of medication, Nicholas began sleeping from 9.30 p.m. to 6.00 a.m. While he was still getting less sleep than the normal amount for his age, this was a major improvement and it made life much easier for his parents. In addition, as is typical of children with neurological impairment, Nicholas seemed to show no lingering drug effects in the morning, and his teachers said he seemed more alert.

Results like these suggest that children such as Nicholas are not sleeping poorly just because their sleep requirements are short. It is also interesting that such children may continue to sleep well even when they are prescribed medication for extended periods, whereas in a normal child the same medications usually become less effective over time and eventually create new sleep problems. When I must recommend medication, I continue to monitor the child carefully, and at intervals we decrease the dosage or stop the medication altogether to see if it is still needed.

Most of these drugs require prescriptions and can only be managed under the care of a doctor. My experience shows that when neurologically impaired children require medication to help them sleep, they often need a fairly powerful drug, and in substantial doses. If a child shows improvement on a mild medication such as an antihistamine, then I am convinced that he can get the same improvement without drugs.

If your child is neurologically impaired and not sleeping well, you may consider discussing a trial of medication with your doctor. But before you decide to give your child a strong sleep medication, do try to identify other possible causes and to regulate his sleep patterns according to the methods outlined in this book. The behavioural approach has been successful with many neurologically impaired children, and it just might be all that your child needs.

PART III

SCHEDULES AND SLEEP RHYTHM DISTURBANCES

CHAPTER 9

Schedules and Rhythms

Children commonly experience sleep disturbances caused by problems in the timing of their sleeping and waking patterns and in their daily routines. Their schedules may be too irregular; they may be regular, but inappropriate in certain ways; or a child may just not be sleeping when her parents *want* her to sleep. If your child's daily patterns are inconsistent, then her sleep at night may be broken. If she naps or eats at unusual times, then she may wake too early in the morning or fall asleep too late at night. If she has become accustomed to sleeping at the 'wrong' hours, then she may be unable to fall asleep as early or sleep as late as you wish.

Many sleep problems can be treated simply by adjusting the underlying sleep schedule. In other cases, an improper sleep schedule is only part of the problem, but still a very important one. If your child isn't tired when you want her to go to sleep, you might rock her or give her a bottle to try to help her settle down, and in the process you may inadvertently teach her to associate these activities with falling asleep. Or, if you have difficulty setting firm limits at bedtime, your child may always stay up too late, and the time at which she gets sleepy may shift. When a child has a sleep problem that includes a disturbance in her sleep rhythm, it will probably not be enough simply to correct her sleep associations or set firmer limits at bedtime: you will have to correct her schedule as well.

To make corrections – in fact, to understand and treat any child's sleep problem properly – you must first understand the rhythm of her sleep-wake pattern. When parents have trouble treating their child's sleep problems, it is often because they haven't considered her schedule. Whenever a family consults me about a child's sleep problem, I always ask when their child goes to bed, when she actually falls asleep, when she wakes in the morning and when she sleeps during the day. I also need to know when she is awake at night and for how long; whether she wakes on her own or has to be wakened in the morning and from naps; whether her schedule changes at weekends and on holiday; and whether her schedule varies when cared for by different adults under different bedtime conditions, or in different sleep locations. Without at least this basic schedule information, it is impossible to make any informed recommendations.

Why is this information so critical? The answer has to do with the body's *circadian rhythms*. The term 'circadian', literally meaning 'approximately one day', refers to changes in an organism's biological systems that cycle approximately every twenty-four hours. Nearly all living things exhibit these rhythms. A branch of science called circadian biology studies them in plants and animals, and discoveries in this field have been truly astounding. Clever and sophisticated experiments have given us a much improved understanding of how circadian rhythms are set and how they control sleep and waking. With these scientific advances, our understanding of sleep and sleep problems in children has improved considerably, and we can use this knowledge to develop rational treatment programmes.

The circadian control of our body rhythms begins before birth, and the same basic pattern of control persists across all ages. The main concepts discussed here apply equally well to adults and children. The regular alternation between sleeping and waking is an obvious example of this circadian pattern, but in fact all of your body's physiological systems follow a daily cycle as well. There are predictable daily variations in hormone levels, body temperature, intestinal activity, urine output and even immune system function. Steroid levels drop at night and rise towards morning; body temperature does the same. The level of melatonin, a hormone secreted by the pineal gland, rises at night in the dark and drops during the day in the light.

None of this happens by coincidence. These cycles are all controlled by the 'biological clock', also called the *circadian,* or *central, pacemaker.* This pacemaker consists of a group of cells located in the hypothalamus, a primitive area of the brain that, in addition to its circadian effects, also directly governs minute-to-minute changes in hormone levels, appetite, blood pressure and other basic functions. In humans, the circadian pacemaker tends to run a little slow: if we allowed it to run freely, it would take about ten minutes longer than a standard twenty-four-hour day to complete one cycle. Yet we normally operate (or should operate) on an exact twenty-four-hour day. We manage that by re-setting the pacemaker every morning, just as you might reset your watch every day if it tended to run slow.

In humans, the only proven way to adjust the clock (other than with certain medications) is through exposure to light. Light travels into your eyes and stimulates your retina; some of that information is relayed directly to the biological clock in the hypothalamus, in effect telling the clock the correct time. If the clock's current internal setting is incorrect, it starts to adjust in the appropriate direction. That is why your body normally runs according to your local time, and why you can adjust your schedule when you travel to a different time zone. (The reason it takes several days to adapt to a new time zone is that, except in specialised laboratory settings, our biological clocks cannot make large adjustments all at once.) Light affects the clock differently depending upon what 'time' it is inside your body when the exposure occurs: light at midday has very little effect, but light after sunset or towards morning makes your body think the day ends later or starts earlier, and so the clock adjusts in the corresponding manner.

Activities, meals and napping can affect your clock's setting, but only indirectly, by changing the hours you are exposed to light.

If you stay up later than usual after an evening nap, or if you get up extra early one morning for an appointment, you will be exposed to light at times when you would normally be asleep. And if you are used to eating in the middle of the night, you will definitely be exposed to light at the wrong time.

Certain regular and predictable aspects of our daily schedules develop through habit or necessity, regardless of the circadian pacemaker's setting. For example, although we generally feel hungriest near our typical meal times, if we force ourselves to eat at different times we will eventually learn to get hungry at those times instead, even if the rest of our daily schedule – including when we sleep – is unchanged. To a degree, even nap times can be changed independently of night-time sleep hours.

If meals, napping, and daytime activities do not follow any regular schedule, our physiological rhythms become disorganised and unco-ordinated, and feelings of hunger and sleepiness begin to occur at unpredictable and inappropriate times of the day. If we don't sleep regular hours at night, this disorientation worsens: now these rhythms no longer function in concert at all, as they should. Our bodies do not seem to know whether it is time for a snack or a big meal, for a brief evening nap or an early bedtime. Some of our circadian rhythms may be set for sleep while others are at levels associated with waking.

'Jet lag' is the same phenomenon in another guise. When you first travel to a different time zone, your body's clock remains set to the time zone you left. You try to conform to the new schedule, staying awake and active during the daylight hours and sleeping when it is night there. But your body, unable to reset its internal clock instantly, wants to wake and sleep at times based on the clock at home. As your rhythms adjust to the new time zone, they may do so at different rates; thus, for a while, not only are they at the wrong setting but they are also out of sync. You feel drowsy and unwell during the day and you sleep poorly at night.

If you follow the new schedule consistently, your circadian clock and all the physiological systems under its control will eventually adjust. But if you don't keep to a regular schedule – perhaps while travelling or even routinely at home – your rhythms may never work in harmony. If you are a shift worker, the symptoms are probably familiar: you have to try to sleep when you feel wakeful and get up when you want to sleep. If you change shifts too frequently, your sleep rhythms cannot stabilise: at home you may continually suffer from sleep problems, and at work you may never feel fully awake.

SLEEP PHASES

The term *sleep phase* refers to the period of time that starts when you (or your child) become sleepy enough to fall asleep for the night and ends when you wake spontaneously in the morning after getting all the sleep you need. If, because you don't get enough sleep during the week, you are tired enough to fall asleep unusually early some nights or to sleep extra late in the morning, it may be difficult to determine your sleep requirement and your sleep phase exactly; they will be easier to determine when you are on holiday. However, it is usually easy to make a very good estimate of how much daily sleep children need and what times of the day and night they are capable of getting it (see Chapters 1 and 2).

If you want to get a real sense of how your sleep phase affects you and the way you feel, stay up all night reading a book. The evening will probably go by without trouble. However, after a while you will begin to feel sleepy. This point of 'sleep readiness' often comes on quite suddenly. Now your eyes no longer stay open of their own accord – in fact, it becomes a struggle to keep them open and focused – and it becomes difficult to pay attention to your reading. You may feel cold and want to get under a blanket. If you gave in and allowed your eyes to close, you would probably be asleep within a minute or two. These signs mean that you have passed from your wake phase into your sleep phase, or (using different terms that mean the same thing) from your *wake zone* into your *sleep zone*. Now it's easier to fall asleep than to stay awake.

If you fight off the sleepiness, you may find that after half an hour or so you briefly feel more awake; but soon the sleepiness

returns again, even more powerfully. This alternation between periods of (relatively) heightened and lessened alertness, known as the
'basic rest-activity cycle', continues all night and through the day as
well, but the overall tendency is to grow sleepier during the night
and to become more alert towards morning. If you stay awake until
perhaps 4.00 a.m., you will probably feel terrible. All your body
rhythms are set for sleep. Your temperature and steroid levels are
low, you may be a little nauseated and the thought of staying awake
for the entire upcoming day is awful. But if you manage to remain
awake a few hours more, until the point in the morning at which
you would ordinarily wake up spontaneously – the end of your
sleep phase and the start of your wake phase – you will notice a surprising improvement: all your body rhythms are switching back to
'wake'. (Hunger is a good sign that you have reached this point.)
After a shower and some breakfast, you probably won't feel all that
bad, even though you have had no sleep at all.

What you're experiencing is the effect of your circadian system.
Your body moves into 'wake' mode whether you have slept or not.
If you are like most people, you can tolerate a single sleepless night
without great impairment. In fact, you probably won't go to sleep
much earlier than usual the next night (that is, your sleep phase will
not shift earlier to compensate for the lost sleep), and that night you
probably won't sleep much more than usual.

The key point to remember is that it is hard to sleep in your
wake phase and hard to stay awake in your sleep phase. This idea
will be important in Chapter 10, when we start to discuss sleep
schedule problems.

THE CIRCADIAN SYSTEM AND THE FORBIDDEN ZONE FOR SLEEP: WHY YOU CAN STAY AWAKE UNTIL BEDTIME – AND SLEEP UNTIL MORNING

If you were to graph your level of alertness while you stayed up all
night, the result would be a rough U-shaped curve: you get progressively sleepier, then start to feel more awake towards morning. On a
normal night when you're sleeping, the pattern is a little different:

there is a 'bump' of lightened sleep and (potentially) increased alertness in the middle of the night (see Figure 9 on page 203). That's why it's often easier to get up to use the toilet at 3.00 a.m. than it is an hour after falling asleep or an hour before your usual wake-up time.

The pattern of alertness during the daytime is similar. Rather than following a simple inverted U curve, or even just declining from morning to night, alertness during the day follows roughly a mirror image of the night-time pattern, with a 'dip' in the middle of the day corresponding to the night-time 'bump': you do become fully alert soon after waking, and you do get progressively sleepier as the day goes on, but you go through a stretch of especially low alertness in the mid-afternoon (again see Figure 9). Children on a one-nap schedule take their nap at this point or become cranky. Adults can nap for an hour or so at this point, too, if they let themselves (as is routine in siesta cultures); if not, they will still probably take a relaxing break from whatever work they are doing. Even if you don't nap, you'll begin to feel more alert as you move past this midday dip, and you will soon be wide awake again. (If you usually stay up relatively late at night, the dip may not actually hit until after dinner.)

In the evening, during the few hours before the start of your sleep phase, you enter the *forbidden zone for sleep,* an especially interesting period in which sleep is nearly impossible. If you tested your ability to nap at various times of the day, you would find it the most difficult to fall asleep during these evening hours: on the contrary, at those times you feel more awake, alert and focused than ever. The same applies to your child. In fact, awareness of the forbidden zone turns out to be critical for understanding and treating certain common sleep problems in children.

All parents see the effects of the forbidden zone on children, though they may not understand what they are seeing. When your child seems sleepy in the afternoon or around dinner-time but gets a surprising second wind just when you want to send her to bed, it might seem strange. This is the forbidden zone at work: the longest period of sustained wakefulness occurs at the end of the day, not in the morning – that is, *before,* not after, the longest period of sleep. That is why your child seems so energetic all of a sudden, ready for fun or just about anything except going to bed. Even in a four-month-old who naps three times a day, the evening nap is the shortest and will be the next one to be dropped altogether.

Why is this so? Don't we get sleepier the longer we stay awake and less able to stay asleep the longer we do sleep? We do, in part, and this effect is caused by the so-called *homeostatic drive,* one of the two main factors influencing sleepiness and alertness. If that were the only cause of sleepiness, we would get progressively sleepier across the day, and the drive to sleep would decrease progressively while we sleep at night. We would have trouble staying awake until dinner-time and difficulty staying asleep until morning. Since we exhibit neither of these patterns – and, in fact, we can function reasonably well during the day after getting no sleep at all the night before – there must be other causes of increasing and decreasing sleepiness across the day and night.

The other major influence is the *circadian drive,* a direct effect of the biological clock. The circadian system works in opposition to the homeostatic drive, trying to make us more wakeful as the day progresses and sleepier as the night goes on. The balance between the two enables us to function at fairly consistent levels all day and sleep fairly well all night (see Figure 9). However, near the end of the day the wakeful component of the circadian system temporarily dominates, causing the forbidden zone or second wind. (As we saw before, the circadian drive is so strong that it can overcome the homeostatic drive and keep you alert during the day even after a full night without any sleep.) At the start of the sleep phase, the circadian system switches to 'sleep' mode; now that both systems are working in concert, pushing us towards sleep, it becomes hard to stay awake.

Other factors also affect sleepiness and alertness. Age and developmental level, more than anything else, determine one's night-time sleep requirement and the number of consecutive hours one can remain awake. (That is why an infant needs several naps during the day, while an older child or adult needs fewer or none.) Losing sleep

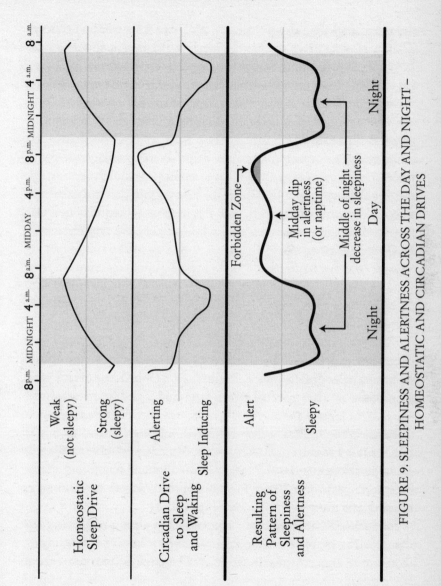

FIGURE 9. SLEEPINESS AND ALERTNESS ACROSS THE DAY AND NIGHT – HOMEOSTATIC AND CIRCADIAN DRIVES

night after night builds up a 'sleep debt', which essentially enhances the homeostatic drive so that the level of alertness is lowered over the whole day. Napping during the day does the opposite, removing some of the drive to sleep. That allows young children to make it through the day, but it also makes it easier to stay up late and more difficult to fall asleep at night, especially for older children and adolescents. Medication can increase the drive to sleep (sedatives and antihistamines, for example) or the drive to stay awake (coffee and other stimulants). Illness can have similar effects: fever usually makes you sleepy; pain usually keeps you awake. Psychological and cognitive factors affect sleep, too: depression sometimes increases sleepiness, especially in children, while anxiety can interfere with the ability to fall asleep.

SETTING THE BIOLOGICAL CLOCK: HOW DO YOU KNOW WHAT TIME ZONE YOU ARE IN?

Recall that exposure to light sets your biological clock and adjusts the timing of your sleep phase. Bright light near bedtime delays your sleep phase, so that you fall asleep later and wake (spontaneously) later. Bright light in the morning has the opposite effect, causing you to wake earlier and fall asleep earlier. If you are exposed to bright light within your sleep phase – that is, after you would usually fall asleep or before you would usually wake spontaneously – its effects are especially strong. (Exactly what happens depends on the timing, intensity and duration of the light exposure.)

For example, suppose your current sleep phase runs from 9.00 p.m. to 6.00 a.m. Now imagine that you begin staying up until midnight every night, sitting in front of a bank of bright lights from 9.00 onwards. Also imagine that you put on a blindfold when you go to bed and wear it until 9.00 in the morning. You are now getting three extra hours of light at night and three extra hours of darkness in the morning. Over the next several days, your sleep phase will *delay* – move later – by those same three hours. Soon you will be unable to fall asleep until midnight, and you will not wake spontaneously until 9.00 a.m. In effect, that is precisely what happens when you travel from London to Rio de Janeiro, cross three time zones and get exposed to evening and morning light three hours later than you're used to.

Now consider the opposite experiment: this time you wear the blindfold from 6.00 to 9.00 in the evening, and get up at 3.00 in the morning to sit in front of bright lights for three hours. Now the night-time darkness starts three hours earlier than you're used to, and so does the light in the early morning. Within a few days, your sleep phase will *advance* – move earlier – by those three hours. Soon you will be falling asleep at 6.00 p.m. and waking at 3.00 a.m. This type of change, of course, is what happens when you travel from Rio de Janeiro to London.

Actually, your biological clock normally undergoes small adjustments of this kind every day. As we saw earlier in this chapter, our circadian clocks naturally run slow: left alone, they will run on a cycle about ten minutes longer than a true twenty-four hours; in practice the cycle is closer to twenty-five hours, probably because we are regularly exposed to electric lights after the sun goes down – not as bright as sunlight, but still bright enough to have an effect – and not exposed to light while we sleep (indoors) in the morning. The result is that we have a tendency to go to sleep and wake up almost an hour later every day. In fact, many of us do just that at weekends and while on holiday. Come Sunday night or the end of a holiday, it's difficult to go to sleep at our usual weekday time, and the next morning it's harder than ever to get up for work or school.

So why doesn't our sleep schedule constantly drift later and later? It's because most days, like it or not, we *have* to get up at the same early time, and when we do, we are exposed to light. That morning light pushes our schedule earlier, usually enough, or almost enough, to counteract the drifting tendency. It keeps us running in place. But when we're free to sleep late every day (as a toddler may be), or even just at weekends and on holiday, we do start to drift. As we will see later in the book, this drifting is behind one of the most commonly seen sleep problems.

Individual Differences:
Are You a Lark or an Owl?

In any discussion of sleep schedules, it's important to take individual factors into account. The forbidden zone seems very powerful for some, less so for others. This difference may be explicable in part by the traits of morning and evening preference, which divide people into the types known as 'larks' and 'owls'.

Owls are people who get energized at night. Their second wind is strong, and the late night is often the most pleasant time of their whole day. Owls feel most alert at that time; they can think clearly, study effectively and play well. Staying up late is easy for them. But owls have a problem in the morning: waking up and starting the day, even after a full night's sleep, is painful and difficult, like climbing out of a deep hole. Owls don't like to get up, and they avoid early-morning activities whenever they can. It's easy for an owl to become phase-delayed (as discussed in Chapter 10).

For larks, the second wind is less forceful. As night falls, larks feel as if they are sliding into the same deep hole that owls wake up from each morning. Finding it unpleasant to stay up late, larks may pass up evening activities or leave them early. But they wake up without any trouble early in the morning, usually feeling great. They want to get right up and start doing things. For larks, morning is the best time of the day and evening is the worst. They are less likely than owls to develop a phase delay; on the contrary, their sleep phase may be earlier – more advanced – than they (or their parents) desire (see Chapter 10).

People do not necessarily fall entirely into either of these categories, but most have a tendency in one direction or the other, and in many the preference is quite strong. Although this is an innate preference that does not change over time and cannot be taught, owls can follow an early schedule, and larks a late one, if circumstances demand it – albeit probably not happily. In fact, larks and owls show genuine biological differences; for example, in owls, body temperature reaches its lowest point of the night nearer the time of morning waking than it does in larks. A specific gene has even been associated with the lark trait.

'Larkness' and 'owlness' exist as traits even in young children. A toddler who is an owl is especially energetic at night. She wants to be part of anything going on anywhere. She can stay up later than usual without difficulty. If her bedtime isn't pleasant, or if its timing is not enforced regularly, the entire process of going to bed may deteriorate and her schedule may become delayed or grow variable and unpredictable. The one problem she is unlikely to have is that of early wakings.

A toddler who is a lark, on the other hand, will probably like going to sleep early. If for some reason you don't put her to bed on time, she may grab her teddy bear and go to sleep on her own at bedtime, wherever she happens to be and regardless of anything going on around her. Bedtime for such a child is unlikely to be a problem, but she may be wide awake and ready to go at five o'clock in the morning.

Society, Sleep Deprivation and the Adolescent

We live in a sleep-deprived and phase-delayed culture. From adolescence until retirement, few people get enough sleep. How many of us wake up in the morning because we've slept enough? How many of us can get up on time without an alarm or someone waking us? How many people would not sleep later if they could? How many don't sleep later at weekends and on holiday than they do on workdays or school days?

The reasons for our cultural sleep deprivation are complex, and there are no easy solutions. First of all, we are exposed to light for several hours between sunset and bedtime. Morning sunlight works to keep us from drifting, but it can't always completely cancel out the effect of all that artificial light we get at night. If we are also chronically sleep deprived, though – if we stay up too late and always get up earlier than we would like – the combination of

morning light and sleep deprivation can be just enough to counteract the phase-delaying effect of the evening light. This pattern is
usually not seen before adolescence, since that is when youngsters
first gain the freedom and ability to stay up late.

Second, the electronic world continues nonstop, day and night.
The days are long gone when the only thing on television from late
evening until morning was a test pattern. Programmes aimed at adolescents and young adults continue until the early morning hours.
Teenagers give up sleep for the programmes they enjoy. (Younger
children will also give up sleep for television, but more often at the
other end of the night, getting up early to watch cartoons.)
The Internet is always on, video games are always available and the
telephone always works. Nowadays all of these activities are acces-
sible no matter where you live; in many places restaurants, pubs,
cinemas and arcades stay open very late as well.

Third, sleep is not a high priority for most people: when faced
with a choice between sleep and another activity, most will choose
the other activity. It is ingrained in our culture that you should be
able to get by on little sleep most of the time and catch up occasionally. It's a rare adolescent who willingly leaves her friends at nine -
o'clock to go home and sleep. (Not many adults do, either.)
Conscientious adolescents may feel that it is more important to finish their homework than to go to sleep early, and most of their parents and teachers would agree.

People wrongly believe that even when they are tired their abilities to work, learn and drive are unimpaired. Study after study
has shown otherwise; yet, though most people understand that it
is unsafe to drink and drive, few realise that driving under the influence of sleep deprivation can be just as dangerous. (When is the
last time you handed over your car keys because you got only six
hours' sleep the night before?) The news is full of stories about
teenagers whose lives were lost when they fell asleep at the wheel
and drifted into oncoming traffic or continued straight when the
road curved. More teenagers die in car accidents than from any
other cause. In the United States, more than 100,000 car accidents
and 1,500 deaths each year occur because of drowsy driving, and

most single-vehicle accidents not caused by alcohol are due to lack of sleep. The drivers in about half of these accidents are teenage boys or young men. Furthermore, the effects of alcohol and sleep deprivation are cumulative: just one beer can have a devastating effect on a seventeen-year-old who has slept only five hours.

Adolescence in our culture is a recipe for sleep-schedule problems and sleep deprivation. Even without taking cultural factors into account, adolescents' night-time sleep is shallower and less restorative than the sleep of younger children, and the ability to nap during the day comes back. Thus, even under the best of conditions, a teenager is sleepier in the daytime than she was as a child. At the same time, she is better able to fight off sleep and stay up late. She also develops the ability to 'oversleep', that is, to sleep longer at one stretch than she really needs, or at least to repeatedly return to sleep until the late morning or into the afternoon. (Preteens generally get the amount of sleep they need and then get up.) Finally, some evidence suggests that adolescents have an *inherent* sleep-phase delay: they naturally fall asleep and wake later in the day, relative to light exposure, than younger children do.

Compounding the problem, in most places secondary school starts earlier than primary school. In some areas, students who take the bus have to get up as early as 5.30 a.m. To get the usual requirement of nine hours' sleep, they would have to be asleep by 8.30 p.m. I find it is pointless even to suggest that idea to most sixteen-year-olds.

In short, adolescents often stay up late and get up early during the week, and they become chronically sleep deprived over time. On Fridays and Saturdays they stay up later than on weeknights, and they sleep late the next morning to make up some of their previously lost sleep. That increases the phase delay, so during the next week they fall asleep even later, get less sleep and have more difficulty getting up in the morning for school than before. Because they are now further behind in their sleep, they sleep still later at the next weekend. As the cycle continues, the discrepancies between weeknights and weekends become more and more pronounced. A teenager may be falling asleep at 1.00 a.m. during the week and getting up at 6.00 a.m. for school after five hours of sleep or less, while at weekends she may sleep from 2.00 or 3.00 a.m. until mid-day or later, getting ten to fourteen hours of sleep. The amount of sleep teenagers get can easily double at the weekend, and they may get up more than six hours later then than during the week.

When a youngster's natural wake-up time is midday, as may be the case if she sleeps until then at the weekend, then not only does she go to school badly sleep deprived, but most of her class time falls at hours when her body's physiological functions are still set for sleep. Her ability to pay attention, learn, think and retain infor-mation is severely compromised. Since a teenager who has to be awake by six in the morning is hard-pressed to get enough sleep at night, at least in our culture, a reasonable remedy would appear to be starting the high school day later; and, at this writing, initial re-sults of research being conducted to test that hypothesis suggests such changes are beneficial. But although a later starting time is almost certainly a good idea, at best it will only help partially. It won't change the underlying problems.

I see no easy way to combat all the social forces that make sleep deprivation so common in adolescents. Education can help: we must recognise the importance of sleep and be willing to arrange our schedules to allow for it. It may not be possible to keep a teenaged child on a perfect schedule, but by helping her to understand the im-pact her schedule has on her sleep and on her daytime performance, we may be able to minimise the problems. I've worked success-fully with many teenagers using that approach. When a teenager is receptive – not all of them are – we can help her to cut down the weeknight-to-weekend sleep differential, to fall asleep earlier on school days, and in general to feel better, function better and be hap-pier during the week.

These days our culture prizes physical fitness and health, and much energy is devoted to diet and exercise (even when it means getting up early and sacrificing sleep to go running). If we valued proper sleep as an equally important component of well-being, we would be moving in the right direction.

SPECIFIC SLEEP PROBLEMS AFFECTING
DIFFERENT PARTS OF THE SLEEP CYCLE:
A SUMMARY

When we refer to a 'sleep schedule problem', we may mean either a specific symptom (such as early-morning wakings) or the responsible underlying physiological problem (such as a sleep phase shift). In the three chapters that follow, we will look at the various types of schedule problem in detail. But keep in mind that problems discussed elsewhere in this book also may primarily affect specific parts of the sleep cycle. Therefore, before we begin, it may be useful to first see an overview of the main causes of all common sleep problems that affect the various parts of the sleep cycle, with reference to the chapters where each problem is discussed.

FIGURE 10. COMMON CAUSES OF SLEEP PROBLEMS
AT DIFFERENT TIMES OF THE DAY AND NIGHT

Bedtime Difficulties

1. Inappropriate sleep-onset associations (Chapter 4)

2. Limit-setting problems (Chapter 5)

3. Anxiety (Chapter 7)

4. Colic (Chapter 8)

5. Late sleep phase (Chapter 10)

6. Time in bed is too long (Chapter 11)

7. Short sleep requirement (Chapter 11)

8. Last nap is too late (Chapter 12)

9. Excessive napping (leading to short night-time sleep) (Chapters 11, 12)

10. Irregular sleep-wake schedule (Chapter 11)

11. Evening noise and activity (Chapter 11)

12. Evening television (causing children to give up sleep) (Chapters 5, 11)

Night-time Wakings

1. Inappropriate sleep-onset associations (Chapter 4)

2. Excessive night-time feeding (Chapter 6)

3. Limit-setting problems (Chapter 5)

4. Anxiety (Chapter 7)

5. Medical disorders (Chapters 8, 17)

6. Sleep terrors, confusional arousals, sleepwalking, nightmares and bed-wetting (Chapters 13, 14, 15)

7. Time in bed is too long (Chapter 11)

8. Short sleep requirement (Chapter 11)

9. Excessive or too frequent napping (leading to short or fragmented night-time sleep) (Chapters 11, 12)

10. Irregular sleep-wake schedule (Chapter 11)

11. Night-time noise and activity (Chapter 11)

12. Night-time television (Chapters 5, 11)

Early Wakings

1. Early sleep phase (Chapter 10)

2. Time in bed is too long (Chapter 11)

3. Early feedings (leading to early hunger) (Chapters 6, 10)

4. Early-morning nap (interfering with the last stretch of night-time sleep) (Chapters 10, 12)

5. Excessive napping (leading to short night-time sleep) (Chapter 12)

6. Irregular sleep-wake schedule (Chapter 11)

7. Short sleep requirement (Chapter 11)

8. Morning light, noise, activity (Chapter 11)

9. Morning television (causing children to give up sleep) (Chapter 11)

Difficulty Napping

1. Too much sleep at night (Chapter 12)

2. Short sleep requirement (Chapter 11)

3. Too many naps or 'naplets' (Chapter 12)

4. Drifting/splitting naps (Chapter 12)

5. Interrupted naps (noise and stimulation) (Chapter 12)

6. Inappropriate sleep-onset associations (Chapter 4)

CHAPTER 10

Schedule Disorders I:
Sleep Phase Problems

Now that you understand how sleep rhythms are regulated (see Chapters 2 and 9), we can discuss how schedule factors cause or complicate sleep problems, and we can develop strategies to correct them. As you will see, many of the problems caused by improper schedules are closely related to each other and they can be dealt with by similar strategies.

SLEEP PHASES

Why Understanding Sleep Phases Is Important

By now you know that your child's ability to fall asleep or stay awake varies over the course of the day and night. If you try to put your child to bed during a waking phase, he may seem unwilling to go to sleep, when the truth is he is simply not sleepy. Likewise, if you try to wake him up during a sleep phase, he may seem unwilling or almost unable to get up, when in fact his body is not ready to be awake.

These scheduling issues affect all of us, not just children. Suppose you usually fall asleep easily at 11.30 p.m. and wake fully rested, without an alarm, at 7.30 a.m. – in other words, that your sleep phase runs from 11.30 p.m. to 7.30 a.m. Now consider what will happen if you try to change your schedule:

- *If you go to bed early,* before the start of your sleep phase – say, at 8.00 p.m. – you will have difficulty falling asleep. Even if you doze, you will certainly not sleep through the night.
- *If you try to wake early* – say, at 4.00 a.m. – you will have great difficulty getting out of bed. You'll be very sleepy, and you may feel terrible for several hours, but by 7.30 (when you're used to waking up) you will start to feel ready to face the day.
- *If you go to bed late,* after your sleep phase begins – say, at 2.00 a.m. – you will fall asleep easily, but you will wake up close to your normal waking time. You will get less sleep than usual, and you may feel tired during the day.
- *If you try to sleep late,* into your waking phase – say, until 10.00 a.m. – you will probably find it impossible. At best, you will doze on and off for the last few hours.

Children have similar difficulties if they try to go to sleep or get up at times that do not coincide with the beginning and end of their sleep phase. If your child's sleep phase does not occur when you want it to, or (for an older child) when *he* wants it to, then he will tend to fall asleep and wake up too early or too late.

Although the amount of sleep a child needs is determined by his individual biology, the specific times *when* he sleeps can change to a large extent according to personal preference and social necessity. Some families prefer early schedules, while others prefer later ones. You need only decide where the sleep phase should fall and take the proper steps to move it there. But just as you can't travel between two time zones every couple of days and expect to keep adjusting, you can't change sleep phases from day to day.

In particular, you cannot have one phase for weekdays and another for the weekends.

If you are comfortable with one end of your child's sleep phase but not the other, then it probably won't help to move the sleep phase as a whole. For example, if your child falls asleep at the hour you want but wakes too early, then moving his sleep phase to allow him to sleep later may also cause him to stay awake too late at night. Issues like this one are discussed in the next chapter.

How to Identify Your Child's Sleep Phase

Before making any decisions about your child's sleep, you need to know where in the twenty-four-hour day his sleep phase falls. If you do not know when he is capable of sleeping, you cannot establish reasonable rules or make reasonable changes.

Usually, the start of a child's sleep phase is simply the time at which he falls asleep most nights. That means when he actually falls asleep, not when you *want* him to go to sleep or when you put him to bed. This time is fairly consistent for most children. If your child's 8.00 p.m. bedtime is always followed by two hours of struggling, calling for you and coming out of his room until he finally falls asleep at 10.00, or even if he just lies awake in bed until then, then 10.00 is probably the start of his sleep phase. Conversely, if he falls asleep on the sofa every night at 7.30, half an hour before his bedtime, or if you have to fight to keep him awake after that point, then you know that 7.30 is probably the start of his sleep phase.

There are other clues to look for. Suppose your child always resists his 8.00 bedtime and struggles for two hours until usually falling asleep at 10.00. If you are out late with him one evening and don't get to put him to bed until 9.30, he may struggle as before, but now for only for thirty minutes, and he still falls asleep around 10.00 as usual. If you put him to bed at 10.00, he falls asleep quickly without much struggle at all, and if you're out later than that, he falls asleep on the way home. Now you can be sure that 10.00 is the start of his sleep phase.

Children can keep themselves up past the start of their sleep phase if they need something. Suppose your child falls asleep at 10.00, which is also when you go to bed. Is 10.00 really the earliest he can fall asleep, or is he waiting for you? You can easily find out. If he falls asleep by 8.30 whenever you go to bed (or stay with him or take him into your bed) at 8.00, then his sleep phase starts no later than 8.30. But if he still stays up playing, talking and laughing until 10.00, then 10.00 really is the start.

Even if your child falls asleep at times that vary from night to night, you can probably identify an hour by which he is almost always asleep. Then you know he is *able* to fall asleep by that time, at least; in other words, his sleep phase starts at or before that time, certainly no later. The important thing is that you have identified a time when you know he is capable of sleep.

Now you need to locate the end of the sleep phase. If your child always wakes for the day spontaneously at 7.00 a.m., then that is probably the end of his sleep phase. But if you have to wake him every morning at 7.00, and especially if that is difficult to do, then you know that at seven he isn't yet ready to wake up 'naturally'. At what time does he wake on days when you don't get him up? That should be the end of his sleep phase.

Here, too, there are more clues. If your child always wakes at 7.00, comes to your bed and goes back to sleep there until 8.00, then 8.00, not 7.00, is the end of his sleep phase. If that happens sometimes but not consistently, then you at least know that his sleep phase can end no earlier than 7.00. The exact time will become clearer as you work to correct his sleep schedule.

Similarly, suppose you regularly wake your eight-year-old for school, with difficulty, at 7.00 a.m. You're expecting that at the weekend you'll be able to see how much later he sleeps when left alone – but on Saturday morning, he wakes *by himself* at 7.00. How his sleeping brain 'knows' it is the weekend is uncertain, but for the purpose of identifying his sleep phase, it makes no difference. You need to look at what he does after he gets up. If he slinks into a dark den, turns on cartoons and curls up under a blanket until 8.00, when, finally looking 'human' and no longer like a zombie, he throws off the blanket and announces that he wants breakfast, then his sleep phase ends at 8.00, not 7.00. He would sleep until 8.00 if there were no cartoons.

Weekends, Holidays and Naps

You've seen the importance of observing your child's weekend schedule (above and in Chapter 9). It's equally important to learn about his holiday schedules and naps. This information will help you to identify his sleep phase and give you a better idea of his sleep requirement. Once you know when he can sleep, when he actually does sleep and how much sleep he needs, you can determine how short of sleep he is on weeknights and how much make-up sleep he gets at weekends. You need to have this information before you can decide what the causes are of his poor sleep and what changes you need to make in his schedule to correct them.

When you note your child's weekend and holiday schedules, always be sure to distinguish between times where the wakings are spontaneous (where he gets all the sleep he wants) and those where he is wakened early, thanks to you, a sibling or an alarm, for example. On holiday he shouldn't have any lost sleep to make up, as he might at the weekend, so if he wakes spontaneously every morning, then you can accurately estimate the amount of sleep he needs each night to function normally during the day.

If your child still takes naps, note when they occur, how long they last and whether or not he wakes on his own. Include all of his daytime sleep, including in the car or pram or by the television, not just formal naps. Parents often tell me their child 'never naps', without mentioning that he falls asleep two or three times a day in the car on errands.

Naps can follow regular patterns or vary widely. A three-year-old may nap at day care but never at home. He may nap at 1.00 p.m. at day care but skip that nap at home, instead falling asleep at 4.00 on the sofa or in the car. If the timing and length of your child's naps show a lot of variation, you may find it helpful to chart them (see the next section, below).

Finally, add up the number of hours of sleep your child usually gets at night, during the day and over a full twenty-four hours. If he sleeps a different amount or at different times at weekends and on holiday, calculate them separately.

Charting Sleep Patterns

It's a good idea to keep track of your child's sleep patterns. You can use the chart in Figure 5 on page 77. If your child's night-time sleep habits or daytime naps are irregular, it may be difficult to tell what is happening without a chart. Once you have a record on paper, you may notice, for instance, that he always falls asleep late on nights that follow late-morning wakings – perhaps every Saturday and Sunday. Or you may see that he always has trouble at bedtime if he napped after 4.00 p.m. Also, parents tend to remember the worst nights and forget about the better ones, especially if they are sleep-deprived themselves, so even if you're not aware of any great irregularity in your child's schedule, what the chart reveals may surprise you.

When plotting your child's 'awake' times, count only those times you are certain he is really awake. If he calls to you repeatedly between 1.00 and 3.00 a.m. but there are stretches of thirty or forty-five minutes in between when you don't hear him, don't assume he was awake for two solid hours (even though it probably feels that way to you).

Finally, it is particularly important to chart sleep patterns while you are working to change them. Only with this record can you look back and actually see the improvements.

SLEEP PHASE SHIFTS

It's important to recognise that there is no such thing as an in-herently unhealthy or 'bad' sleep phase: the hours we sleep are determined by preference or by scheduling requirements, not by biological necessity. So when we talk about an 'early' or 'late' sleep phase, we really mean early or late enough to be inconvenient or disruptive.

Early (Advanced) Sleep Phase

Your child is said to have an early sleep phase if he naturally falls asleep and wakes at earlier hours than you (or he) would like (see Figure 11 on page 223). That is most likely to happen if he is inherently a lark.

Victoria was a nine-month-old girl with this problem. Her parents wanted her to sleep for ten hours a night, from 8.30 p.m. to 6.30 a.m. Victoria did get ten hours of night-time sleep, but she got them between 7.00 p.m. and 5.00 a.m. Her parents were particularly unhappy about the early-morning wakings. On several occasions they kept Victoria up until 8.30 p.m., with great difficulty; she woke at 5.00 a.m. anyway, unhappy from loss of sleep. Her parents saw no point in continuing that approach.

Victoria obviously had an early sleep phase, but her parents' attempts to change it by moving only her bedtime had not worked. We needed to look at the rest of her schedule. Since she woke at 5.00 every morning, her parents were feeding her at that time. They gave her lunch at 11.00 and supper at 4.30 p.m. She napped for an hour at 8.00 a.m. and again at midday, after lunch. In short, her entire schedule was shifted too early, not just her wake-up time. If *everything* in her daily routine could be moved one or two hours later, the problem would go away. That was what we had to do.

If we had kept trying to move Victoria's night-time sleep later without adjusting the rest of her schedule, we would have faced a couple of potential problems. First of all, because she was being fed at 5.00 a.m. – not unreasonably, given when she was falling asleep – she had learned to be hungry then. If we only made her bedtime later, she might still wake at 5.00, no longer because she was done sleeping but because she was hungry. So we needed to help her learn not to get hungry until later. Second, her early-morning nap was a possible trouble spot: if we didn't adjust it along with her bedtime, it could start to function as her last sleep cycle of the night, broken off from the rest of the night by a short period of undesirably early wakefulness. We needed to move that nap later so that it would stay separated from Victoria's night-time sleep and allow her to begin sleeping later in the morning.

I explained to Victoria's parents that moving her bedtime later for one night would not re-set her biological clock, which was the main reason she woke up at 5.00 even when they had kept her up late the previous night. The schedule shift required gradual and consistent changes. I asked Victoria's parents to shift all the parts of her schedule that they could control – her first feeding in the morning, lunch and supper times, nap times and bedtime – moving them fifteen minutes later every day. They could then expect that her morning wakings would gradually move later as well.

This strategy worked effectively. After six days, Victoria's schedule had been pushed later an hour and a half: now she was sleeping from 8.30 p.m. to 6.30 a.m., as her parents desired. She napped now at 10.00 a.m. and 2.00 p.m., and she ate her meals at 7.00 a.m., midday, and 6.00 p.m.

Changing a child's entire schedule is not always necessary. For example, if his sleep phase is too early for you, but his feedings and naps do not fall especially early, then you can gradually adjust his bedtime alone. Regardless, if your child is still at the age of napping, he should keep doing so, but don't let his naps last longer than they did before: as you move his bedtime later, you want him to make up the lost sleep at the end of the night, not in the daytime.

If, despite a later schedule, you are still having trouble getting him to sleep late enough, keep moving his bedtime even later, a little at a time – while being sure you don't let him extend his naps or have an early-morning nap or feeding. His bedtime may have to be temporarily moved later than you want in order to force his wake-up time later to the desired hour, but at some point it will happen. Once it does, you can begin to gradually move his bedtime earlier again, as long as he continues to wake up when you want.

It may help to provide your child with lots of light in the

evening, and to keep his room dark in the morning until the time when you want him to wake. Blackout shades and curtains can be useful. Children whose rooms let in bright sunlight early every morning may simply be unable to move their sleep phase later until this light is blocked.

Late (Delayed) Sleep Phase

Your child is said to have a late sleep phase if he naturally falls asleep and wakes later than you (or he) would like (see Figure 11 on page 223). That is most likely to happen if your child is inherently an owl. But, as explained in Chapter 9, all of our sleep phases tend to drift later due to certain biological drives and exposure to artificial light at night. As a result, a late sleep phase is one of the most common sleep problems to occur at any age.

If your child wakes on his own every morning at the desired hour but seems to have difficulty falling asleep on time, then he may simply not need as much sleep as you think (see 'The too-long-in-bed problem' in the next chapter). If he falls asleep easily at the desired bedtime but has difficulty waking in the morning, he may need *more* sleep than you think, and his bedtime may have to be moved earlier. But if both ends of his sleep phase are too late, so he has trouble falling asleep at the desired bedtime *and* then either has trouble waking in the morning or sleeps later than you would like, this section will help you.

A late sleep phase can occur alone or in combination with other sleep problems, so many different situations can arise. The examples that follow all share the basic features of a late sleep phase.

Adam was an eighteen-month-old who never went to sleep when his parents wanted to put him to bed, at 7.30 p.m. If they tried to rock him to sleep, he just squirmed and tried to get out of their grasp. They would try again every half hour or so without success, until finally, around 10.00 p.m., either he would let them rock him to sleep or he would fall asleep on his own on the living room floor; once he was asleep, they would move him to the cot. Once or twice a night he would cry and his parents would have to rock him for a

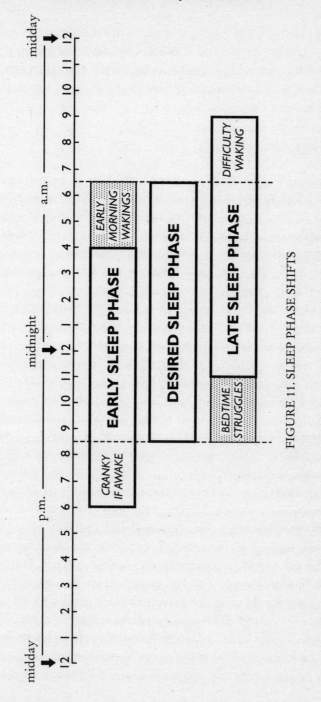

FIGURE 11. SLEEP PHASE SHIFTS

few minutes to get him back to sleep. Adam's mother got up at 6.30 every morning to take care of the other children, but because Adam always fell asleep so late his parents were reluctant to wake him that early. (In any case, whenever they had to get him up before he woke on his own at 8.00, he would wake in a miserable mood.) He ate breakfast soon after getting up at 8.00, he ate lunch at 1.00 p.m. and he took an hour-long nap at 3.00.

Mark, a six-year-old, always resisted his 8.00 p.m. bedtime, saying he wasn't tired. Bedtime was a struggle, and even the evenings were becoming more and more unpleasant. Mark made continual requests for stories, drinks, trips to the toilet and tuck-ins, and he often came out of his room complaining that he didn't feel well. His parents had been told that they needed to be firmer, so they threatened to take away daytime activities he liked and tried locking his door. These approaches only upset him further; sometimes he lay in bed sobbing, and, if anything, he would fall asleep even later than usual. Most nights he grew quiet at around 11.00 p.m., and his parents knew he would be asleep soon. But he had to get up for school at 7.00 a.m., and waking him was difficult: he cried and begged to continue sleeping. At weekends he was allowed to stay up until 9.00, and sometimes his parents were less strict than usual about making him stay in his room, but he still fell asleep around 11.00. On Saturday and Sunday mornings he woke on his own at 8.30, in good spirits.

Lindsey, nine, had no behaviour problems and did not complain about her 8.00 bedtime. But she would never fall asleep until about 10.30, no matter what her parents did, and it was difficult for them to wake her at 6.30 a.m. to catch the school bus. Once put to bed, Lindsey would come out of her room quietly every half hour or so and say she couldn't sleep. She was not frightened. Her mother would sit with her for a few minutes, rubbing her back, and then leave again; she occasionally gave Lindsey some warm milk, and she told her to 'practise thinking pleasant thoughts'.

Lindsey sometimes asked, 'What's wrong with me? Why can't I fall asleep?' She did not attend sleepovers because she was afraid she would remain awake long after everyone else had fallen asleep. The family doctor prescribed an antihistamine that did seem to help her fall asleep more quickly, but her parents did not want to medicate her every night. Eventually they began allowing her to read in bed, which she often did for hours. At weekends, they usually let her stay up until 10.00; she would then fall asleep much more easily than on weekdays, and she would wake on her own the next morning around 8.00.

Each of these children had a late sleep phase, although each also had different complicating factors.

Adam's sleep phase ran from 10.00 p.m. to 8.00 a.m.; his nap, at 3.00 p.m., was also late. His parents had inadvertently conditioned him to fall asleep while being rocked (which is why he needed to be rocked again when he woke during the night). It would be easy to break this association with a progressive-waiting programme, as described in Chapter 4, but if his parents started such a programme at the 7.30 p.m. bedtime they were hoping for, they would have to let him cry for two and a half hours before he would even be capable of sleeping. That would be not only unhelpful but cruel.

I told Adam's parents to set his bedtime at 10.00 – the usual time when he actually fell asleep – and then (only then) to work on eliminating the rocking. At the same time, they were to wake him fifteen minutes earlier each morning until he was getting up at 6.30 along with his mother and the other children. His nap was to move from 3.00 to 1.30, also in daily fifteen-minute increments. Once he was falling asleep quickly at 10.00 his parents could also begin moving his bedtime earlier, again in fifteen-minute increments, as long as he continued to fall asleep quickly and as long as he still had to be wakened in the morning. Soon he was sleeping from 8.30 p.m. to 6.30 a.m. and napping for an hour at 1.30 p.m. He was falling asleep on his own without being rocked, he was no longer waking during the night and he was waking on his own in the morning. Ten hours of sleep at night were plenty for a child his age, and his parents now understood that pushing his bedtime earlier to 7.30 p.m. was unrealistic.

Mark's nightly struggles would have suggested a limit-setting problem (see Chapter 5), except for the crucial fact that his parents had been trying to get him to fall asleep during his forbidden zone, when he could not sleep at all (see Chapter 9). Shutting him in his room at that time could not and did not help. Indeed, it only made matters worse by leaving everyone upset, tense and angry. Mark's sleep phase ran at least from 11.00 p.m. to 8.30 a.m. – nine and a half hours – but he was only getting eight hours of sleep on school nights.

Mark probably expected to dislike any suggestion I made to his parents, thinking it would be punitive. Instead, I told him that there was nothing wrong with him and that he was just going to bed too early. I said I thought he should stay up until 11.00, and I asked if that would be okay with him. A big grin slowly covered his face, although he tried to hold it back, and he looked nervously over at his parents (who, by the way, were not smiling). I asked him if he thought that with the 11.00 bedtime he could stay in his room quietly, and he said he could. We encouraged this co-operation with a sticker chart and a chance to earn small rewards (see Chapters 5 and 7). Mark's parents were initially less than thrilled at the idea of the late bedtime, but they consented when I pointed out that he was not falling asleep before 11.00 anyway and that the change was only temporary.

Mark's parents agreed to make themselves available to him in the evening. They would read him a bedtime story at 10:45 p.m. and say good night at 11.00. Mark was to be awake and out of bed (dressed and given breakfast, and, most importantly, exposed to light) at 7.00 every morning, weekends included, and at weekends he would not be allowed to watch television immediately after getting up. Because he would now be getting up regularly at 7.00, his parents soon could start moving his bedtime earlier again (probably within a few days, as long as he was falling asleep quickly).

This approach was a success from the first night on. The bedtime struggles vanished, and without them Mark found it hard to stay up until 11.00. Evenings became pleasant again. He earned his prizes without difficulty, and his self-esteem improved. His parents gradually moved his bedtime all the way back to 9.00, and his total sleep time increased to nine and a half to ten hours every night.

Unlike Adam and Mark, Lindsey presented no behaviour problems, but her nights were nevertheless unpleasant, and so was her feeling that there was something wrong with her, that she was 'different'. Her sleep phase ran at least from 10.30 p.m. until 8.00 a.m., nine and a half hours, and like Mark she was getting only eight hours of sleep on school nights. It was certainly better for her to read in bed than to lie awake in the dark for hours, but it did little for her sense of failure and it did not get her any more sleep.

I reassured Lindsey that she was completely normal and explained the delayed sleep phase problem to her and her family. I suggested that she should read in the living room in the evening if she wanted, but not for so long in bed. We moved her bedtime to 10.00 and allowed her to read in bed for half an hour; she was to turn the lights out by 10.30. Her parents would wake her at 6.30 every morning. Lindsey started falling asleep quickly, and we were able to begin moving her bedtime earlier. She ended up sleeping from 9.00 p.m. to 6.30 a.m. – a more realistic bedtime than her original one, 8.00, but still early enough to allow her a full nine and a half hours of sleep before she had to get up for school.

All of these children's sleep phase problems were taken care of without struggles or unnecessary limit-setting, threats, demands or medication. They were resolved simply by fixing their sleep schedules.

Treating a Late Sleep Phase

As the examples above show, the easiest way to treat a child's late sleep phase is first to put him on a schedule that matches the current setting of his sleep phase – that is, one that fits the current times he is falling asleep and waking up – then to move his bedtime a little earlier each day as you gradually advance his sleep phase by carefully controlling his wake-up time. The key points to remember are:

- Control evening and morning light
- Start with a late bedtime
- Adjust (and enforce) morning wake-up times, naps, and mealtimes
- Gradually move bedtime earlier

The following detailed guidelines should help you to plan your child's treatment.

1. Identify your child's current sleep phase, as described earlier in this chapter.

2. Set his bedtime initially at the start of his current sleep phase, or a little later. Allow your child to stay up until the time he normally falls asleep so that, when he does go to bed, he will fall asleep fairly easily. If you are not sure of the correct time, err on the late side. It's important to reaccustom your child to falling asleep quickly: that way bedtime will become pleasant rather than full of bickering, anxiety and frustration. If your child is old enough to understand what's going on, he will be relieved to learn that you are not angry with him, there is nothing wrong with him and the sleep problem was not his fault.

3. Avoid unnecessary bright light in the evening; ensure bright light in the morning.

4. What you do next will depend on whether or not your child sleeps as late as he wants on most days or usually has to be wakened.

   a. If he sleeps late every morning, you can either accept the late sleep phase (but now with a late bedtime as well as a late waking, assuming the late schedule isn't a problem for either of you), or gradually move his whole sleep phase earlier.

      If you want to move his sleep phase earlier, then once he is falling asleep quickly at his new (later) bedtime – which should happen within a day or two (if it isn't, you may have to temporarily move the bedtime even later) – begin to gradually shift his wake-up time earlier. Every day, wake him fifteen minutes earlier than you did the day before. Don't start advancing his bedtime quite yet – *you must begin with the morning wake-up time:* you cannot make a child fall asleep, but you can make him get up. Once his wake-up time has been moved up by thirty to sixty minutes, so that he is mildly sleep-deprived each night, you can then begin moving his bedtime fifteen minutes earlier each night as well. The slight loss of sleep that happens initially (because of the earlier wakings) will help ensure that he still falls asleep quickly at night. Once you have reached the desired morning wake-up time, you may be able to keep advancing his bedtime a little further until he is getting the same amount of sleep that he was getting before you started shifting his schedule.

b. If your child must be wakened on weekdays, such as for school or day care, then you must correct his sleep phase while keeping his wake-up time fixed.

Wake him at the same time *every* morning, including weekends and holidays. He should get up, get dressed and have breakfast, and he should be exposed to plenty of morning light. (Don't let him get up and immediately start watching television.) The early wakings, combined with the later-than-usual bedtime, will leave him mildly sleep-deprived, and he will soon be falling asleep quickly at night. Once that happens, begin advancing his bedtime by fifteen minutes a day. You can keep moving his bedtime earlier as long as he continues to fall asleep quickly. If he starts waking on his own at the correct time, then his sleep phase is now where you want it, and he is probably getting all (or almost all) the sleep he needs. About the only way you can push his bedtime much earlier than that is by continuing to move his wake-up time even earlier.

5. If your child regularly takes age-appropriate naps, keep letting him nap while you adjust his sleep phase, but don't let the naps run longer than usual. The sleep you are cutting out in the morning should be made up at the earlier bedtime; it should not be moved to the daytime.

6. If, like his sleep at night, your child's naps and meals are shifted later than they should be for the schedule you are trying to achieve, you may have to move them earlier as well. Advance them at the same rate at which you advance bedtime and waking.

7. You *must* start by setting your child's bedtime at least as late as the time he regularly falls asleep, even if that is later than you like or later than you yourself want to stay up, and you must be available to take part in your child's evening activities. It won't be long before his bedtime has moved to an hour that suits you better.

8. If your child has other sleep problems, such as limit-setting difficulties or inappropriate sleep associations, you can correct these problems either while you are working on his sleep schedule or separately. Regardless of your choice, address the other problems *only* if you are certain that your child is being asked to sleep at times you know he is capable of doing so. If you aren't yet sure where his sleep phase falls, you would do better to adjust his schedule first and tackle the other problems later.

How a Late Sleep Phase Develops

There are many ways for a child to develop a late sleep phase. In addition to the predisposing biological and environmental factors described in the preceding chapter, anything that interferes with falling asleep – illness, excitement, travel and fears are typical examples – can result in a sleep phase shift if the child sleeps later than usual the next morning. If he doesn't sleep later, the sleep phase will not shift. But if he does, and especially if he is allowed to continue sleeping later on the mornings that follow (as may happen in homes where everyone does not have to be up and out by a certain hour), a problem can develop. Even sleeping in just at weekends can be enough to persistently delay a child's sleep phase – in fact, that is the most common cause of late sleep phases in school-aged children.

Although late sleep phases are a frequent cause of problems, they are relatively easy to treat – at least until adolescence – because the schedules of young children are (or should be) entirely under their parents' control. However, once a child has entered adolescence, the situation becomes more complex (as described in the next section).

SLEEP PHASE SHIFTS IN THE ADOLESCENT

Early (Advanced) Sleep Phase in the Adolescent

Advanced sleep phases in adolescents are almost unheard of. As I explained at the end of the previous chapter, so many forces (biological, academic and social) push a teenager's sleep phase later that it is extremely rare to find an adolescent who consistently falls asleep too early and wakes well before he needs to get up for school. Adolescents who have strong lark tendencies may have earlier sleep phases than their peers – they may not like to stay up past 11.00 or sleep past 8.00, say – but even their sleep phases are likely to be late-shifted with respect to school hours. Still, these youngsters usually have an easier time than most because they get up for school closer to the end of their sleep phase and are consequently less sleep-deprived.

Late (Delayed) Sleep Phase in the Adolescent

Adolescents are particularly likely to have late sleep phases, and their sleep phases are more difficult to correct than those of younger children. Teenagers frequently stay up late on weekend nights and then sleep until midday or later, so their sleep cycles can shift profoundly (as discussed in 'Society, Sleep Deprivation and the Adolescent' in the preceding chapter). As a result, they are often severely sleep-deprived during the week, when they most need to be alert.

It is often very difficult for a parent to assume control over an adolescent's sleep cycle. A teenager may not be willing to maintain a regular sleep schedule even if he understands its importance. Pressure from friends is very strong in these years, and most adolescents love to stay up late watching television, playing on the computer, talking on the phone or listening to music. Finally, as we saw in the previous chapter, biological factors as well as social ones are working against him: he is now physically able to stay awake very late or even all night, and he probably has to get up earlier for school than he used to. Adolescents may also have an inherent tendency towards late-shifted sleep. All of these factors push teenagers to lose sleep during the week and to sleep later at the weekend, and thus these youngsters tend to develop progressively greater delays of the sleep phase.

Connor, a fifteen-year-old, had been having trouble falling asleep early and waking for school for many years, but over the summer before I saw him the situation had developed into a major problem. By the time school had started in the autumn, he was unable to fall asleep until 3.00 or even 4.00 a.m. on weeknights, even though he went to bed at 11.30 the night before. He would pass the time listening to the radio and occasionally he would get up for a snack.

Needless to say, he had great difficulty getting up for school in the morning at 6.30. His parents were becoming angry, and sometimes their attempts to wake him turned into battles. Despite these problems, Connor made it to school most days and usually just on time or a few minutes late. On weekend nights Connor often stayed up very late watching television, and he wouldn't even get into bed until 3.00 or 4.00 a.m. He would sleep through weekend mornings, staying in bed as late as 1.00 in the afternoon, and he did the same on days when he missed school.

Connor was an average student. Although he didn't particularly like school, he did want to attend and graduate. He was upset by the considerable trouble he had falling asleep at night, and he hated getting up in the morning feeling so tired after only three hours of sleep. He often fell asleep in his morning lessons, and even when he was able to stay awake he had a great deal of difficulty paying attention.

Connor was surprised and pleased when I told him that I knew what was wrong and that there was a solution to his problem. He found it reassuring that I sympathised with his difficulties and understood that he wasn't lazy, and he was particularly relieved when I confirmed that he truly *couldn't* fall asleep early (at least, not yet). The problem was that his sleep phase had shifted dramatically, much more so than the sleep phases of the younger children described earlier in this chapter: it was delayed by five or six hours, running from about 3.30 a.m. to 12.30 p.m.

Connor could have corrected his sleep phase by getting up early seven days a week and never napping, even in school, and I did offer this approach. This is the same technique we saw used successfully for the younger children, and the guidelines given above would have applied. But that approach is easiest to use when there is a shift of only one to three hours. For a six-hour shift like the one Connor needed to make, it will be much harder (think of flying from Chicago to London). In practice, teenagers like Connor – who are already having considerable difficulty getting up on time for school and who are already unable to stay awake during the school day – may find it very hard to follow a programme that temporarily cuts down even further on their nightly sleep. Until the shift was complete, Connor would be getting much less sleep than he needed, even on Friday and Saturday nights. He would be extremely tired, his motivation likely would flag and he might be unable to resist occasionally sleeping late, especially at the weekends, or falling asleep during the day, in or after school. If he lapsed in any of those ways, the treatment would not work.

So I also offered a different approach that is sometimes useful with extreme sleep phase delays, namely that he correct his sleep phase by going to bed *later* each night, until he had gone all the way round the clock to the times he wanted to be sleeping – say, from 11.00 p.m. to 6.30 a.m. After that it would be critical for him to keep getting up early every day, even if he stayed up late at weekends, in order to keep his sleep phase in place. (It would be easier for him to follow through with the plan, and therefore more likely for him to succeed, if he was allowed to stay up late some nights as long as he still got up by 6.30 on weekdays, no later than 7.30 at weekends.)

Regardless of which method he chose, Connor had to agree to assume control over his own bedtime and waking. In particular, he needed to take responsibility for getting up in the morning, like most adults. As things stood, his parents had the task of waking him each morning, while Connor was actually trying to go back to sleep. Instead of working together, he and his parents were working at cross-purposes, and this only led to fights. So Connor bought a clock radio and set it to a loud morning talk show; and, at the other end of the room, he put a backup alarm clock that would not stop ringing until he got up and turned it off.

Connor chose the second option, the one that would move his sleep phase round the clock: his plan was to go to sleep and get up three hours *later* each day according to the following programme:

Connor's Initial Sleep Schedule 3.30 a.m. to 12.30 p.m.

One week round-the-clock programme	Bedtime	Waking
Saturday	7.00 a.m.	3.00 p.m.
Sunday	10.00 a.m.	6.00 p.m.
Monday	1.00 p.m.	9.00 p.m.
Tuesday	4.00 p.m.	midnight
Wednesday	7.00 p.m.	3.00 a.m.
Thursday	10.00 p.m.	6.00 a.m.
Friday	11.00 p.m.	6.30 a.m.

Connor's Final Sleep Schedule 11.00 p.m. to 6.30 a.m.

The first day he would go to sleep at 7.00 a.m. and get up at 3.00 p.m. The next day, he would go to bed at 10.00 a.m. and get up at 6.00 p.m., and so on. After six or seven days he would arrive at the schedule he wanted, with all his sleep moved back into the night-time where it belonged. Oversleeping by an hour or two was acceptable for most of the transition period, since it would push his schedule later and speed up the process, but in the last couple of days he would have to be careful not to sleep past 6.30 a.m. He agreed to chart his sleep patterns so that he and I could follow his progress.

Most teenagers find this adjustment fairly easy to make; as they go through the transition they will be falling asleep quickly, getting enough sleep each night, and waking without difficulty. Hopefully, any unpleasant feelings they have come to associate with lying awake at bedtime will diminish. Besides, this programme follows the natural tendency of their circadian rhythms instead of fighting it. Within a week, they should be sleeping and waking at the desired times. From then on, if they keep their morning wakings under control (see 'Settling for Improvement in the Adolescent's Schedule' on page 236), their sleep patterns will remain regular and gradually grow more stable.

During the transition they may have to miss one or two days of school, but absences can be kept to a minimum by starting the programme in the early hours of a Saturday morning (as we did with Connor, overleaf). By Tuesday or Wednesday, they won't be going to sleep until after school. Once their sleep schedule is adjusted, their attendance should be better than it was before.

Certainly, if your teenager's sleep phase is late-shifted by less than four hours, it makes more sense to try the other approach first, moving an initially late bedtime earlier little by little while keeping the morning wake-up time consistently early seven days a week and avoiding naps. (Even with bigger phase delays, many youngsters choose this option since they already have to get up early five days a week.) This approach involves sleep loss and requires some self-discipline, so you cannot do it *for* a teenager. You can explain to him the whys and hows, but he must *want* to make the change, and he must be willing to get himself up each morning. If this approach is not successful, you can always fall back on the round-the-clock approach that shifts bedtime progressively later.

Other Ways to Shift the Clock

There are some other tools available to adolescents to try and counter the forces that push their sleep phases later. Exposure to bright light in the morning, as we have already seen, moves the setting of the biological clock earlier and with it the timing of the sleep phase. Having a teenager get up half an hour early every morning to sit in a brightly lit room, with his eyes open, will definitely help to advance his sleep phase, and this method is both safe and effective. (Exposure to bright morning sunlight is ideal, but in the winter adolescents often have to get up before there is much light outside. Ordinary room lighting will help, but not as much as a bank of bright fluorescent lights made especially for this purpose.) However, getting adolescents to give up that extra half hour of sleep every morning is usually not realistic. It makes sense nonetheless to get room lights on and shades up as soon as possible in the morning. Hiding from morning light will only worsen the problem.

Some people find it useful to take the hormone melatonin in the afternoon or evening. Melatonin levels are a marker of the setting of the biological clock, rising at night when the sleep phase starts and dropping in the morning when it ends. Melatonin does not induce sleep directly (at least not very strongly), but it may make falling asleep easier by 'tricking' the brain into responding as if the sleep phase had already started. It may also help shift the biological clock earlier in the same way that morning light does. Several studies have shown that these effects may indeed benefit some youngsters. To avoid daily use of this agent, some researchers recommend using melatonin only late on Sunday afternoons, to help counteract any phase delay developing over the weekend. (Several studies suggest that a dose in the afternoon is more effective for adjusting the biological clock than one in the evening.) However, even though it is available over the counter, melatonin is a hormone with a number of different effects (among them effects on sexual function, at least in animals), and there is almost nothing known about its long-term use in adolescents.

Using sleeping pills to induce sleep before the start of the sleep phase generally does not work well, since they do nothing to re-set the biological clock, but their use for one to two weeks may help to make it easier to start getting up early every day. Other than that, avoid such drugs except for very occasional use since they may be dangerous and can be habit-forming. The same goes for using stimulants to help stay awake in the daytime after getting too little sleep the night before. If the underlying sleep phase problem is not corrected, medications will be helpful only briefly, if at all. Discuss any and all such treatments with your GP.

Settling for Improvement in the Adolescent's Schedule

Whether you fix a sleep phase delay by shifting it forward or pushing it back, the real challenge is to keep it from moving again once fixed. The difficulty is that you may be able only to minimise the problem, not to solve it completely. If a teenager has to be up for school at 6.00 a.m., then to get nine hours of sleep he must be asleep by 9.00 p.m. That is simply not practical in our culture. Even a conscientious student who comes home, eats, does his homework and goes to bed without watching television or talking on the phone is unlikely to get to sleep much before 10.00 or 11.00 p.m. But if he can at least fall asleep quickly when he does go to bed, he will still get more sleep than he would with a delayed sleep phase.

While roughly nine hours of sleep at night is an ideal amount for a teenager, getting seven hours is much better than getting four, five or six – but it is still not quite enough. If a student gets up at the same time seven days a week, he may *never* get enough sleep, especially if he also goes to sleep later at weekends than during the week, as he probably will. To permit some repayment of his sleep debt, we have to allow for him to sleep later on one or both weekend mornings. We only need to be sure not to let his morning sleep last so long that his sleep phase begins to drift again. If that happens, he will fall asleep even later than before and his sleep debt will only increase. If we must allow teenagers some make-up sleep at weekends, perhaps an hour or so, the trick is that it not be so much that they start to fall asleep later on weeknights. Their weekday and weekend wake-up times will still differ, but by only one or two hours, not four, five or six.

A 'Desired' Late Sleep Phase in the Adolescent

Some teenagers actually want a late sleep phase, although they may not be willing to admit it, even to themselves. It is important that you be able to recognise this problem, because the kinds of schedule change described above will not alleviate it. On the surface, this pattern resembles the sleep phase delays we've already discussed, except that the phase delay is long-standing, the child says he cannot wake in the morning, the parents say they are unable to wake him and his school attendance is very poor. (When he does go to school, he probably gets there quite late.) Actually, in these cases there is usually nothing wrong with the child's sleep itself. Sleep studies have shown that such youngsters sleep normally and have a normal ability to wake up. In fact, even at home the child *can* wake in the morning if there is something important that he wants to do – just not for school.

Anna was fourteen years old. Like Connor, she had a very late sleep phase, but with several important differences: rather than just finding her difficult to wake in the morning, her parents often could not wake her at all; unlike Connor's occasional absence or tardy arrival, she never made it to school on time and usually did not go at all; and instead of falling asleep later and waking later over summer holidays, as children usually do when they are out of school, she fell asleep and woke earlier (during summer she slept from 1.00 a.m. to 10.00 a.m., but during the school year she usually fell asleep at 5.00 a.m. and woke at midday). When her school made special allowances for her to come in at 12.30 p.m. for a half day, she soon became unable to wake before mid-afternoon or to fall asleep before 7.00 a.m. When I saw Anna, she had missed most of Year 10. Her parents did try to get her up each morning until they had to leave for work, and Anna usually went back to sleep after they left.

Although Anna's problem had only become so severe after she started secondary school, she had always fought going to school and always had a large number of absences. Her family situation was tense, unhappy and unsupportive; she was depressed, she had no close friends and she hated school. Being 'unable' to wake until the afternoon allowed her to miss a great deal of school and kept her apart from other children her age. That was really what she wanted. Anna had convinced her family – and herself – that she wanted to have a more normal sleep schedule but couldn't. That was partially true: her sleep phase had genuinely shifted so that she couldn't fall asleep early, but she also didn't want to do anything to change it.

The techniques described earlier in this chapter would fail with Anna because she would never co-operate. Just to be sure, we tried moving her schedule progressively later round the clock, as we had done with Connor, but she did not follow through at all. Although she had initially complained that she couldn't fall asleep before 5.00 a.m., now she said she was unable to stay up *after* 5.00. But she never really tried: before 5.00 even arrived, she would already be in bed with the lights out.

Youngsters like Anna need more than direct treatment of their 'sleep problems', because their sleep isn't really the problem. A child who really does not want to attend school may be glad to have a plausible reason why he 'can't' go. If the underlying problem is not solved, the child's sleep schedule will never be corrected. Anna's real problems were depression, isolation, low self-esteem and, above all, a dislike of going to school. If she could have given up school altogether and taken on another daily activity instead – one she liked and looked forward to – her sleep problems would largely have corrected themselves.

For children like Anna, I always recommend psychological evaluation and counselling. Often family therapy is useful, because the problems are often connected to the child's relationships with other family members. It is not unheard of for a child to feel obliged to stay home during the day to care for a parent who is depressed and isolated; here the parent is actually subtly encouraging the child to maintain a late sleep phase. Since in this case neither the parent nor the child really wants anything changed, my recommendation for counselling is often turned down.

Not all children with a 'desired' late sleep phase are depressed. Nor do they all dislike school, perform poorly in class or have major problems at home. Nevertheless, they are all using their sleep 'problem' as a way to avoid something else in their life, often at great cost to their ability to get by in school. All of them have underlying problems that must be understood and resolved before they can function normally again.

A 'desired' late sleep phase is usually not easy to treat. The longer it has been going on, and the more school the child has missed, the harder it will be to turn things round. However, when the underlying problems have been satisfactorily addressed, the sleep problem may resolve itself. If the youngster is placed in a setting he likes (for example, if he switches from a high school he hates to a vocational programme or college he loves), he may become motivated to get up instead of to stay in bed. In that case, the sleep problem will go away.

At first, Anna and her parents were quite reluctant to accept counselling. After a few months they finally agreed to give it a try, although they found it difficult to discuss their family's troubles openly. Very gradually, they began to understand many of the problems whose existence they had previously denied. Although many issues remain to be settled, the family has made much progress. Anna still does not like school, but she attends regularly. She is not outgoing, but she has made a few tentative efforts towards making friends and is noticeably happier. Relationships within her family have improved. Although Anna still tends to stay up until about 1.00 a.m., her sleep phase is now much closer to normal.

CHAPTER 11

Schedule Disorders II: Other Common Schedule Problems

Not all sleep problems related to a child's sleep schedule involve a shifted sleep phase. This chapter deals with three topics: schedule-related problems that occur despite a regular schedule, problems that can arise when the schedule is irregular or inconsistent and ways to minimise problems when travelling across time zones.

PROBLEMS IN REGULAR SCHEDULES

Besides shifts in the sleep phase, which were discussed in the last chapter, there are a number of other ways in which even a basically regular schedule can give rise to problems. Since some of these problems can have more than one cause, and since a given cause can lead to more than one kind of problem, there will be some degree of overlap in the sections that follow.

The Too-Long-in-Bed Problem

Parents' ideas of how long their children ought to sleep are often based less on biology than on misinformation or wishful thinking. Some families set a single 'children's bedtime' without taking into account that each of their children may have different sleep requirements (due to age differences or just normal variation among individuals) or that their children may not all get the same amounts of daytime sleep. Their expectations may be based on what their friends and neighbours tell them; everyone seems to have a friend or neighbour whose infant or toddler supposedly sleeps far more than their own child does. But these claims are often the result of faulty observations and assumptions. Sometimes parents think that their child sleeps more hours in a day than is, in fact, physiologically possible. The truth is that some children do stay in bed for long hours without calling or crying, but it does not follow that they are asleep the entire time: they may wake at night and look about, play quietly or just think.

Most children past the early months of life sleep no more than eleven to thirteen hours in total, including naps. They rarely sleep more than eleven hours at night; if they are napping a couple of hours during the day, they probably won't sleep more than nine or ten hours at night. (The more they nap, the shorter their night-time sleep is likely to be.) Most school-aged children, having given up naps altogether, sleep between nine and eleven hours at night. So, when parents tell me they are having trouble getting their infant or toddler to sleep twelve hours at night (say, from 7.00 p.m. to 7.00 a.m.) along with two hours of napping, I have to tell them that fourteen hours of sleep in a day is not likely. We can adjust their child's sleep so that he has an early bedtime or a late waking, I explain, but not both.

When you make your child stay in bed at night for more hours than he can sleep, any of several problems can appear. Like phase shifts, to which they have some similarities, these problems can exist alone or in combination with other problems.

Imagine that you have a child, of any age, who can sleep for no more than ten hours at night. If you expect (or hope) that he will get twelve hours of sleep at night, you may be in for trouble. Supposing you set his bedtime at 7.00 p.m. and expect him to sleep until 7.00 a.m., what will you see? Several scenarios can develop, depending on whether the beginning, middle or end of the night is affected (see Figure 12 on page 244). Your child might experience all three problems on the same night or at different times, sometimes having trouble going to sleep, sometimes waking too early and sometimes lying awake in the middle of the night for long stretches. If your child is young, he may even show a fourth scenario: actually sleeping all twelve hours at night but then being unable to nap during the day.

As you will see, all forms of the too-long-in-bed problem are solved by correcting the timing and distribution of sleep. Whether the night-time problem appears as trouble falling asleep, waking too early or an extended night-time waking, the child generally is getting the amount of sleep he needs at night and no more. You can move that sleep round, but you cannot reasonably expect to get him to sleep longer at night, unless you can cut down on excessive daytime napping. (But only eliminate *excessive* napping; don't make your - child's normal-length naps overly short in an attempt to maximise his night-time sleep. Children are flexible about how their sleep is divided, but only up to a point.) Similarly, if your child's only sleep problem is an inability to nap easily or well, then to get more daytime sleep you may have to shorten his night (see Chapter 12).

Trouble Falling Asleep at Bedtime

Suppose your child always takes two hours to fall asleep after his 7.00 p.m. bedtime, and after he finally falls asleep at 9.00 p.m., he sleeps through until 7.00 a.m. His sleep phase runs from 9.00 p.m. to 7.00 a.m., and that means his night-time sleep requirement is ten hours. The period from 7.00 p.m. (when you want him to fall asleep) to 9.00 p.m. (when he actually does) falls in his forbidden zone, the one time he absolutely cannot sleep (see Chapter 9). This problem resembles a delayed sleep phase, except that the child still wakes at the desired time in the morning. What actually happens in those two hours varies from child to child (as with Adam, Mark and

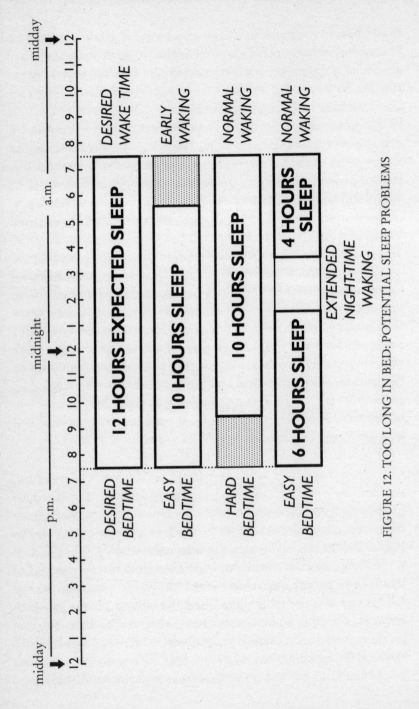

FIGURE 12. TOO LONG IN BED: POTENTIAL SLEEP PROBLEMS

Lindsey from the previous chapter, who were also being put to bed in their forbidden zone). Your child might cry quietly, demand your attention or lie in the dark imagining things. You might only occasionally be aware that he's awake, or you might spend those two hours rubbing his back to quieten him.

If you see any such pattern in your child, treat the problem by giving him a later bedtime (at least initially). His bedtime should come at the start of his sleep phase so that he can fall asleep quickly. (In our example, bedtime would move to 9.00 p.m., and the child would still sleep until 7.00 a.m.) That should solve the schedule part of the bedtime problem and any other associated problems can now be addressed.

You won't need to do anything more if evenings are now pleasant, your child falls asleep quickly and you know now that he is getting enough sleep. But if you want him to fall asleep earlier – so you can have some time to yourself in the evening, perhaps – use the same approach we discussed in the preceding chapter for fixing a delayed sleep phase: gradually move the morning waking earlier, then follow suit with the bedtime. (Remember, you must keep to the same schedule seven days a week, and don't let longer naps during the day take up the lost morning sleep.)

Waking Too Early in the Morning

Suppose your child falls asleep easily at 7.00 p.m. as desired but wakes every morning at 5.00 a.m., ready to start the day. His sleep phase runs from 7.00 p.m. to 5.00 a.m., again indicating a ten-hour sleep requirement. It's unfair and unrealistic to force him to stay in bed until 7.00 a.m. and hope he will go back to sleep. The problem is much like an early sleep phase, differing in that only one end of the sleep phase is earlier than desired, not both – since he usually falls asleep at a desirable hour – and the solution is the same: to eliminate the early waking, you must make bedtime later. You can do this by gradually adjusting the schedule later until your child is sleeping the particular ten hours you prefer (from 8.00 p.m. to 6.00 a.m., from 8.30 p.m. to 6.30 a.m., or from 9.00 p.m. to 7.00 a.m.).

Long Middle-of-the-Night Wakings

Seth was a two-year-old boy who woke up for two hours in the middle of the night, every night. He went to bed without difficulty at 7.00 p.m., he woke at 6.30 a.m., and he took a two-hour nap after lunch. He liked his cot and went to sleep at night and at nap time without problems. But at about 1.00 a.m. he would wake and start to cry. His parents thought that if they went to comfort him they would only reinforce bad habits and encourage the wakings, so they looked in on him only occasionally to make sure he wasn't ill. Every night he cried off and on for one and a half to two hours before going back to sleep. Even though his parents were firm and consistent, this pattern continued for several months. Finally Seth's parents tried bringing him into their bed when he woke up. Now he was happier, at least if he could keep one of them up to play with him. But he did not go back to sleep any faster – in fact, when he did finally get sleepy, he would ask to go back to his cot. At last, his parents started bringing him into the living room when he awakened. His mother would put on a DVD, give him some toys, and try to doze on the sofa until he was ready to go back to sleep. He - wasn't crying now, at least, but his sleep was no better, and neither was his mother's.

If a child takes one nap a day in addition to his night-time sleep, his overall sleep is divided into two separate segments. On a two-nap schedule there are three segments, and so on. In young children, the number of sleep segments is fairly flexible: they can move without much difficulty from a two- to three-segment schedule or from a three- to four-segment schedule. Also, children get their deepest sleep at the start and end of the night (see Chapters 2 and 9); their sleep in the middle of the night can be quite light. (Remember, this is true of adults, too. If you wake in the middle of the night, you may notice that you feel more awake than you will when your alarm goes off a few hours later.)

We've already seen that when a child is put to bed for more hours than he can sleep he may have trouble falling asleep, or he may wake up too early in the morning. A third possibility is that he may find himself wide awake at some point in the middle of the night. In that case, a child is still getting his required night-time sleep, but in two segments instead of one. This form of the too-long-in-bed problem is usually seen in children still taking naps; it is sometimes seen in older children, but it is uncommon once they reach school age. If your child follows this pattern, you should re-alise that he can't be in pain, even if he is crying when he wakes at night, if whenever you pick him up he becomes happy and wants to play. If you take him into your bed, he won't lie down and go to sleep; like Seth, he wants your attention. But he is fine if you get up and play with him, or (like Seth's mother) put on a DVD for him, lie on the sofa and let him play by himself. After a long period of wakeful activity – perhaps lasting thirty minutes to three hours – he goes back to sleep.

In my experience, when a child is consistently awake for a long time in the middle of the night and is happy if he is allowed to do what he wants during that time, the reason is almost always that he is in bed for more hours than he can sleep. It is easy to respond to this situation with the wrong approach. Strategies of setting strict limits, checking at intervals and simply refusing to respond are all likely to fail, as they did with Seth. Those approaches all presume that the child is capable of sleep at that time. In fact, nothing you do in the middle of the night can solve this problem. The child is *not able* to sleep at that time of night; he is not even sleepy.

To eliminate a long night-time waking, add up the hours of ac-tual sleep your child gets at night and adjust his bedtime and wake-up time so they are separated by the same number of hours. For instance, if your child gets ten hours of sleep out of the twelve hours he spends in bed, that means setting his bedtime and wake-up time ten hours apart. That can be done by putting him to bed two hours later, waking him up two hours earlier, putting him to bed one hour later and waking him one hour earlier, or any other combination that may be convenient, as long the time between bedtime and wake-up time is ten hours. Initially it is better to underestimate the number of hours than to overestimate it, and if your total does turn out to be a little too low, then once he is sleeping through the night you should be able to extend night-time sleep a little without re-creating the problem. If he naps, don't let the naps run any longer than usual: you want to move sleep from the ends of the night to the middle, not into the day. (On the other hand, if your child's naps are too long, you would do well to shorten them to a normal length and move some of that sleep into the night as well; see Chapter 12.) Only after you have shortened his time in bed is it reasonable to eliminate the middle-of-the-night activities.

Seth, as we saw, was spending eleven and a half hours in bed at night and another two hours during the day – thirteen and a half hours in all. Since he was awake for one and a half to two hours each night, he was getting a total of eleven and a half or twelve hours of sleep – a normal amount for his age. He was waking at night because he simply couldn't sleep thirteen and a half hours in a day. To fix the problem, we moved his bedtime two hours later, keeping his wake-up time and nap times fixed, and then (and only then) eliminated the night-time DVDs. Seth's night-time wakings stopped completely within a few days.

Most children with this problem behave at night the way Seth did. However, some youngsters are quiet and apparently happy when they wake, so their parents – who hear them at night only occasionally – may assume that these children are asleep more than they really are. Other children wake but remain too sleepy to get up and play; they may lie in bed restlessly or even doze off and on for long stretches before fully returning to sleep. Some children even take to rocking or head-banging to fill up the time (see Chapter 16). Even if your child is quiet during these long wakings, correcting the problem is still probably a good idea, assuming you even know it exists. Just because he is willing to entertain himself for long periods at night doesn't mean he should have to, and, in any case, one day this willingness may cease and a big sleep problem may seem to de-velop suddenly, out of nowhere. All forms of this problem – once you are aware of its cause – can be handled in essentially the same way, by correcting the schedule.

Nap Problems

If a young child sleeps well at night for more hours than most children his age, then unless he has an unusually long sleep requirement, he may not have enough sleep drive left to nap well in the daytime. This variation on the too-long-in-bed problem is discussed in the next chapter.

Short Sleep Requirements

Parents often tell me that their child 'has never needed much sleep': he sleeps only a few hours at night, during the day or both, they say. This is usually a misperception. There is, of course, variation in sleep requirements, but the range is surprisingly small (see Figure 1 on page 10). It's very rare to find a normal nine-month-old who *really* needs only eight hours of sleep at night and one hour during the day, or a four-year-old who needs only seven or eight hours in total. A child who truly has a short sleep requirement may be asked to spend more time in bed than he can sleep and, for that reason, the too-long-in-bed problems described in the previous sections could certainly develop; but, for most children, a short sleep requirement is almost never the actual explanation of these or any other sleep problems. So I usually start by assuming the child has a normal sleep requirement and normal sleep ability, and see if I can prove myself wrong.

Often, when I add up the parents' reports of their child's day and night-time sleep hours, it becomes clear that the child actually gets a normal amount of sleep. Sometimes parents have an inflated idea of what 'normal' sleep really is. In many other cases, the child is getting more sleep than his parents think he is. If they have to get up three times a night to get him back to sleep, they may end up very sleep-deprived and assume their child is, too. If they have to go to their child every hour, they may assume incorrectly that he never sleeps between their visits (they may not even realise that they themselves fall asleep between his calls). Finally, it's often the case that the nights they remember most clearly are their child's most difficult nights, when he really did not get very much sleep; nights when he slept well are easily forgotten.

When home life provides too little regular structure, with inadequate or inappropriate parental control and poor limit-setting, inconsistent schedules, anxiety or general chaos, total sleep time may truly be shortened. But it doesn't follow that the child is truly a short sleeper and is getting all the sleep he needs. If we can help the family to restore order and a sense of support and control, normal hours of sleep (and a much happier child) will usually re-appear.

How much sleep is enough? Requirements vary from person to person, of course, but if a child is getting enough sleep, he functions well during the day, without signs of sleepiness. He wakes spontaneously, or at least easily, in the morning and from naps. He will not appear sleepy, except, of course, before naps and at bedtime, and he will not act overtired at other times (see Chapter 1), except perhaps at the afternoon 'dip' (see Chapter 9). His behaviour, attention span and mood will not improve markedly when he happens to have slept longer than usual the previous night.

For us to say that a child's total sleep requirement truly is short, he must sleep less than most children his age no matter what the circumstances. A child who gets a normal amount of sleep in his preferred circumstances does not have a short sleep requirement. If he falls asleep quickly when you rub his back, if he sleeps through the night when you stay with him, if he goes back to sleep when you take him into your bed after he wakes or if he naps readily in the car, and if he gets a normal amount of sleep when you do these things, then the problem lies not in his sleep requirement but rather in his habits, associations and fears, his ability to keep himself awake when circumstances are not to his liking, and the limits you are or are not setting for him. (For help with these problems, see Chapters 4 through 7.) Similarly, if he is obviously happier and better behaved on days when he has had more than his usual short sleep, then his sleep requirement is probably normal.

If your child really is one of the rare individuals who require unusually little sleep, and there is no underlying medical or psychological problem, do not medicate him to try to get him to sleep more than he needs to. Nor should you insist that he stay in bed longer than he can sleep. This situation can be difficult for you as parents, because your child may have to go to bed later, get up earlier or nap less than would be convenient or restful for you. Still, if his time in bed is shortened to match his ability to sleep, most of his sleep problems (other than the short sleep) should resolve themselves, and those that persist will now be treatable.

Environmental Disturbances: Noise and People

Problems can occur when a child is wakened early by light or noise that he perceives as a sign that morning has arrived. You can block sunlight from entering the room, but street sounds are harder to control. Some children wake when they hear their parents getting up and simply will not go back to sleep. It's not hard for these children to wake an hour or two early; by then they have completed most of their night-time sleep, and that component of the drive to sleep (the homeostatic factor) is weaker than it was earlier in the night.

These environmental disturbances can affect a child's sleep-wake rhythms. If your child is regularly awakened and exposed to early light, he may develop an early sleep phase. If the morning disruptions are frequent enough, he will begin to anticipate them and wake spontaneously just before dawn or just before the family gets up. This can be a challenging problem. Some parents resort to sneaking out in the morning and showering at night or when they get to work.

If you are struggling with this kind of situation, there are some steps you can take. You may be able to reduce the disturbances themselves. Use blackout blinds and perhaps curtains to block out light; insulating curtains will also help to mute sounds from outside. You may have to shut the windows as well. Sometimes it is helpful to move the child to a quieter bedroom, perhaps switching rooms with a sibling who sleeps more soundly. Although I usually recommend against the use of gadgetry, machines that produce constant soft background noise, such as fans, humidifiers or 'white-noise' generators, can help to mask occasional loud noises from outside, especially those occurring in the early morning. (Unless these machines seem to offer the only solution, though, I recommend avoiding them: children need to learn to sleep under natural conditions, and if they become dependent on the background sounds from these machines, they may have trouble sleeping in quieter surroundings.)

You can also try shifting your child to a later sleep phase, following the guidelines given in the preceding chapter. The rationale is that if you showered at an earlier point in his sleep, perhaps at 3.00 a.m. instead of at 5.00 or 6.00, he would be too sleepy to get up. Fortunately, you can get the same effect by moving your child's sleep schedule later instead of moving up your own morning schedule. Now the morning disturbances will fall earlier in his sleep phase, when he has had much less sleep, and he will be more likely to sleep through them.

Evening noise can be a more difficult problem than morning noise. It can be hard for a child to fall asleep when people are laughing and yelling in the next room. The house need not be silent – it's okay to watch television at a low volume, for example – but do keep things relatively quiet long enough for your child to fall asleep. Once he is sound asleep he will soon be difficult to wake, at least for several hours. As long as his bedtime is properly set and he is ready for sleep, this need not be a major burden.

Sometimes a parent comes home just as a child is going to bed or before he has fallen asleep. The parent may want to spend some time with the child, and the child, wide awake again and excited at seeing the parent, may want to stay up later. If this parent always comes home around bedtime, the child may try to stay up every night and wait. The best solutions are for the parent to come home either early enough to spend some time with the child before his bedtime or (less ideally) late enough that the child is already sound asleep, or to shift the child's sleep phase earlier or later to get the same result.

Usually there is less noise and activity to disrupt sleep in the middle of the night than at the ends, but they may be present. For instance, suppose a child always has to be moved late at night, perhaps when he is brought home after falling asleep elsewhere. Usually that will not cause a big problem – children either sleep through the move or return to sleep promptly afterwards. But if the child regularly wakes and cannot return to sleep easily, then it may help to bring him home earlier or later, or to shift his sleep phase so that the disruption occurs in a part of his sleep cycle when his sleep is less easily disturbed.

Also, if a child is on an exceptionally late or early schedule, a parent's arrival late at night or departure early in the morning can coincide with the child's normal period of relatively light sleep that comes in the middle of his night. If the noise usually awakens the child then, you can use the same techniques that you would try if this happened earlier in the evening or later in the morning: trying to be as quiet as possible; considering moving your child's sleep schedule to make him less likely to wake at these times; or, if necessary, using a fan or other source of continuous background sound to help mask the parent's activity.

The Television (or Computer or Phone) Problem

Young children are often willing to trade sleep for cartoons. If they are free to watch television immediately upon waking, they will probably choose to get up early for cartoons over returning to sleep for their last sleep cycle. (Although they may doze in front of the television, this sleep will be of poor quality.) As mentioned in the preceding chapter, even children who are difficult to wake for school are somehow able to get up for cartoons at the weekend. It is never a good idea to go right from bed to television. Besides being a habit that can directly cause insufficient sleep, it is also one that can leave a child (and his biological clock) confused about when morning really starts, and this, in turn, can lead to irregularity and unpredictability in his sleep schedule (see next section). For these reasons, it is best not to allow your child to watch any television for the first hour or two in the morning, at least until an hour late enough to allow him to completely finish sleeping. It's a particularly bad idea, and an unnecessary temptation, to let your child have a television in his room – if he has one, now is the time to remove it. If cartoons are no longer available to him on weekend mornings, he will probably choose to stay asleep.

Older children often have a similar problem, but at the other end of the night: they stay up late to watch television, use the computer or talk on the phone. The late-night shows they watch and the web sites they surf are likely to be even less appropriate for them than some of the cartoons can be for younger children. Unlike as with a book, which becomes difficult to read when you are sleepy (and which you can put down today and pick up again tomorrow), you can watch television even when you are bleary-eyed with fatigue, and most programmes are designed to keep you watching to the end, with teasers encouraging you to watch the next programme. Talking on the phone doesn't even require you to keep your eyes open. If you fight off the first wave of sleepiness to see the end of a programme or to keep talking, you may have a half hour or so until the next wave hits, and by then another show or another subject may have caught your interest.

Just as television should not be a child's first activity in the morning, it should not be his last activity at night. Set a time at which the television is turned off. Make similar rules for the computer and the phone. (While your child gets used to this change, others in the house may temporarily have to give up some television as well.) Reading or listening to stories is a far better activity with which to end the day. Again, letting your child have a television in his room is particularly unwise. Even an older child should not watch television alone in his room at night: late-night programmes are geared for adults and may stimulate emotions in the child he does not yet fully understand and may find upsetting, confusing or frightening. If you don't supervise his viewing, you may be unaware of what he is being exposed to.

Don't make late-night television a special weekend privilege, either. If there are shows you'd like to allow your child to see that are on too late, get in the habit of recording them and watch them (ideally together) at a more reasonable time on another day.

Some children get up to watch television in the middle of the night. This is not terribly common, but it can happen if you allow it, especially if the television is in the child's room. Even very young children know how to turn the television on. Children who exhibit this behaviour usually fall asleep watching television; when they wake during the night, they want to resume their viewing. This development becomes more likely if the child is free to make up the lost sleep by sleeping late in the morning or by napping excessively or at the wrong hours in the daytime.

Needless to say, middle-of-the-night television should not be allowed for any reason. The child should not have access to a television during the night – it should be impossible for him to watch television at night without you knowing about it. If necessary, unplug your televisions at night or keep them in rooms where you can control access. Finally, as described earlier in this chapter, enforce a proper bedtime, morning wake-up time and daytime naps so the 'hole' in the middle of the night can close up.

IRREGULAR AND INCONSISTENT SLEEP-WAKE SCHEDULES

Many of the children I see have difficulty sleeping because their sleep-wake patterns are irregular. They fall asleep early one night and late the next, they wake at odd hours and they never nap at the same time two days in a row. Mealtimes are equally inconsistent.

If you are not sure whether this description fits your child, chart his schedule (using Figure 5 on page 77) for a week or two. You may be surprised by what you find. If his schedule is irregular, then in all probability his circadian rhythms are also disrupted (see Chapter 9). His body temperature may be rising when he goes to bed and falling when he gets up, the opposite of what should be happening. He may be hungry between meals or when he should be sleeping, and not hungry at mealtimes. He may be active when he should be napping, and sluggish when he should be playing. He may have difficulty falling asleep at bedtime – if he *has* a bedtime – and he may wake during the night.

It is important to realise that this problem differs (at least in part) from the bedtime difficulties and night-time wakings described in Chapters 4 through 7. There may be stretches of time – hours, even – during which your child cannot fall asleep, or return to sleep, no matter what you do. Like a child either sent to bed in his forbidden zone or kept in bed more hours than he can sleep, he is unable to sleep because his sleep-wake rhythm is in the waking phase. However, when a child's schedule is disorganised, these wakeful periods can appear at different times night to night. For the same reasons, periods of daytime sleepiness or grumpiness can appear un-predictably from day to day.

Children's daily rhythms can only be established and maintained in a consistent twenty-four-hour pattern if they are regulated by events that occur at the same times every day. Although regular ex-posure to light is the only stimulus known to directly control our biological clocks, other regularly occurring events can affect the amount and timing of exposure we get. If your child naps late in the day, he may be able to stay up later at night and be exposed to light later than usual; this extra light adjusts his clock later. If he misses

a nap and falls asleep early, the opposite may occur: he gets less evening light and his clock moves earlier. If his meals are irregular, poorly timed hunger signals may leave him awake and exposed to light at an inappropriate hour.

If your child does not have reasonably consistent daily routines, his system has no way to know when he should be asleep and when he should be awake. The result is that his sleep-wake patterns dete-riorate. If he sometimes goes to sleep at 9.00 and sometimes at 6.00, then when he goes to bed at 6.00 his body does not know whether to expect a late nap or an early bedtime, and therefore whether he should sleep one hour or ten. His sleep pattern becomes disorgan-ised into irregular fragments, none of which even approximate the ten or more continuous hours of sleep a young child should have at night. Whereas normal night-time sleep is interrupted only by brief arousals and the return to sleep is rapid, the child without a clear schedule may sometimes wake at night completely, for long periods, and his daytime naps may sometimes be unusually long.

James, for example, was a four-year-old boy whose sleep problems were difficult to characterise because they were so erratic. He
had no formal bedtime and no regular bedtime routines. He went to
sleep at any time between 7.00 and 11.00 – whenever he got sleepy,
which depended to some extent on if and when he had napped that
day. He fell asleep sometimes in his own bed but more often wherever he happened to be, usually in the living room with the lights
and television on.

When James fell asleep on the early side, he sometimes woke an
hour or two later and would not go back to sleep for several hours.
Other times, he would sleep for nine or ten hours and then find
himself wide awake at 4.00 or 5.00 a.m. On the days that followed
these early wakings, he usually took a long nap and then stayed
wide awake until 11.00 p.m. He might still wake early the next
morning, but he would be grumpy and might doze off and on during the day or even fall asleep so deeply that his parents could not
wake him. When he did nap, it could be as early as 9.00 a.m., as late
as 6.00 p.m., or anywhere in between, and his naps could be as short
as thirty minutes or as long as four hours.

James's unstructured sleep habits mirrored a lack of structure
in his home, which was not caused by family problems or any lack
of caring on his parents' part. It was a style commonplace in his
family's community: irregular mealtimes and bedtimes were quite
usual and unremarkable in the family and among their friends.
These irregularities did not bother James's parents in the daytime,
but they were concerned about his wakings at night. They did not
see the connection.

When the family sought my help, I learned that, in addition to
the absence of a consistent schedule, James had no customary routines to guide him in getting ready for bed and falling asleep. It was
clear that his parents needed to establish a bedtime ritual that
was pleasant and consistent. But better bedtime routines alone, even
if they came at the same time each night, would not solve James's
sleep problems. He also needed more order in his haphazard daily
schedule.

The fundamental problem was that, without any regular cues to guide it, James's twenty-four-hour sleep-wake pattern had become badly disrupted. Although this problem sounds severe, the solution was actually simple and straightforward.

Correcting an Irregular Schedule

Setting up and sticking to a regular schedule is a necessary step toward solving this kind of sleep problem, whether the irregular schedule is the main problem, as it was with James, or just one factor complicating other problems. If the irregular schedule is the only problem, that may be all you need to do.

For the first few weeks, keep your child on a fairly strict timetable for going to sleep, getting up and eating. Once things are going well, you can try being more flexible, within reason. But remember, if your child's schedule has been unstructured in the past, it can revert easily if you are not careful.

If you are not sure how long your child can sleep at night, start with the smallest amount you are sure he can achieve. It is much better to err on the lower end than the higher, because that will make it easier for him to sleep at the times you set, making it in turn easier for you to enforce the new schedule. If your child is at an age when he should still be napping, add suitable naps to the schedule as well (see Chapters 2 and 12). If you are not sure whether he needs a nap, try eliminating it; if you are not sure whether he needs one nap or two, try starting with just one. When his sleep settles into a regular pattern, it will become clear whether he needs more sleep; if so, you can gradually lengthen his time in bed at night, add new naps or lengthen existing naps.

James's parents agreed to set up a daily schedule for him that included a regular bedtime and wake-up time. There was to be no daytime sleep, as he was too old for regular naps. They instituted a bedtime routine that they felt would suit them. In addition, they agreed to provide his meals at the same times every day, whether he was hungry or not, and not to feed him at other times, except for appropriate snacks. Although these decisions were out of keeping with the relatively unstructured way of life they were accustomed to, they willingly accepted the changes once they understood that James would sleep better at night and probably feel better during the day.

Since James was usually asleep by 9.00 p.m. on days when he did not nap, we decided to start his bedtime there (we could certainly have started later if we weren't sure about that time). He would go to bed every night at 9.00 after a story or a quiet game; if he was still asleep at 6.00 a.m., his parents would wake him for the day, dress him and give him breakfast. He was not to sleep during the daytime at all – if he did fall asleep, his parents were to wake him as soon as possible, within ten or fifteen minutes at most. James probably needed a total of more than nine hours' sleep, but I wanted to start with a sleep schedule I knew he could achieve. Once he was sleeping well on this schedule, then we could begin moving his bedtime earlier or his wake-up time later, in adjustments of fifteen minutes, as long as he was falling asleep quickly at night and had to be wakened in the morning.

His parents also began making sure that he always slept in his own room, not in the living room. When he wakened during the night they would go to him, but they wouldn't allow him to get up and play, since that would only reinforce the habit of waking. They were to insist that he stay in bed at bedtime and after wakings during the night, even though at first he had trouble falling asleep at some of these times. They could sit with him, but quietly, without much conversation.

Once James's sleep rhythm had normalised and he could consistently fall asleep quickly, which I told his parents to expect within a week or two, they were no longer to stay with him when he woke. (However, I asked that they delay this step until it became clear that, except for brief wakings, he was in fact able to sleep the full time his schedule called for.) We planned to enforce this rule with the methods discussed in the chapters on associations and limit-setting (Chapters 4 and 5), but these measures proved unnecessary: James was never especially demanding even when he was awake, and he had never really associated his parents' presence with falling asleep, anyway.

The family was able to follow through because they now understood the importance of a good daytime structure. Because they found it helpful to chart his sleep patterns, they continued to do so for two months, well beyond the few weeks I had asked for. Like most parents, they found it easier to stay consistent when they could see their child's progress in black and white. James resisted the changes for the first week, but his parents held firm and were careful to be supportive. Soon both he and his parents began to look forward to the period before bed; it became an opportunity for a closeness they had not enjoyed before. By the end of the second week James was falling asleep easily at a regular bedtime and sleeping through the night. It soon became apparent that he could sleep longer than nine hours, so his parents gradually shifted him to a schedule that ran from 8.30 p.m. to 6.30 a.m.

Disrupted schedules usually happen because parents have not understood the importance of consistent daily routines. Occasionally, though, the disorganisation and loss of structure stems from underlying family problems. When issues such as marital strife, physical or psychiatric illness, death, separation and divorce are involved, parents may be unable or unwilling to enforce a normal schedule for their children. In these situations, I always urge the family to seek counselling.

TRAVEL

Parents often wonder what to expect and what to do when travelling with children to different time zones. Understanding the effect such travel has on your child's sleep pattern and learning to plan for it should help to avoid worry and limit problems.

Neither children nor adults can adjust instantly from one time zone to another. However, children do find the transition easier to make than adults do: the homeostatic drive to sleep (which makes you get sleepier the longer you stay awake) is very powerful in children, especially young children, and it can even overcome the stimulating effects of the circadian drive (which helps you to wake in the morning, keeps you awake all day and gives you a 'second wind' in the early evening). If your child is not permitted to sleep when he expects to, he will be better able than you will be to make up the lost sleep at times when he would normally be awake.

Suppose you travel west by three time zones. Your child will want to go to sleep and wake three hours 'earlier' than usual according to the new local time. If you keep him up until the local clock says it is his usual bedtime, then instead of waking three hours earlier than usual (local time) the next morning, he will sleep until closer to when the local clock says it is his usual wake-up time. Conversely, if you travel east, your child will go to sleep and want to wake 'later' than usual, but if you wake him in the morning three hours earlier than he would like, when the local clock says he should be waking, then that night he will be able to fall asleep much earlier than the night before. In both cases, if the changes don't happen the first day, they certainly will by the second or third. (As always, it's important to limit daytime napping to the usual amount, so sleep lost at one end of the night will be moved to the other end.)

When travelling across time zones with children, most people make the necessary changes without even thinking about them because of expectations driven by activities, meals and other obligations.

If you are travelling west (one to three time zones):

- Try to keep your child awake until the 'correct' bedtime in the new time zone. If the change is too large to accomplish on the first night, do it gradually over two or three days.

- Be aware that you may have to get up early with your child for a day or two (if he usually wakes at 7.00 a.m. in London, he may wake at 4.00 a.m. on the first day in Rio de Janeiro). It's not fair to leave him crying for three hours in the morning just because he hasn't fully adjusted to the new time zone. In any case, you will probably wake up early yourself for the same reason.

- Allow only the usual amount of napping. Initially your child will want to nap too 'early' in the day. Try to delay his naps as much as you are delaying his bedtime.

- Consider moving bedtime and nap time somewhat later than usual beginning a few days before you travel. That will reduce the adjustment you have to make once you arrive, and it may prevent the very early wakings.

- If the trip is short, you could choose to let your child continue to operate according to his home time zone, especially if you're only travelling one or two time zones or if your child usually goes to sleep and wakes up late. Thus, if he sleeps from 10.00 p.m. to 8.00 a.m. at his home in Helsinki, he would sleep from 8.00 p.m. to 6.00 a.m. while in London. Naps should be adjusted similarly. When you return to New York, he can go right back to the usual schedule without any re-adjustment.

If you are travelling east (one to three time zones):

- Your child may not be able to fall asleep until 'later' than usual for the first day or two, and there is no point in making him try; you do not want him lying in bed wide awake and frustrated on his first night in a new place. If he usually goes to sleep at 8.00 p.m. in Rio de Janeiro, he may not be able to fall asleep until 11.00 p.m. in London. (In fact, it would be counterproductive to let him fall asleep at 8.00 on the first night in London because, since that's only 5.00 in Rio de Janeiro, he could treat that sleep as only a late nap and then be awake much of the night.)

- Wake your child at the 'correct' wake-up time in the new time zone. If the change seems too large to accomplish the first morning, do it gradually over two or three days.

- Allow only the usual amount of napping. Naps, like bedtime, may initially tend to run late by the amount of the time change. Try to move the naps earlier, to match the earlier wake-up times.

- If the trip is short, you could choose to let your child continue to operate according to his home time zone. Thus, if he sleeps from 8.00 p.m. to 6.00 a.m. at his home in Rio de Janeiro, he would sleep from 11.00 p.m. to 9.00 a.m. while in London. Naps should be adjusted similarly. Once back in Rio de Janeiro, he can go right back to the usual schedule without any re-adjustment.

If you are travelling across more than three or four time zones (for instance, between the UK and the USA or Asia):

- Children handle these larger changes more easily than their parents do. Although the details can be confusing, most parents find that their children adapt quickly on their own. There is no need to make elaborate plans.

- You cannot force your child to sleep when he is not sleepy, but you can keep him awake when he should be awake in the new time zone. He will self-correct quickly, making up the lost sleep at proper times for the new time zone. If you wake him when he is sleeping at the 'wrong' times, he will want to sleep at the 'right' times. The rest will take care of itself. If that is all you remember, you will be successful.

- Simply be aware that if you travel east, your child may fall asleep much later than usual at first and have to be wakened in the morning; travelling west, he may want to fall asleep earlier than usual and you may have to keep him awake. In either case, the times he wants to sleep or stay awake may seem erratic for a day or two; he could be up much of the first night and want to sleep much of the first day. These problems should all resolve themselves within a few days.

- The changes are particularly easy to make for a young child who still naps: he already sleeps both in the daytime and at night, getting his sleep in several widely separated time segments. Instead of having to shift his sleeping schedule by six to twelve hours, he may only need to adjust by a few hours, if that. If you limit his sleep in the daytime, he will quickly increase the sleep he gets at night. If the original nap periods now fall at night, they can lengthen, and perhaps combine, to become the new night-time sleep, and if the original night-time sleep period now falls in the day, that sleep can shorten and perhaps split to become the new nap or naps.

- If your child is too old for regular naps, he (like you) will have to shift his schedule the full amount; still, as long as you do not let him sleep during the day (or at least limit it as much as possible), his inability to get enough sleep the first night (or two) will be enough to force his sleep into the next night and, when this happens, to put him on a correct local schedule.

CHAPTER 12

Naps

All children nap, at least up to a certain age. When people tell me that their child 'never napped', it may be that the naps were always difficult, short or unpredictable, or that the child could never be put down for a formal nap. But it cannot be true that he never slept during the day, even if just for a few minutes here and a few minutes there. The same parents, typically, will report that their child actually did sleep during the day, but 'only in the car' or 'just in the pram on the way back from the playground', or 'not at home, but every day at day care'. Charting your child's sleep patterns (see Figure 5 on page 77) may reveal that he is getting daytime sleep that you were unaware of.

In the newborn, sleeping and waking occur in shorter and longer periods spread over the whole twenty-four-hour day. By the time a baby is three months old, day and night should be well differentiated, with most sleep occurring at night; the daytime should be settling into an increasingly predictable pattern of wakeful periods and naps. By three or four months, a baby should be taking three naps a day: long ones in the mid-morning and the mid-afternoon, and a short one in the evening. The evening nap is usually given up at around six months of age.

Most children give up one of the two remaining naps around the time of their first birthday, or within the next few months. Although some children seem to drop a nap one day and never go back to it, most first go through a few weeks of intermittently skipping one nap or the other, or at least having trouble falling asleep at one of them (see 'Trouble Giving Up a Nap: Transition Problems' on page 280). And most children do not simply drop one of the naps; rather, they replace both of the naps with a single new one at an intermediate time. For instance, a child who was napping at 10.00 a.m. and 2.00 p.m. will likely switch to a single nap after lunch. Even though a nap is lost, the child's total sleep time usually changes little – either the new nap is longer than either of the original two were, or the child sleeps longer at night to compensate. At this point, getting the child to fall asleep may well become easier at bedtime as well as for the remaining nap, because he is now staying awake for longer stretches between periods of sleep. Staying awake longer increases the drive to sleep, and that makes falling asleep easier.

The final nap will disappear eventually as well, but when it will happen is less predictable than it is for the others. Most children stop napping altogether between their third and fourth birthdays, but some two-year-olds have already given up their last nap, and some children continue napping until the start of nursery school. Similar to the dropping of his second nap, your child may give up his last nap fairly suddenly, abruptly starting to stay awake all day, or he may gradually have more difficulty falling asleep at nap time, so that some days he falls asleep and some days he doesn't.

Napping habits and tendencies differ widely among individual children. Some children love their naps and always go to sleep willingly, while others, preferring to stay awake having fun, fight each and every nap. Some children can miss a nap or nap at the wrong time without any apparent impact on their mood, behaviour or schedule: they are fine the rest of the day, and they go to sleep at the usual time that night. Others will be miserable all day, and their night-time sleep will be affected: if they skipped a nap they may go to sleep for the night earlier than usual, and if they napped unusually late they may not be able to fall asleep at their usual bed-time. For a few children – happily, not very many – any change in the nap schedule seems to disrupt both daytime and night-time sleep for as long as a week.

Similarly, children vary in their tolerance for napping in different places and under different circumstances. Some children are very flexible: they nap equally well in the cot, in bed, in the car or in a pram. Other children's naps are more rigidly dependent on a partic-ular setting or condition: if a child sometimes naps in the car, for in-stance, he may have difficulty napping anywhere else. Parents of these children sometimes resort to such unfortunate habits as driving their youngsters around every day at nap time, occasionally even parking the car in the driveway and leaving the child there to finish the nap with the motor running. Fortunately, most children are at least somewhat flexible regarding the specific times and cir-cumstances of their naps. Just how much variation your child can tolerate can be determined only by trial and error.

It is usually easier to treat a sleep problem that occurs at night than one that occurs during the day, because children get sleepier and sleepier as the night goes on until they finally must fall asleep. If you are helping your child learn to associate new habits with falling asleep at night, you will succeed if you wait long enough, even if he is stubborn. However, during the day the drive to sleep comes and goes. After a midday dip in alertness, your toddler's circadian sys-tem wakes him up and moves him towards his 'forbidden zone', when he will be wide awake (see Chapter 9). If you are trying to enforce new patterns at nap time, you may not succeed completely, especially if your child is nearly old enough to give up the nap in question anyway. You cannot – or, at least, you should not – keep a toddler in bed or in his cot all day waiting for him to fall asleep. (Teaching new patterns at nap time is easier in infants, since their drive to sleep during the day at each of their nap times remains very strong.)

If you are having trouble with your child's naps, or if you're worried about them, there are a number of possible factors to consider, in addition to the causes of sleep problems discussed in other chapters, and a number of things you may be able to do.

PROBLEMS WITH THE LENGTH
AND TIMING OF NAPS

Solving many common napping problems is merely a matter of adjusting nap times, or altering the lengths of naps or of night-time sleep. Think of naps not as isolated sleep periods, unrelated to other naps and night-time sleep, but rather as part of a full day's schedule, in which each sleep period influences all the other ones: night-time sleep affects naps, naps affect night-time sleep and naps affect other naps. As you will see, children are adept at moving periods of sleep round. Although the total amount of sleep they get does not change much, the hours when they sleep can and do.

'Hidden' Naps

Because children are able to divide their sleep into a variable number of segments and to move sleep between day and night, the line between night-time sleep and daytime naps can become unclear. Where you draw the line can affect how you interpret your child's schedule, and in turn how you approach his problem.

An example of this situation might be a five-month-old who, at first glance, goes to sleep at 6.00 p.m. after a feeding, gets up at 7.30 a.m., and naps twice a day. This child is a bit young to have only two naps, and thirteen and a half hours is an unusually long night for almost any child. Furthermore, on this schedule his sleep is disrupted. After going to bed for the night he regularly wakes up fussing at 7.30 p.m., and it takes an hour for his parents to settle him, nurse him again and get him back to sleep. He may nurse briefly one or two more times during the night. At 5.30 a.m. he wakes again for an hour, then he goes back to sleep until 7.30, when he gets up for the day. His morning nap, at 10.00, is short, and he has trouble falling asleep then; his afternoon nap, at 2.00, is more successful.

One way to view this problem is to see the child as having a broken thirteen-and-a-half-hour night and two daytime naps, suggesting that the cause of his sleep difficulties is that he is in bed too long at night and his total time in bed is more hours than he can sleep (see 'The Too-Long-in-Bed Problem' in Chapter 11). But there is another, related way to look at this child's schedule. According to this other interpretation, he sleeps only *nine* hours a night, from 8.30 p.m. to 5.30 a.m., and, in addition to his mid-morning and mid-afternoon naps, he naps for an hour and a half in the evening (from 6.00 to 7.30 p.m.) and again for another hour in the early morning (from 6.30 to 7.30 a.m.). Now the situation appears quite different: instead of a child who naps too little and suffers from disrupted sleep at night, we see a child who takes *too many* naps – four a day – and consequently has trouble falling asleep at night and wakes early in the morning. Although both interpretations are valid, viewing the problem the second way may make it easier to understand and to find a solution.

If your child regularly wakes up for a while either after a short period of sleep early in the night or before the final stretch of sleep in the morning, it may be useful to think of these wakeful periods as dividing a late-night or early-morning nap from his main night-time sleep period. Now if you more completely separate these naps from the night-time, by moving the late nap earlier or the early nap later – even if it seems to make the night shorter than you had hoped for – both night-time sleep and naps likely will improve (see 'Too Much Napping During the Day and Too Little Sleep at Night', 'Too Many Short Naps: The "Naplet" Problem', 'Napping Too Early', and 'Napping Too Late' below).

Too Little Napping During the Day and Too Much Sleep at Night

A child who has difficulty napping in the daytime commonly sleeps very well at night, regularly getting perhaps eleven hours or more. During the day it is hard to get a child of this sort to nap, and, when he does nap, often it is for no more than thirty minutes.

If this description fits your child, he may be getting almost all his required sleep at night. Most young children with the same overall sleep requirement as your child will sleep fewer hours at night (nine and a half hours, say) and nap longer during the day (possibly taking a two-hour nap, or two one-hour naps). But because your child sleeps so well at night, he feels little drive to sleep during the day.

If the only 'problem' is that your child's naps are brief, you may not need to do anything. However, often children function poorly on such short naps even if they are sleeping an adequate amount overall. They are not sleepy enough to nap longer during the day, but at the same time they are too sleepy to behave well and are likely to be grumpy instead. Other reasons to change this pattern can be that the brief naps are inconvenient or that you have difficulty getting your child to fall asleep even for those naps he does take.

If you're in any of these situations, you may have to start reducing your child's sleep at night. Try cutting back his night-time sleep by thirty to sixty minutes – even by as much as two hours if necessary, though it's rarely appropriate to shorten the night to less than nine hours. You can make this change all at once or gradually over several days, and you can do it by making his bedtime later, waking him up earlier or both. Don't worry if you have to shorten the night too much at first to get results – you can always add some time back later. Remember, you are not trying to eliminate any sleep, just to shift some of it from the night to the day.

Too Much Napping During the Day and Too Little Sleep at Night

If your child sleeps a great deal during the day, you may be worried that something is wrong. Even if you're glad that he takes such long naps, you might be troubled if he also sleeps too little at night. You may think that his poor night-time sleep is causing him to sleep longer during the day, but the reverse is more probably true: the excessive daytime napping is probably interfering with his sleep at night.

For instance, when parents report that their infant or toddler sleeps only six and a half or seven hours at night, they are also likely to describe daily naps totalling four to six hours, an unusually large number. Even when this child gets only four hours of daytime sleep, he is still sleeping ten and a half or eleven hours total. If he gets six hours of daytime sleep, his parents are very lucky that he can get anything close to seven hours at night.

Even if this kind of schedule doesn't pose a problem for you, it's not appropriate. Children rarely need to nap longer than two hours at a time, and most children taking multiple naps get no more than three or four hours of sleep during the day, at least after the first three or four months of life.

The solution is easy: cut back some of your child's sleep during the day so that he has to sleep more at night to compensate. (Simply keeping him in bed longer at night won't help unless he's not sleeping enough overall.) If your child takes too many naps for his age (for example, a ten-month-old still taking three naps, or an eighteen-month-old still taking two), you will have to eliminate one or even two of them (also see 'Too Many Short Naps: The "Naplet" Problem' on page 272). If he takes an appropriate number of naps, but they are too long, they can be gradually shortened: for example, a single four-hour nap can be shortened by fifteen to thirty minutes a day until it is only two hours long. A pair of three-hour naps can be cut back the same way until they each last two hours, or an hour and a half if that works better for you and for him. Don't allow your child to sleep at other times during the day, anywhere, until the new nap routine is firmly established. You may have to avoid errands and unnecessary car trips for a week or two. If your child is cared for by someone else during the day, be sure that he or she doesn't allow naps to run too long; the more your child sleeps during the day, the less work that person has to do, so it may be tempting.

Short Sleep Day and Night

If your child needs much less total sleep than most, then even if he is sleeping as little as eight or nine hours at night, that may still be almost all the sleep he needs for an entire day, and there may be little sleep left to allow him to nap. Keep in mind, however, that this is an uncommon problem (see 'Short Sleep Requirements' in the preceding chapter). If your child really does need unusually little sleep and you do not want to shorten his night-time sleep further to get better naps, you may have to accept this situation – with a short night and only short or occasional naps – and hope that his night will lengthen a bit once he gives up his daytime sleep altogether. On the other hand, if he is grumpy, irritable or otherwise having trouble getting through the day without a nap, after having stopped napping at an early age, you may have no choice but to shorten his night to try to get the nap back, at least until he is able to function normally in the day without it.

Long Sleep Day and Night

If your child sleeps at least ten or eleven hours at night despite napping three hours or more during the day, you obviously do not need to shorten his naps. Some children are just long sleepers (a tendency that sometimes runs in families). But if after the early months your child is still an *extremely* long sleeper, getting fifteen hours of sleep or more over twenty-four hours, you may want to discuss the matter with your GP. Certain neurologic or metabolic disorders that cause unusual sleepiness may show symptoms starting even in infancy (see Chapter 18).

Remember that the appearance of a long sleep requirement can be deceiving. Even if your child stays quietly in his room for eleven to thirteen hours at night, it does not necessarily mean he is asleep all that time. Often, such children are actually awake for periods of up to an hour or so at a time during the night, and their total sleep time is quite normal. They are simply content to play quietly until they go back to sleep. (These wakings can suddenly turn into a problem if, starting one night, a child decides that playing alone is no longer fun – see 'Long Middle-of-the-Night Wakings' in Chapter 11.) When the child's naps are shortened, or his time in bed at night is reduced, these long wakings disappear.

To see if that is the case, look in on your child a few times a night for several nights to see if he sleeps as much as you think he does. Or you can try shortening his naps, or his time in bed at night, and see what happens: if after several weeks he is obviously unhappy and grumpy during the day, and if he has to be wakened in the morning and from naps rather than waking spontaneously, then he probably has a genuinely long sleep requirement.

Too Many Short Naps: The 'Naplet' Problem

Excessively long daytime naps can shift too much sleep from the night to the day, as discussed above. However, nap-related problems can arise even when a child gets a normal amount of daytime sleep or less. Even very brief periods of sleep, or, as I call them, 'naplets', can significantly lessen the drive to sleep later in the day and at night. During naps, as at night, children reach deep sleep almost immediately. Since this deep sleep is the most restorative part of the sleep cycle, the first ten minutes of a one-hour nap reduce the need for sleep more than the last ten do. In short, even a brief nap can have a significant impact on a child's sleep schedule. (Even in adults, a quick nap after dinner often interferes with the ability to fall asleep at night.) Also, a child who takes too many naps will not have much room in between them for wakefulness, and – unless the child is borrowing from his night-time sleep as described above – the short periods of waking assure that the naps that follow will be short as well. The wakings will be too short to allow good naps, and the naps too short to allow good wakings. The result is that his naps will be short, frequent, probably inconsistent, unpredictable and troublesome.

Consider a ten-month-old with this problem. Instead of napping twice a day as he should, with three or four hours of wakefulness preceding each nap, he takes four naps a day, one every three hours between 8.00 a.m. and 5.00 p.m., and most of his naps last only fifteen to thirty minutes. Or consider a twenty-month-old who is still taking two naps, at 10.00 a.m. and 2.00 p.m., each lasting thirty to forty-five minutes and each preceded by thirty minutes of crying.

He should be falling asleep easily after staying awake for about six hours before his single nap after lunch. Similarly, if a thirty-month-old takes one 'official' nap after lunch but falls asleep several times each day for ten minutes at a time (in his pram or in the car, for example), then getting him to fall asleep for his official nap will be difficult and that nap too will be short.

Children like these need to have their 'naplets' eliminated and their daytime sleep consolidated into the right number of naps of appropriate timing and length. The ten-month-old who takes four naps a day may need to cut down to two. Perhaps his 8.00 a.m. nap can be moved to 9.30 or 10.00 a.m. (either all at once or in gradual steps of fifteen or thirty minutes a day). Now that he is awake longer before that nap, he will probably fall asleep easily, and the nap will probably last a little longer than before, so he can be kept awake until 2.00 p.m. and have his second nap then. This nap, too, will start more easily and last longer than before. Then he must be kept awake longer until bedtime, which will also become progressively easier. The two naps now permitted will gradually lengthen, probably to at least an hour each.

The twenty-month-old taking two short naps can be handled in a similar way. His morning nap can probably be eliminated, and his mid-afternoon nap moved one or two hours earlier, to right after lunch. Alternatively, the morning nap can be moved thirty minutes later each day until it falls after a temporarily early lunch, and the second nap can then be eliminated. Either way, he is now napping just once a day and staying awake longer before his nap time. He, too, will start falling asleep more easily, and his nap will lengthen.

The thirty-month-old child can keep his regular nap after lunch, but his 'naplets' must be eliminated. The easiest way to do that is to keep him out of the car and pram for a week or two to keep him from dozing. If that's impossible, then the car trips and pram rides should ideally be scheduled after the 'official' nap, so that even if he falls back asleep then, he will only be extending his single nap. If his parents do not have that flexibility, they might be able to leave him with a family member or babysitter while they run errands until the new schedule has been established and the problem resolved.

Once the child is no longer taking naplets, he should be able to fall asleep more easily at nap time and sleep longer. After the new pattern is well established, he may be able to stay awake on short car rides that don't coincide with his nap time, and if he does sleep in the car occasionally, it may no longer be disruptive.

Napping Too Early

An early-morning nap can prevent a child from sleeping late enough in the morning, at the end of his night. The early nap, in this case, actually makes up the last sleep cycle of the night, split off from the rest of the night by a period of intervening waking and perhaps even a feeding. Even a late-morning nap, if it's the only nap of the day, can cause trouble – but now on the evening end because the stretch between the end of the nap and the start of the night may be too long, and the child may have a great deal of difficulty towards the end of the day. Some days he may fall asleep in the late afternoon or early evening, which can adversely affect that night's sleep (see the next section).

Such problems can easily be corrected by gradually shifting the morning nap later, as described in the section above, and if necessary by also moving the child's first feeding later so that the morning hunger signals move sufficiently late so as not to wake him before his need for sleep is met. On a two-nap schedule, delay the nap until mid-morning; on a one-nap schedule, delay it until after lunch.

Napping Too Late

If your child naps in the late afternoon, let's say from 4.00 to 6.00 p.m. each day, he may be unable to fall asleep until 10.00 or 11.00 p.m. If you try to make his bedtime earlier, you will likely face real struggles. Most families recognise the problem and make the nap earlier or shorter. If you want to move the nap significantly earlier – for instance, if your child is used to napping at 4.00 p.m. and you want him to nap at 1.00 or 2.00 p.m. – it will be easiest to make the change gradually. Move his nap time (and his bedtime, too, if it is later than it should be) ten or fifteen minutes earlier each day until he is sleeping at the desired times. If he still has a nap in the morning, you may need to move it earlier as well – if it occurs in the late morning – or, if he's old enough, eliminate it altogether in order to move the late-afternoon nap earlier. If his afternoon nap and his bedtime are both late, and he also wakes late in the morning, you will have to move all three earlier together (see 'Late (Delayed) Sleep Phase' in Chapter 10).

Prematurely Eliminated Naps and the Problem of Being Overtired

Since too much napping can make it difficult for a child to fall asleep at night or cause him to wake early in the morning, one might think that decreasing or eliminating naps will always lead to easier bedtimes and better sleep, but that is not necessarily the case. Simply making a child sleepy does not always make him sleep better – in fact, it may have the opposite effect, at least in the short run. Being overtired puts stress on a child; he is likely to become irritable and overactive, and his behaviour may worsen. In this state, children often have a hard time relaxing at bedtime: they may struggle against going to sleep and stay awake longer than they should. Even if an overtired child does fall asleep promptly, he may wake more often at night than a less tired child, and he is more likely to have sleep terrors and other partial arousals (see Chapter 13).

Gabriella, a two-and-a-half-year-old girl, refused to go to sleep until at least 10.00 p.m. Her parents told me that in the past she had been sleeping for several hours in the late afternoon every day, which was why she had been going to sleep so late to begin with, but they had cut out the nap in hopes of achieving an 8.00 bedtime. At that point several new problems had developed. Gabriella was still sleepy in the late afternoon: her parents had to work hard to keep her awake, and she was unhappy not to be allowed to go to sleep. If she happened to be in the car at the time, she would always fall asleep, and she would then be difficult to wake, so her parents could not enforce the new schedule consistently. Dinners were unpleasant because Gabriella was always irritable. After dinner, just when it was time for her to go to bed, she got her second wind: she became very energetic, and putting her to bed at 8.00 was impossible.

Gabriella's problem, when I saw her, was not that she didn't need much sleep, it was that she wasn't getting enough: she was overtired. She still needed an afternoon nap, but at a more appropriate hour than the naps that had been disrupting her bedtime. We restored the late nap she had been accustomed to but limited it to ninety minutes; after that we gradually shifted her nap time and bedtime earlier. Gabriella now naps for an hour and a half after lunch and goes to sleep for the night by 8.30 p.m. Now that she is getting the proper amount of sleep at the proper times, she has become much happier during the day and settles down easily at bedtime.

A younger child can develop a similar problem if his second nap is eliminated too soon. Even older children who no longer need a nap may have bedtime difficulties and disrupted sleep on nights when they go to bed overtired. As a general rule, if you wait until your child seems extremely sleepy before you put him to bed each night, you are probably waiting too long. That is particularly likely if his behaviour worsens near bedtime and if you have to wake him in the morning. Infants are often ready for bed at night before they look sleepy at all. Try moving your child gradually to an earlier bedtime, early enough that he won't become overtired but not so early that it takes him longer to fall asleep. That will make it easier to maintain a pleasant nightly bedtime ritual, and you may find that he sleeps better.

Interrupted Naps

Naps can be interrupted in many ways: a sibling comes home from school and makes noise; a child falls asleep at the babysitter's before being picked up and brought home; or (most commonly) a child falls asleep in the car but wakes as soon as the trip ends. If a nap is shortened only slightly, the interruption may make no difference. But problems can arise when the nap lasts long enough to prevent a return to sleep after the interruption but is still too short to meet the child's needs.

Some interruptions are easy to avoid. A sibling can play outside or watch a DVD until the other child finishes his sleep. A nap can also be started a little earlier so that the interruption won't cut it so short, or a little later so that it begins after the potential interruption. Alternatively, shortening the child's night-time sleep period by thirty to sixty minutes may increase his drive to sleep during the day enough that the interruption won't wake him at all. (For instance, even if he falls asleep at the babysitter's house, he may now be sleepy enough to tolerate the move home without waking.) This is not an ideal solution, but if his total sleep time is unchanged or even increased, it can be useful on a short-term basis.

Short naps in the car can be more challenging to solve. If your child falls asleep in the car, you certainly don't want to have to keep driving around for an hour just to let him complete his nap. If it's early in the day and he is asleep only very briefly, it may not interfere with his proper nap later in the day. But if he has been asleep for even ten minutes, he may not go back to sleep either straight away or later when he should be napping. The ideal solution would be to keep him from falling asleep in the first place; unfortunately, - it's very difficult to keep a child awake in the car anywhere near his nap time and drive safely at the same time. If someone can watch your child during your midday errand, it should avoid the problem. If not, then you may be able to move his nap earlier, so that he starts napping at home and either finishes before you have to leave or else goes back to sleep in the car. Moving the nap may require waking him earlier in the morning and perhaps putting him to bed earlier at night.

Naps can also be interrupted by hunger. A child who is put down for a nap before an upcoming feeding, rather than after it, may wake too early because he needs to eat. Feeding him before the nap may allow the nap to run longer.

Inconsistent Schedules

When a child's bedtime, wake-up time, nap times and mealtimes vary from day to day, children cannot develop the consistent internal rhythms that should control sleep and the rest of their daily cycles. On a biological level, these children's systems do not know when and how long they should be napping. You cannot give your child different nap times every day and not expect to have trouble. Before good nap patterns can emerge, you must set and enforce a consistent and regular schedule throughout the day and night.

Problems caused by inconsistent schedules and ways to deal with them are discussed in Chapter 11.

Drifting/Splitting Naps

When a child is still on a multiple-nap schedule, the timings and lengths of his naps can vary considerably from day to day even if he is being kept on a generally consistent schedule overall. So can the times when he falls asleep at night and wakes in the morning. If the child's sleep patterns are charted for several weeks, a pattern to the changing schedule may become apparent (see Figure 13 on page 279). For example, a 10.00 a.m. nap can split into two short naps close together; these two segments may then move a little further apart each day. The segment that moves earlier can eventually merge with the end of the night-time sleep in the morning, causing the child to wake later than usual for a day. The segment that moves later can likewise merge with the afternoon nap, which will then start earlier and last longer than usual that day. Or the final period of night-time sleep may break off from the end of the night, appearing first as an early waking followed by a very early nap; over a few days, this new nap may drift progressively later until it merges with the mid-morning nap. As a third example, part of an afternoon nap can split off and eventually merge into the beginning of the night-time sleep, leading to a temporarily early bedtime. It is also possible that the hours when a child goes to sleep at night and wakes in the morning will change little or not at all, even as naps shift round.

On Loan

ITEM(S)	DUE DATE
Solve your child's sleep	14 Mar 2018
0333 40277	

Your current loan(s): 1
Your current reservation(s): 0
Your current active request(s): 0

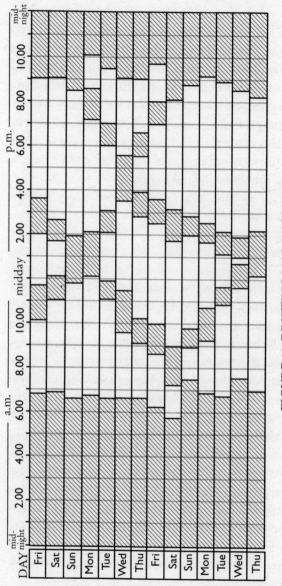

FIGURE 13. DRIFTING NAP PATTERNS

It is fascinating to see these patterns charted on paper, but not so fascinating to live with them. Although the rhythms controlling these drifts are complex, they are simple to control: all you have to do is to keep your child on a sufficiently regular nap schedule and avoid letting him pick different nap times each day. Remember, our biological rhythms work best when controlled by regular and predictable daily signals; they do not work as well when allowed to run freely.

Trouble Giving Up a Nap: Transition Problems

A three-year-old trying to give up napping altogether may nap on some days and not on others. Often that's not a problem; however, sometimes a child gets caught in the middle of the transition, making the days when he does not nap, or the nights after he does, very difficult. On the days when he is not sleepy enough to nap, he's not really able to go without the nap either, perhaps because he has not yet moved some of the lost sleep into the night. He regresses and becomes grumpy in the afternoon. He may manage to nap when circumstances are perfect – for example, if he happens to be in the car at the right time, or if he's required to lie down for rest time at day care, under pressure from peers and staff to lie quietly – but then if he does nap, he may not be sleepy at his usual bedtime at night and he might stay awake up to several hours later than he should.

Usually the transition lasts a matter of weeks. If it persists longer than that, you need to help it along. Cutting out the nap altogether is usually easier than reinstating it regularly. Try eliminating it completely for a week or two and see if your child is able to make the adjustment.

Once the transition period is over and the child has spent a few weeks consistently without napping, these difficulties will have vanished. He is still likely to have a low point around his former nap time, when he will not want to do much other than cuddle or sit on the sofa and watch a DVD for an hour. (If there is such a thing as a good time to let your child watch television or DVDs, this is it.) Don't expect much from him at this point in the day.

The same situation applies to younger children making the transition from two naps to one. Some children drop their afternoon nap but keep their remaining nap in the morning, instead of moving to a single nap after lunch; others nap sometimes in the morning and sometimes in the afternoon. The problems that result are described above in the sections on 'Napping Too Early' and 'Napping Too Late'. The solution is to progressively adjust the remaining nap time until it becomes an after-lunch nap, or, if the child is napping at inconsistent times, to enforce a single midday nap time.

Your child may be ready to give up a nap a little sooner than you expect. For example, say you have an eleven-month-old who still naps at 10.00 a.m. and 2.00 p.m., and one of the naps has become a challenge (not necessarily the same one every day): it takes you forty-five minutes to get him to sleep, and he sleeps for only thirty minutes. Since he is having trouble on a two-nap schedule, and since he should be giving up that second nap within a few months anyway, you might try putting him on a single nap after lunch and seeing if it's easier for both of you. If you feel that he is still too young to give up the second nap, you might try shortening his night-time sleep by thirty to sixty minutes so he can move some more sleep to the daytime.

NAP TIME SLEEP ASSOCIATION PROBLEMS

A child can associate the same kinds of activity with falling asleep at nap time as he does at night: being rocked, having his back rubbed, sucking on a dummy or drinking from a bottle (see Chapter 4). Usually nap time associations can be changed along with night-time ones. Sometimes habits apply only to naps – for example, falling asleep in the car. If your child is not ready to stop napping, you can change these habits without much trouble. As always, the key is to be consistent. For example, to teach your child to nap at home instead of in the car, or in the cot instead of in your arms, you must not allow him to fall asleep the way he's accustomed to for a while. Put him in his cot or bed at nap time. If he doesn't fall asleep in thirty minutes, declare the nap or 'quiet time' over and wait until the next nap time to try again. Do not then let him fall asleep in your arms, car or pram. But if, while waiting for the next nap time, he falls asleep on his own on the floor or sofa, at least he did so without his old habits being reinforced, so it's still a sign that he is learning to fall asleep without the old expectations. Don't let his bedtime or wake-up time change. He may not nap at all for a few days, but unless he needs less sleep than you think he does, the naps will come back.

You may find that you can get a nap started with your child alone in his cot, without the circumstances he's used to, but that he then wakes from the nap early in a grumpy mood. If you let him be, he cries and doesn't go back to sleep. If you provide the circumstances he wants – rock him, say – he will fall back to sleep, complete the nap and then wake up happy. If that doesn't take long, it may not bother you. But if he has to be rocked for a long time, or if it's inconvenient to rock him, it may be better to take him out of the cot when he wakes the first time and refuse to rock him back to sleep. Even if he is grumpy at first and his nap is shortened, at least he is learning not to expect to be rocked at that time. If he falls back to sleep while playing, so much the better, because he did it on his own. After a week or so he will probably start going back to sleep by himself in the cot. If not, he may begin to sleep a bit longer at night to compensate, and he should no longer wake in a bad mood.

Napping (or Not) at Home and at Day Care

Children commonly nap at day care or nursery school three to five times a week and are expected to nap at home on the other days. Many children handle the day-to-day difference without trouble. However, a child who always naps at day care may still refuse to nap at home. Even that may not be a problem unless his behaviour deteriorates when he doesn't nap. Usually this child is at least three years old, possibly old enough to give up the nap altogether. He might have an easier time on a schedule with no naps at all than on one that changes from day to day, if that is an option at his day care or nursery school. If it's not, then this problem – an extended version of a transition problem associated with the giving up of a nap, as described above – may just take some time to resolve. Instead of trying to force your child to nap at home, insist only on a 'quiet time' (a story, listening to music, watching a DVD, quiet play). Thus no demands will be made of him at the low point of his day, and without the stress of fighting over a nap, some days he may even fall asleep.

A child who has completely given up naps may have trouble if he is required to lie down at day care with his peers. Most day care centres handle this situation appropriately: typically all the children lie down, but after about fifteen minutes, children who are still awake or have already woken up are allowed to get up and enjoy a quiet activity. However, some centres require all children to lie down for an hour or more even if they don't sleep at all. That is not a good idea: it's unkind to make a child lie awake for an hour each day with nothing to do. (It may be nice for the day care providers, but certainly not for the children.) If that's the practice at your day care centre, speak to the workers. If they are unwilling to reconsider, you may want to look for other care.

YOU MAY HAVE TO ACCEPT WHAT WORKS

Even some children who love going to bed at night resist going to their room at nap time. You may never win this battle. If you keep it up, your child may start to dislike his room so much that you will begin having trouble at night as well. If he will nap under other conditions that are both practical and suitable, such as in the living room listening to a story or watching a DVD – *not* sitting in a parked car with the motor running – then you are probably better off leaving well enough alone and going with what works.

PART IV

INTERRUPTIONS DURING SLEEP

CHAPTER 13

Partial Wakings:
Sleep-Talking, Sleepwalking,
Confusional Arousals
and Sleep Terrors

I. What They Are and
Why They Happen

Marcy, aged four, often moaned, babbled semi-coherently and moved about her bed restlessly about two hours after falling asleep, but she always went back to sleep on her own after a few minutes. Lisa, eighteen months old, was a happy baby; yet every night, a few hours after falling asleep, she began crying and rolling about in her cot, seemingly unable to be comforted. Noah, nearly three, would sleep peacefully for two or three hours and then begin thrashing about and yelling bizarrely, calming down only after fifteen to twenty minutes. Christopher began to walk in his sleep at age six, quietly and calmly, with a blank expression on his face; by the age of eight, he had also begun sitting up in bed and screaming in apparent fright. Maria, a twelve-year-old, jumped out of bed and ran round her room or thrashed frantically on the floor. David, seventeen, would suddenly leap out of bed after two or three hours and run around as if terrified, so wildly that he actually injured himself.

Despite the apparent differences in their behaviours at night, all of these children were experiencing variations of the same kind of event: incomplete wakings from deep, *dreamless* non-REM sleep. The characteristics and significance of such arousals vary with age and certain physiological, behavioural, habitual and psychological factors. While sleep-talking (like Marcy's) is so common that it can hardly be considered abnormal or even a problem, the less common phenomenon of sleepwalking has always been seen as a disorder, worrisome to parents and fascinating to sleep specialists and poets. Sleep terrors – episodes like those exhibited by David – are perhaps the most dramatic of all sleep disorders; they are certainly the most frightening to family members who witness them. Most people know little about sleep terrors, even though they are fairly common. Less intense than sleep terrors, but even more common and often longer in duration, are confusional arousals, which take the form of periods of confused thrashing (like Noah's) and can appear equally frightening.

We will return to these children and their stories at the end of the chapter – once we've explained the nature of partial wakings like theirs – and then discuss how each child was treated.

Parents often misinterpret these partial wakings, or 'confusional events', as bad dreams or even as epileptic seizures. In fact, not only are they unrelated to dreams and seizures (see Chapter 14 for more information on distinguishing confusional events from nightmares), but they are also quite different from full wakings and call for a different response from the parent, at least during the event itself. In a typical full waking, a child might ask for a dummy or a back rub; if that behaviour becomes a problem, the appropriate response is usually to set limits and teach the child new habits and expectations. By contrast, a child experiencing a confusional event is not truly awake or fully conscious of her actions. Firm parental responses during the event will be of no benefit: there is no point in enforcing limits on a child who is unaware that limits are being set. (If the child wakes fully afterwards, then the confusional event is over, and parents may handle problems at this time as they would at any other night-time waking.)

Thus, the causes and treatments of the sleep problems discussed in this chapter often differ from those involved with habits, associations, limits and fears. Surprisingly, however, there is also sometimes a considerable overlap: what happens during a child's full wakings may actually be responsible for some of her partial wakings, or the full and partial wakings may have similar causes, and in these cases they ultimately require similar treatments.

The Normal Transition from Deep (Stage IV) Sleep Towards Waking

We know with certainty that episodes like those described in this chapter could not possibly occur during dreams. Because of the near-paralysis of REM sleep, you cannot sit up, thrash about, walk, scream, run round or otherwise act out your dreams; instead you remain safely in bed. But in non-REM sleep you can move, and in fact you usually do, at least a little bit, especially during the transitions between sleep cycles. Ordinarily these movements are minor and brief, but even when they are more dramatic, violent or extended, they are still examples of the same phenomenon. Thrashing, sleepwalking and screaming are closely related to the quieter behaviours that occur normally at the end of a period of deep sleep – they are just more intense, complex and long-lasting.

Stage IV is the deepest stage of sleep. In this state the body is on auto-pilot, with heart rate, respiration and other functions controlled in a stable and regular manner. People wakened from Stage IV report no dreams and have little or no memory of ongoing thoughts. Generally it is difficult to wake someone from this stage, even with words ('Fire!' 'Help!') or noises (crying, crashes) that will produce a swift, powerful reaction in just about any other state. This is particularly true for children, who often can't be wakened from Stage IV sleep even with vigorous stimulation. As we saw in Chapter 2, a child who has fallen deeply asleep in the car or at a neighbour's house can often be carried back home, undressed and put to bed with only a slight arousal and no memory of being moved.

As you will also recall from Chapter 2, sleep begins with a descent into Stage IV. This transition happens rapidly in children, more gradually in adults. At the end of the first sleep cycle, usually sixty to ninety minutes after falling asleep, the sleeper shifts to a lighter stage of sleep and perhaps even wakes briefly. In children, this arousal is usually followed quickly by another rapid descent into Stage IV sleep as the second sleep cycle begins (adults may have a brief and unremarkable dream first). The second sleep cycle ends much like the first, and the rest of the night is mostly spent alternating between lighter non-REM and REM sleep. Before waking for good in the morning, children often descend once more into Stage III or Stage IV sleep; although deep, this sleep is still easier to wake from than are the Stage IV periods earlier in the night.

The transition from deep Stage IV sleep back towards waking begins suddenly. Even when we observe a child in the laboratory, we see no indication that a change in state is about to occur. Suddenly and without warning, the child moves. She may turn over in bed, and often she will briefly open and close her eyes before descending again into deeper sleep and beginning the next sleep cycle. Typically she won't wake completely, and if she does, the waking will be brief and the child will not become fully alert. During the transition out of deep sleep, the child's brain waves show a mixture of patterns including some from deep sleep, some more specific to the transition towards waking itself, and even some from the drowsy and waking states.

Although the state transition starts suddenly, the full change from one state to the next takes time to complete, especially in children. During this transitional phase, a child is in a state of partial waking, somewhere between deep sleep and full waking, with some of the characteristics of both. Usually this phase is brief: the child wakes slightly, turns over, pulls up the blanket and goes back to sleep with little or no awareness of waking or nearly waking. But sometimes it does not go so smoothly. She may begin to wake, then start to walk, thrash, scream or run. It is these 'confusional events' that parents so often find alarming.

MORE INTENSE TRANSITIONS: A SPECTRUM OF CONFUSIONAL EVENTS

Confusional events happen most frequently at the end of the first or second sleep cycle, between one and four hours after falling asleep. They always occur during a partial waking from non-REM sleep. Most of these episodes – certainly the more intense and long-lasting ones – arise from Stage IV, but mild episodes in young children can arise out of lighter sleep, even from Stage II, which is still fairly deep sleep throughout the toddler years.

In young children, up to age five or six, confusional events are so common that most are typically considered 'developmental', meaning that the events only reflect the normal maturation of a child's sleep systems. Probably all toddlers at least occasionally have fairly intense episodes. It is hard to be sure how often these events occur because their characteristics are so varied, and because they probably often go unrecognised in children that young (particularly if the events are mild or brief, with only a few minutes of confused restlessness or perhaps a single momentary shout).

Although all the confusional events discussed here usually end with a quick return to sleep, they sometimes recur only a little while later. Several confusional events can follow in succession, separated by a mere few minutes of sleep, before calm, sustained sleep finally returns.

In a very mild period of confusion, a child may moan, mumble incomprehensibly and move about restlessly for several minutes, as Marcy did each night. She may also lift her head, grind her teeth and even sit up briefly and look about in a confused manner before returning to sleep. Most sleep talking occurs during this kind of mild partial non-REM arousal rather than during a dream.

If the arousal is a bit more intense (see Figure 14 on page 295), there may be an episode of calm sleepwalking: your child may begin to crawl about the bed as if in search of something, or she may even get out of bed and walk around quietly. Although her eyes are open and she can make her way round the room or house, she has little actual awareness of the world about her. She may come to you, wherever you are, but she probably won't seem to recognise you. She may stop and stare, but 'through' you, not at you. She may seem to be looking for something, and she may mumble phrases that are difficult to understand. She may walk downstairs and even try to leave the house. If she is very calm, she may respond to simple questions ('Are you okay?') with one-word answers. If you tell her to go back to bed she may comply on her own, or she may let you guide her back to bed. Once back in bed, younger children usually return to sleep without ever becoming completely awake. Older children and adolescents may become alert briefly – possibly to their embarrassment, if they find themselves in unexpected places with people staring at them – but they, too, usually return to sleep promptly.

If an older child's partial arousal is still more pronounced, she may jump out of bed and hurry about the room or house. Perhaps she will feel along the wall for the doorway leading out of her bedroom, almost as if she can't see. She may appear upset, confused and disorientated, perhaps even frantic. She may yell alarming things, such as 'No, no! Stop it', but although she may seem very upset, she will not seem to be really terrified. During such episodes of agitated sleepwalking, your child is unlikely to respond to your questions. She will not recognise you, and if you try to hold her she will only become more upset and push you away. You won't be able to wake her, but after a period of usually not more than forty minutes (typically between five and twenty minutes) she'll calm down, wake briefly and go back to bed on her own or let you lead her there. She will remember little or nothing of the episode, and she certainly - won't report having had a dream.

Toddlers and young children are unlikely to sleepwalk in this agitated way, but the more intense of their confusional arousals can seem even stranger and are often quite frightening for parents.

If your child shows this kind of behaviour, she may moan, then begin to cry, sob or even scream. She may then thrash wildly about the bed with her eyes open and her heart pounding. These disturbances can continue as long as forty minutes, even an hour on rare occasions. The thrashing and rolling may be unlike anything you have ever seen her do during the day or in her other night-time wakings. You might think at first that she is having (or has just awakened from) a bad dream, but she doesn't calm down when you enter the room and she might even seem unaware that you're there. She isn't comforted when you try to hold her, and she may arch, twist and push you away. If you try to wake her by shaking her or putting cold water on her face, the thrashing may only get worse. Many parents say that during these episodes their child seems 'possessed', because of her strange facial expression, wild thrashing and unresponsiveness to their attempts to help. Some parents become so alarmed, perhaps believing their child is very ill or possibly having a seizure, that they rush their child to hospital, only to have the episode end before they get there.

These episodes of screaming and thrashing are commonly referred to as 'night terrors' or 'sleep terrors' by families and some GPs. But since the child does not really appear terrified so much as agitated, confused and upset during these episodes, the term 'confusional arousal' is more appropriate. The label 'sleep terrors' should be reserved for those even more intense events where the child appears and acts extremely frightened, as described below.

As the confusional arousal nears its end, your child will most likely stretch, yawn and lie down again or let you tuck her back into bed. If she wakes more fully at this point, she will be perfectly calm and will just want to go back to sleep, which she will do quickly if you don't insist on keeping her awake. She will have no memory of the episode, either then or when she wakes in the morning. If she does wake fully when the event ends, she will, of course, not remember dreaming. *You* may be upset, but she will be fine.

Infants at least as young as six months of age can experience similar partial wakings in the form of long periods of crying during which they cannot be comforted or calmed. These episodes don't seem so strange to parents, partly because any thrashing is less intense than it would be in an older child, and partly because they are difficult to tell apart from the occasional periods of uncontrollable wakeful crying that are commonplace in infants. Many parents simply assume their baby has had a bad dream. It's an easy mistake to make, especially if the child is too young to say otherwise.

An interesting variant sometimes seen in toddlers and school-aged children resembles a temper tantrum. It is not, of course, a real tantrum (since those begin when a child is awake), and it may well occur even in children who are not prone to temper tantrums in the daytime. Once such an event is under way, however, it may be difficult to distinguish from a waking tantrum. Your child may stomp about angrily, seeming upset and confused, and run away from you. She may make demands, but she will seem unsure of what she wants; for instance, she might request an object and then throw it away as soon as you give it to her. These events last from ten to forty-five minutes before ending as peacefully as the other kinds of partial wakings.

The most pronounced confusional events, less common but more intense than those we've covered so far, are the aforementioned 'sleep terrors'. These arousals occur most often in adolescents and preadolescents, although younger children can have episodes with many of the same features. Generally, a full sleep terror event, unlike a more typical confusional arousal, starts very suddenly without a gradual build-up. The child lets out a bloodcurdling scream and sits bolt upright in bed. She is sweating and her heart is racing, as in a confusional arousal, but in this case she looks truly terrified. She may yell phrases that suggest fear or danger: 'It's gonna get me!', 'Leave me alone!', 'Stop it!', or, most commonly (as in confusional arousals), 'No! No!' These episodes often end within one to five minutes, without the extended thrashing shown by younger children; afterwards, the child wakes briefly and quickly returns to sleep. If she wakes fully, she is unlikely to remember anything frightening, although she might report a vague memory that may or may not fit the words she uttered during the episode itself. She might say,

FIGURE 14.
SPECTRUM OF BEHAVIOUR IN CHILDREN AT THE END
OF A PERIOD OF STAGE IV SLEEP

Listed in order of increasing intensity *

Normal termination of Stage IV (brief body movements; perhaps eye-opening, mumbling, chewing)

Sleep-talking

Calmly sitting up in bed, looking about, blank expression

Calm sleepwalking (semi-purposeful; child may appear to be looking for something and/or may walk towards parents or light; actions may seem to be aimed at fulfilling a need such as hunger or the urge to urinate)

Agitated sleepwalking (confused, jumpy and upset; child appears to be trying to get out of the room or away from something)

Confusional arousal (extended period of confused wild thrashing, moaning, yelling, kicking, screaming; may be prolonged, child may act bizarrely or seem 'possessed')

Sleep terror (screaming with appearance of fear or panic; child may leap out of bed and run wildly, as if away from something; increased chance of accidental injury)

---

* *The confusional arousal, common in young children, does not fit neatly into one place in this table, since it has its own severity spectrum and can vary from mild to intense and from brief to long-lasting, with the child anywhere from semi-responsive to completely unresponsive.*

'Something was going to get me', but she will not be able to describe the memory in any of the detail that you would expect if she had actually been dreaming.

In the most extreme sleep terrors, which are fortunately quite rare, a child may jump out of bed and run wildly, as if trying to get away from someone or something. She appears to be in a real panic. She may knock over furniture or even people, break lamps or windows or fall and injure herself. This phase usually lasts less than a minute, though the child may remain confused for some minutes longer.

What a Confusional Event Feels Like

When you watch a confusional event unfold, you are seeing the simultaneous functioning of your child's waking and sleep systems. The waking system is trying to activate, and the sleep system does not 'want' to yield control. Both processes are going on at the same time, so the child shows elements both of being awake and of being asleep at the same time.

This phenomenon is not really as strange as it may seem at first. Consider a similar event in a more familiar context: suppose that an hour after you fall asleep you are awakened by a loud crash. You 'wake up' instantly, your heart racing, but for a few seconds you will still be partially asleep and not thinking clearly, unable to figure out what's happening or whether you need to do anything. The feeling of those first few seconds, in which you are agitated but still confused and not fully alert, is probably more or less what children experience during a confusional arousal or sleep terror. (However, you will be closer to full waking than your child is during a real confusional event, so there are differences: you might be genuinely frightened; your behaviour, while possibly comical, won't be truly bizarre; and you will probably remember the episode in the morning.)

To take a milder example, suppose you set an alarm to wake you in the middle of the night to give your child medicine. When the alarm goes off, you get up and automatically walk into the bathroom, but instead of getting the medicine, you use the toilet, start to return to your bedroom and then stop, vaguely aware that there's something else you're supposed to be doing. If somebody were watching you at this point, they would see you look about with a blank or dazed expression, unsure what you are looking for, where to look or why you are even out of bed in the first place. This experience is probably similar to what a child experiences during a quiet sleepwalking episode.

Adults don't ordinarily have true confusional events, largely because their Stage IV sleep is lighter than a child's, so they wake more easily in the middle of the night. But in each of these examples, if it was more difficult than normal for you to wake up – perhaps because you hadn't slept the night before, or because you had taken a sleeping pill or had some alcohol before bed – the loud noise could conceivably trigger a full confusional event: that is, you might behave especially bizarrely and might not remember the event in the morning.

WHY CONFUSIONAL EVENTS HAPPEN: THE BALANCE BETWEEN SLEEP AND WAKING

Given the confused and often upset appearance of a child during a confusional event, it would be easy to assume that scary thoughts of some sort were the cause. In fact, some theories, particularly from the older psychoanalytic literature, maintain that the initial cause of confusional events is a frightening idea, urge or image that suddenly intrudes into 'consciousness' during the deep sleep state, when the child's emotional defences are down, and that the thought triggers the arousal. These theories broadly explain the appearance of a sleep terror, but they have some serious weaknesses. They do not explain how such thoughts can appear in nondreaming sleep. They do not explain why a sleep terror can be triggered by a common, unthreatening sound or why most confusional events are mild and have no appearance of terror. They do not explain why spontaneous confusional events arise near the end of a deep sleep phase, rather than in the middle. And, most importantly, they do not explain why (unlike after a nightmare) the child has no terrifying memory upon awakening fully, only a desire to go back to sleep. (Supporters of these theories may argue that there was a momentarily frightening thought at the onset, but one that then was immediately forgotten. However, evidence based on studies of sleep terrors induced by external stimuli suggests that this possibility is extremely unlikely.)

Actually, all the characteristics of confusional events can be more easily explained if they are viewed as primarily physiological events that just produce the physical appearance of agitation, and (sometimes) even of terror, without any preceding or accompanying scary thoughts. The physiological changes that create this appearance of upset (increased heart rate and blood pressure, bulging eyes, perhaps even screaming) are responses to activity generated deep in the nervous system, without any conscious emotion or thought being involved. That explains why in less intense confusional events such as calm sleepwalking there is often no appearance of fear at all. It also explains why confusional events typically occur when the first or second sleep cycle is coming to an end (when an arousal is due anyway), why the child doesn't remember any clear thoughts when she finally wakes, and why she no longer seems afraid or upset as the event ends, the transition towards waking is completed and bodily functions return to normal.

To understand why confusional events occur at all, the most important thing to remember is that partial wakings are a normal, inherent part of the way our sleep systems function. Everyone has these partial arousals several times every night – specifically, periods of semiwaking confusion that occur at the end of each cycle of deep non-REM sleep – though ordinarily they consist only of brief movements without vocalisations. Confusional events occur when these partial wakings don't go smoothly. Even the most dramatic episodes are only exaggerations of normal behaviour.

As you remember from Chapter 9, the main factors controlling sleepiness and alertness are homeostatic (based on how long you've been awake or asleep) and circadian (based on the current time and the setting of your biological clock). These factors can be strengthened, weakened or otherwise modulated by other important biological factors, as well as by various environmental and psychological ones. Understanding how these factors interact is key to understanding why confusional events, rather than normal partial wakings, sometimes occur.

What a child does when waking from sleep is determined by the activity of her sleep and wake systems at that time. Partly, that depends on what kind of sleep she is waking from – deep or light, REM or non-REM. It also depends on the relative strengths of her drive to sleep and her drive to wake: that is, how sleepy she is at the time of the arousal, how strong the arousal signals are (whether generated internally or externally) and how urgently she feels she must wake.

It may seem strange to talk about a child's drive to sleep or how 'sleepy' she is when she's already asleep, but in fact the drive to sleep waxes and wanes during sleep just as it does during the waking hours. During the day this drive affects how easily you can fall asleep; at night, it affects how hard it would be to wake you up. While you sleep, the strength of this drive depends on several things: how long you were awake before bed, how long you have been asleep, how well you have been sleeping, how sleep-deprived you are, what drugs or medication you have taken and where your biological clock is in its daily cycle. The drive is particularly strong early in the night, after you have been up all day and before you have had a chance to sleep very long.

While you sleep, there are also forces that push you towards waking up, which I refer to collectively as the 'drive to wake'. This drive can be strong or weak at different times, depending on (again) where your biological clock is in its cycle, as well as on levels of external stimulation and psychological factors. In the morning and at the end of each sleep cycle, internal signals from your biological clock strengthen the drive to wake. External stimulation (an alarm clock or someone shaking you, for example) also strengthens the drive to wake, and the more intense the stimulation is (the louder the alarm clock, or the more vigorous the shaking), the greater its effect. The meaning you give to the stimulus makes a difference: a cry of 'Fire!' will probably affect you more strongly than 'It's your turn to feed the baby'. The drive to wake also increases if you have some important reason to wake up – to check on your child in the middle of the night, say, or to get to work on time in the morning.

When there is a proper balance among the forces controlling sleep and waking, you will sleep well at night, move smoothly from one sleep cycle to the next, wake easily in the morning and generally be alert during the day. During deep (Stage IV) sleep early in the night, your drive to sleep should be strong and your drive to wake should be weak, so that your sleep will be uninterrupted. Towards morning, when your sleep is lighter, the drive to sleep should be weaker and the drive to wake should be stronger, making it easy for you to wake up. But if the balance is not as it should be – if one of these drives is strong when it should be weak, or weak when it should be strong, or if your sleep is light when it should be deep, or deep when it should be light – you can be left awake and unable to sleep soundly (insomnia) or asleep and unable to wake fully. The latter is, as we will see, the condition in which confusional events occur: that is, when a child is strongly driven to stay asleep and to wake up at the same time.

At the end of a cycle of light sleep (Stage II, or REM), it's relatively easy for a child to wake up, so confusional events at these times are unlikely. But consider what happens at the natural arousal that follows a cycle of deep (Stage IV) sleep. Since these cycles tend to come early in the night when the child hasn't been asleep for very long yet, her drive to sleep will be strong. If her drive to wake is weak at that moment, as it should be, she will move quietly into the next sleep cycle, stirring, perhaps, but hardly waking, and all will be well. But if the drive to wake is strong for some reason, then her waking and sleeping systems will fight for control: she will struggle to emerge from sleep but won't be able to wake completely. The same thing can happen if something disturbs her in the middle of a deep sleep cycle. In either case, confusional events become much more likely.

Understanding how these forces work is the key to finding the causes of a child's confusional events: we look for things that affect the depth of her sleep, her need or drive to sleep and her drive to wake up. When a child receives a signal to wake up – typically the internal signal that comes at the end of a sleep cycle, but possibly an external one, such as a noise or someone touching her – then anything that deepens her sleep or strengthens her drive to sleep will make it harder for her to wake fully, increasing the chances of a confusional event. Similarly, when her sleep is deep and her drive to sleep is strong, anything that strengthens her drive to wake will also make confusional events more likely.

A variety of factors influence the depth of sleep and the drives to stay asleep and wake. Some of them can affect both drives, even simultaneously. Let's look each of these factors in turn.

Factors That Make Sleep Deeper and Strengthen the Drive to Stay Asleep

Developmental Factors

The fact that young children naturally sleep very deeply explains why confusional events are so common among them. Their Stage IV non-REM sleep is deeper than that of older children, and much deeper than that of adults. For that reason alone, even when the normal internal mechanisms that trigger an arousal at the end of a cycle of deep sleep are strong, they sometimes fail to entirely break the grip of the sleep state, leaving the child half-asleep and half-awake.

Being Overtired or Behind in Sleep

In a young child who experiences confusional arousals only occasionally, the best predictor of such episodes is whether the child is overtired, and, if so, how badly. The cause could be an early waking, a missed nap or a late bedtime; increased daytime activity and inappropriate schedules can lead to overtiredness, too. When young children are overtired, their sleep drive, already strong at the start of the night, is strengthened further: sleep is less 'willing' to give way to wakefulness, and wakefulness less able to wrest control back from sleep.

Factors That Strengthen the Drive to Wake

A Job to Do

Ordinarily, when we wake slightly between sleep cycles, there is no reason for us to wake up all the way or for any length of time. We need only get back into a comfortable position, adjust the pillow and blanket and return to sleep. But if there's anything else we need to do first – such as check the environment for unwanted changes, re-establish the conditions we associate with falling asleep or get control of our thoughts and emotions – we may have to wake completely to take care of it; thus the drive to wake is strengthened, and confusional events become more likely. Children are particularly prone to this problem.

This concept, of having a 'job' to do causing an increased effort to wake, is so important in understanding and treating confusional events in children that we will return to it in more detail shortly.

Sensory Stimulation

Noises, lights and other kinds of sensory stimulation can easily strengthen the drive to wake, since they signal a change in the environment that might warrant investigation. If they disturb a child during or at the end of a period of Stage IV sleep, the additional drive to wake up can lead to a confusional event – in the laboratory, a loud buzzer set off an hour after sleep begins can trigger a sleep terror in susceptible children. Lower levels of stimulation can have the same effect at home: your child may sit up and scream when you make noise climbing the stairs, for instance, or if you cover her with a blanket near the end of her cycle of deep sleep. Even children who don't ordinarily sleepwalk often can be induced to do so at the end of a Stage IV period simply by lifting them up and setting them on their feet.

Factors That Can Strengthen Either Drive

Inconsistent and Chaotic Sleep/Wake Schedules

The drives to stay asleep and to wake are controlled in large part by our biological rhythms (see Chapter 9). When we travel, jet lag can cause our bodies to get confused: these rhythms are no longer rising and falling together at predictable times, and the relative timing of the sleep and wake drives may be affected. As a result, our bodies get mixed messages from different physiological systems, some saying to wake and others saying to sleep.

The same thing can happen to a child on a variable schedule. As a cause of partial wakings at night, this phenomenon is particularly important in young children. Day-to-day changes in bedtimes, waking times or the number or timing of naps can throw a child's underlying biological rhythms out of sync. Her drive to wake may be increased at a time when she should be sleeping, or her drive to sleep may be increased when she should be awake. Thus, for example, the internal signal to wake and end the night's first sleep cycle may come before that cycle is really done – while the drive to sleep is still very strong – and a confusional event becomes more likely.

Sleep Disruption, Illness and Medication

Illness and medication affect the waking and sleeping drives in complex ways. Many illnesses, and the side effects of some medications, directly affect the body in ways that increase sleepiness. On the other hand, the side effects of other medications stimulate the drive to wake up, and some illnesses and sleep disorders (like sleep apnoea) do the same, either directly or by causing pain or discomfort that wakes the child. (For instance, an ill child may wake at night because of throat pain or a dry mouth.) This extra tendency

towards waking leaves a child's sleep disrupted, broken or fragmented, and that loss of sleep in turn increases her drive to sleep as
well. Not surprisingly, some children experience confusional events
only when running a fever, when ill (with or without a fever) or
when taking medication that affects sleep or the ability to wake.

Other Causes of Confusional Events

Inherited Characteristics

Some children who experience confusional events at night have
close relatives with a similar history. We do not know what traits
these children inherited; it may be that family members simply tend
to sleep more deeply than most, or that they have a stronger inherent
biological drive to wake between sleep cycles. In some children, inherited characteristics by themselves appear to account completely
for the confusional events. In others, they may only be predisposing
factors. These characteristics might explain why only some children
with jobs to do during the night walk, thrash, talk or yell in their
sleep. Genetic factors may also partially determine the specific type
of arousal shown by a child – that is, where on the spectrum of intensity they occur, from sleep-talking to terrors.

Other Biological Factors

In a small group of children, frequent arousal events persist at
night even after we have dealt with all identifiable causes. In some of
these youngsters non-REM sleep is continually broken by small
arousals that are identifiable only with special monitoring, like that
done during an overnight study in a sleep laboratory. (You would
not see them just by watching your child sleep at home.) These children's sleep patterns seem to be inherently unstable, although we do
not yet know the biological factors responsible. Although their
night-time arousals may be resistant to behavioural treatments, they
still usually respond well to medication.

The Significance of Having a Job to Do at Night

The problems facing a child with a 'job' to do at night should be largely familiar to you from the chapters on associations, feedings, limits and fears. For example, if a child starting to wake after a sleep cycle finds that the conditions associated with falling asleep have changed, or she has learned that they frequently do, she will try to wake fully to check and, if necessary, to try to get the previous conditions re-established. She may find she is in a different room, that her parents are no longer sitting on her bed, that the rocking has stopped or the dummy fallen out or that it is time for her to change to another bed. If she starts to wake during the night at a time when she is used to eating, she will try to wake fully to ask to be fed. If she spends an hour testing limits by repeatedly calling and coming out of her room before she falls asleep, she will pick up where she left off and start doing the same thing when she starts to wake.

In each of these scenarios, the child has a job of some kind to do – some situation that requires her full attention – and she must wake up to do it. She can't simply slide into the next sleep cycle after a brief brush with the waking state, as she should. You may well have experienced this kind of thing yourself: if you have to get up early but your alarm clock is broken, for instance, you may find that you awaken completely several times during the night to check the time, whereas ordinarily you would just stir slightly and go right back to sleep. Having jobs to do during the night is not good for sleep. They greatly strengthen a child's drive to wake and, as we've seen, that may lead to confusional events.

Consider a child who will only go to sleep at bedtime if her father is sitting in the room. Instead of falling asleep quickly, she keeps checking to be sure he is still there and to go and find him if he isn't. Suppose she wakes every night at 2.00 a.m., checks for her father and, finding him gone, goes after him; then she gets into her parents' bed, where she sleeps the rest of the night. She can switch rooms without trouble because at that hour she is waking from fairly light sleep.

Now suppose that one night she tries to do the same thing when she starts to wake at the end of her first sleep cycle, at 11.00 a.m., after only two hours of sleep. The pattern of room switching may have become so automatic that she tries to leave her bed and head for her parents' room before she is fully awake. Her habitual response is to try to become more alert and switch rooms – that is, her drive to wake is strong. But at this time of night her sleep is very deep, much deeper than at her usual 2.00 waking. It may be so deep that she cannot wake fully enough even to realise why she is struggling to get up. The conflict between her waking and sleeping systems produces a partial arousal, a confusional event.

Exactly what she does may depend upon the strength of the sleep system when she tries to wake. If she is almost able to wake, she may still get to her parents' room, but now by walking in her sleep. It may be even be hard to tell if she is asleep but almost awake, or awake but almost asleep (although this distinction is probably meaningless anyway, since in both cases sleep and wake systems are active simultaneously). If the balance is closer to sleep, she may remain in bed but cry and thrash about; or, she may be able to get out of bed and sleepwalk, but in an upset or very confused manner, heading off in the wrong direction. She is too asleep to know why she is trying to get up. If she did not have this job to do during the night, she would simply slide back into sleep and the confusional event would not happen.

As this example illustrates, confusional events commonly occur only at a child's first or second waking at night; later in the night she will be waking from lighter sleep, so those wakings are likely to be more complete. However, patterns and habits learned at these later, fuller wakings, like this girl's need to check for her father, or another child's habit of calling to have her back rubbed, are often behind the confusional arousals that occur earlier in the night, especially in toddlers and young children of school age. In these situations, a single problem (that of improper behaviour patterns and habits) shows up in different ways at different times of night: as full wakings with specific requests or demands in the middle and end of the night, and as confusional events early on.

At the end of a confusional event triggered in this way, the child's job remains undone, so it is not uncommon for both types of behaviour to appear in a single waking. The waking starts as a confusional event – recognisable because the child's thrashing about seems to have no purpose, and because she doesn't respond well to attempts to help – but when she wakes at the end of the episode, she does not go right back to sleep, as most children do after even intense events. Instead, because she still has the job to do, she may force herself into fuller alertness. From that point forward she is completely awake, and her behaviour may now clearly reflect learned habits and associations of the kind discussed in earlier chapters.

The specific jobs a child can have to do at night vary with age and with factors such as sleeping arrangements, patterns of parental response, recent events and current concerns. School-aged children typically have different jobs to do than do toddlers. An eight-year-old child who is trying not to wet the bed may have a strong impulse to wake fully, get up and use the toilet each time she stirs. And a ten-year-old girl who frequently hears her parents fighting at night may feel the need to wake and listen to be sure they are okay. Also, an older child who is frequently carried to bed after falling asleep in the living room may need to check which room she is in each time she starts to wake – in the same way that a toddler often must do.

Once a behaviour pattern of this sort has been established, it can persist out of habit in sleep even after it ceases to serve a purpose and is no longer reinforced by full waking behaviour. A child who no longer moves to her parents' room at night when she is fully awake may still walk there (or elsewhere) in her sleep, effectively on automatic pilot. In a sense, this habit still functions as a job to do, even though the job no longer really needs doing – she just can't wake fully enough to remember that.

During middle childhood and into adolescence, children may develop another type of job to do at night, that of controlling their own urges and thoughts. Many people find it easy to keep unpleasant feelings in check during the day, when they are wide awake and fully alert, but not so easy when they are asleep and dreaming, drowsy and daydreaming or just waking up. As you wake from deep sleep, you are not in full control of your thoughts and behaviour. If, for any reason, it is important to you to re-gain control quickly, then you may try to become fully alert as soon as possible. As we have seen, that struggle can, at least in a child, be enough to trigger a confusional event.

For example, some children keep their behaviour carefully controlled during the day. When such well-behaved children start to wake at night, they may instinctively work to regain the self-control they gave up during sleep. This task requires the child's attention and effectively strengthens the drive to wake, which, in turn, also makes partial arousal events more likely.

(Such well-controlled children are typically pleasant to be with and easy for a teacher to have in class. This tendency towards control is often just a personality style, but it can become a problem if carried to excess. Some children, for example, choose to keep any feelings they might consider negative, such as anger, jealousy and guilt, inside and unexpressed. Others do so only in class, but feel freer to show their emotions at home. Most children put extra checks on their behaviour at the start of a school year, particularly if they have a new teacher; probably for this reason, confusional events are especially common in September and October. Interestingly, whereas school-aged children who frequently sleepwalk or have confusional arousals tend to be the well-behaved type, children with frequent nightmares are more likely to be ones who act out their feelings and have trouble controlling their behaviour during the day.)

Anxieties and other concerns may also be associated with a need for control and an attempt to wake fully during the night. If you go to sleep after lying awake for a long time troubled by anxieties, for example, you may wake fully and start worrying again whenever you stir at night, instead of just turning over and returning to sleep. Similarly, if an anxious child lies in bed frightened for a long time at bedtime, struggling to avoid certain thoughts or behaviours as she goes to sleep, she may try to wake fully enough to get the same control over those thoughts and actions whenever she stirs during the night. If this occurs on waking from deep sleep, then, despite her efforts, she may be unable to wake fully.

Children may also find themselves reacting to situations outside of their control: a move to a new neighbourhood, a transfer to a new school or especially a personal loss such as a divorce, separation or death in the family. Even an intact family can lack warmth, love and nurturance: parents may be rigid, demanding and uncompromising, setting unrealistically high expectations for their child's behaviour, school performance and athletic success. Older children in such situations are often angry, but, unlike most toddlers, they may choose to keep their anger locked up, probably in the belief that expressing their feelings would only lead to more unpleasantness. A child may blame herself for her parents' separation or for other family problems, and she may carefully avoid giving her parents any reason for displeasure. Such a child is likely to act extremely pleasant and well behaved – if anything, too well behaved. Occasionally her anger will show in passive ways that seem safer to her: she may stay in her room after school and keep silent at mealtimes, or she may not do as well in school as she could. She expends enormous quantities of energy during the day guarding her emotions and keeping them in check. But at night, in sleep, these defences must be relaxed. Whenever she starts to wake, she senses this loss of control and tries to wake more fully to get it back. This job can easily be enough to cause a confusional event.

To get a better idea of how a child's emotional state at bedtime can alter her reaction to a normal partial arousal, and turn a routine end-of-sleep-cycle waking into a confusional event, think about how your own state of mind can affect your reaction to a stimulus while you're awake. Imagine that you are nervously walking through an old cemetery alone on a dark night, when suddenly you hear a twig snap. You will probably jump or cry out in fear – you might even run away without ever learning whether there was really anything to be afraid of. If you heard the same twig break at home in the light of day, it might not startle you at all. But alone in the cemetery, you are already jumpy and on your guard: your state of mind determined your response to the noise.

The analogy isn't perfect, because in this example you are awake and (relatively) clear-headed. But the same idea applies during sleep.

If a twig breaks outside your window while you're comfortably asleep in your own bed, you probably won't be aware of it, and if it wakes you at all, you will not consider the noise important and you'll immediately return to sleep. But if for some reason you were sleeping in that cemetery, or on a battlefield where an attack could come at any time, the same sound of a snapping twig might awaken you instantly in a panic. Confused and terrified, you might jump up and even cry out (as a child having a sleep terror does). But it's not the noise of the twig that made you scream, or even finding yourself in the cemetery or on the battlefield, since you reacted before you had a chance to see or remember where you were. Rather, it was the anxieties that you went to sleep with in the first place that gave the snapping twig significance and caused you to have an increased need to wake to check to see that you were still safe. Going to sleep in the cemetery or on the battlefield, you knew you were letting down your guard in threatening surroundings, and as a result your drive to wake, and thus your response to the noise, is much greater. Your psychological state at the time of falling asleep made the difference.

The causes of calm sleepwalking are similar to those of sleep terrors, but the need to wake may not be so urgent. Think of going to sleep with the window open on a night when thunderstorms are predicted. If a storm starts, the sounds of thunder and rain – which ordinarily would barely interrupt your sleep – will trigger a strong impulse to wake up, but only because you knew the window was open. If you are deeply asleep at that moment, you won't be able to wake fully right away, and you may be too confused at first to remember what exactly you needed to do. For a short while, wandering about befuddled and unsure why you are up, you will be feeling something much like what your child feels when she walks in her sleep.

The same phenomenon is true for children. Any child who goes to bed at night knowing she will have to try to wake later because she has a 'job' to do, whether to check for change or danger or to complete a simple habit or task, may be prone to sleepwalking, confusional arousals and sleep terrors. The solution for these children is (if possible) to take away the jobs that are driving these children to wake up and to help them learn to relax their guard when they go to sleep so that they can take normal night-time arousals in stride. We will return to this idea later in this chapter when we consider treatment methods.

The Variability of Arousals over Time

The intensity of confusional events can be mild (restlessness, sleep-talking, mumbling), moderate (thrashing in bed, sleepwalking, yelling) or severe (wild screaming, appearance of panic or marked agitation, running). They can be very brief in duration (several minutes at most), short (five to twenty minutes) or long (up to an hour), and they can occur only occasionally (no more than once every few weeks), commonly (up to once a week) or frequently (several times per week, even nightly).

A child's night-time arousals may differ from night to night, month to month or year to year. They may progress in either direction along the continuum ranging from quiet arousals to major sleep terrors (Figure 14 on page 295), becoming either more or less severe. But day-to-day changes in a child's life can be subtle and difficult to recognise, and the occurrence and intensity of arousals may change from night to night without any apparent changes in the child's daytime activities or stresses; in fact, symptoms usually wax and wane over weeks and months without any evident psychological or physiological reasons. Therefore, it's not easy to predict on which nights a child's confusional events will occur based only on knowledge of what is currently happening in her life, even when that includes major events such as an upcoming exam, an operation, a football match or a separation from the family. (The main exception is that confusional events are much more common in toddlers when they are overtired.)

It's also possible for daytime changes to affect the pattern of confusional arousals in unexpected ways. For example, if your child's partial arousals are caused in part by a need to keep her thoughts and behaviour tightly controlled, then an apparent change for the worse in her daytime behaviour may actually be associated with a *reduction* in the frequency of these night-time arousals. Because she is allowing herself to express more of her feelings in the daytime, even if inappropriately, she might feel less of a need to guard against them at night.

EVALUATING CONFUSIONAL EVENTS: WHEN TO TAKE ACTION

In deciding how significant your child's partial wakings are and whether you should do anything about them, there are several factors to think about: your child's age; the frequency, length and intensity of the episodes; the extent to which they disrupt other family members' sleep, including yours; what social consequences they may have (at camp sleepovers, for example); the risk of injury; any identifiable triggers (such as being overtired or starting a new school year); and any self-imposed or external psychological stressors. As you evaluate your child's symptoms, consider the possible causes described in this chapter, but remember that you may well be unable to find a good explanation for any *particular* episode.

Without any treatment, the typical confusional arousals of a toddler will usually be outgrown by age five or six. Emotional factors are rarely the cause during these early years, but if they seem to be – for example, if the episodes' onset coincides with a significant event such as a divorce, a death in the family or a family member's hospitalisation – then you may want to consider professional consultation. However, other causes of partial wakings are more common at these ages (jobs to do at night, a regular schedule becoming irregular, being overtired), and these are most often straightforward to treat. When partial waking episodes begin in or persist into middle childhood or adolescence, their significance, causes and course may be different. For example, psychological style and other emotional factors are more likely to be relevant in an older child, especially if the partial waking events are frequent. Partial wakings with these causes usually can also be treated successfully; but, if left untreated, it's impossible to say when they will stop.

Events that are mild and brief are probably of little importance, even if they happen frequently, and they generally need no treatment. Even moderately intense events, regardless of whether they are short or long-lasting, are probably unimportant if they occur only occasionally. But moderately intense events that happen more frequently should be considered significant enough to at least consider treatment. So should more severe events, even if they happen only occasionally. You should also consider treating any events an older child finds embarrassing, particularly if social decisions – such as attending sleepovers and camp – are affected. Keep the context in mind: if confusional episodes happen only when your child is overtired or febrile, they are probably of little concern, especially if the child is young and the episodes are relatively mild. In older children, episodes that happen only at times of temporary anxiety, such as exams or the start of the school year, should probably not worry you either.

If the problem does appear to require treatment and you cannot solve it yourself, you should consult your GP. You should probably also discuss with your GP any events that are extremely frequent, very long-lasting or very intense, especially if they pose any danger to your child or other family members. Don't hesitate to contact your GP even if you are simply feeling uncertain or worried about what is happening.

In very rare cases, medical or neurological problems may be involved: for example, pain from heartburn or ear disease may be triggering the events, or seizures may be causing them or being mistaken for them. Be particularly suspicious and always seek medical advice if your child's episodes are significantly different in character from those described in this chapter – for example, if they occur near morning instead of closer to bedtime; if the episodes are always *exactly* the same; if your child wakes fully just before the beginning of the episode, rather than only at the end, and knows that something unpleasant is about to occur; if she clearly remembers the entire event or its beginning; if her body stiffens and consistently takes on an asymmetrical posture (such as with her left arm extended and her head turned to the left); or if her body jerks prominently and repetitively during the episodes.

Keep in mind that most normal toddlers occasionally have confusional arousals of varying intensity. It is not known how many children have extended thrashing spells, sleepwalking and full sleep terrors, but at least 15 per cent of all children sleepwalk at least once, and extended confusional arousals probably occur in far more children than that. Of course, the number of these children whose episodes are very frequent and intense is smaller, but occasional wild sleep terrors – where the child runs about in apparent panic – are by no means rare.

If your child is a toddler, you may want to see if you can eliminate her confusional events using the methods described below, even if the events are not particularly troublesome or worrisome; it is often easy to identify and treat the causes in toddlers. With older children, you need to consider psychological factors as well as the actual symptoms in deciding whether or not to seek treatment, but take care not to be too quick to ascribe a serious psychological significance to your child's particular night-time partial arousals. In a happy, socially active, academically successful youngster, the episodes may only reflect the child's style of controlled behaviour and thought, which is not necessarily a sign of trouble. If nothing else points to an ongoing problem, there is probably no need to seek psychological counselling. The best guide is to assess your child's psychological well-being in the daytime. If she is having emotional problems in general, she may benefit from psychological help, and if she is also sleepwalking or having sleep terrors at night, it may help with those, too. Bear in mind, however, that significant progress in psychotherapy may not produce an *immediate* improvement at night. Don't judge therapeutic success by, say, how far your child walks in her sleep at night.

As you judge your child's emotional condition, don't place too much weight on things she says while sleep-talking or during other confusional events. The things children say during agitated partial arousals – most commonly 'No, no!' – are automatic vocalisations triggered in low-level areas of the brain, not in the areas that control waking thought. Don't let them worry you: they do not reflect subconscious or deep-seated fears or urges. You can even ignore violent or alarming speech (such as 'Kill him!' or 'I want to die'), *if* she is mostly asleep when she says such things. Do, however, pay attention to what she says when awake. If she is truly depressed, anxious or suffering from another emotional disturbance, it will show in her waking life, not just when she's in a semi-waking confused state.

Because often neither parents nor children discuss these sleep episodes with friends, they are likely to think of the episodes (and the child herself) as strange or abnormal. You should recognise by now that these behaviours are, in fact, common, and that, even without help, preschoolers, at least, will probably outgrow them on their own.

II. Treatment

What You Should Do and What Else to Consider

Most treatment approaches used with young children are not only benign in themselves but also good sleep hygiene practices in general. Applying them is a good idea even if they don't entirely solve the problem of partial wakings

As you begin to determine what to do about your child's partial arousals, first try to identify any factors that make it harder for her to wake out of deep sleep or that make a full waking more urgent. Then eliminate these factors, if possible, or at least minimise them. Having done that, you will probably find that the arousals disappear or at least become milder, shorter and less frequent. Even if they continue, you have at least prepared the way for other techniques.

Depending upon your youngster's age and the details of her problem, you will likely need to use one or more of the following approaches. Specific techniques for dealing with many of these individual issues are also discussed in depth in other chapters.

General Advice

Ensure Adequate Sleep

As we saw earlier, an overtired child will have more, not fewer, partial arousals, because her increased need for deep sleep interferes with her ability to wake at the end of the first or second sleep cycle. For youngsters up to about age six, and sometimes older children as well, simply ensuring that the child gets enough sleep at night may be the only intervention needed. For children younger than three and a half or four years of age, continuing regular naps may be similarly important.

Keep to a Regular Schedule

Try to keep bedtimes and nap times consistent and predictable. That will allow your child's biological rhythms to stabilise and work in harmony so that the arousals at the end of the first and second sleep cycles will be timed appropriately, when deep sleep is 'ready' to give way to a lighter state.

Eliminate Night-time Jobs and Habits

Your child should have no need to wake fully between sleep cycles before going back to sleep. She should not have to call for something (to be rocked, have her back rubbed or get fed), look for something (a parent or a dummy), or check on her surroundings (to determine what room she is in, for instance). She should not have to get out of bed (to switch rooms, change beds, walk about or check that you are home). Methods to accomplish these changes are discussed in Chapters 4 through 7.

Provide a Pleasant Structured Bedtime; Avoid Bedtime Activities That Your Child May Try to Resume on Waking

When we wake during the night, we tend to feel and act as if it were still bedtime. If your child is occupied by any tasks at bedtime other than falling asleep, she may try to continue these activities as soon as she begins to wake up. Thus, it's important that bedtime be a happy time without demands and struggles. A child should not start the night by fighting to stay awake or testing limits; nor should she have to check that you are still rocking her and have not put her in bed or left the room. Otherwise, she will have an increased drive to wake up during the night.

Set an Appropriate Bedtime, Late Enough for Your Child to Fall Asleep Quickly

Setting bedtime at an appropriate time is important for the same reason. If a child has too much time to think, worry or make demands before she falls asleep, then when she starts to wake she may try to continue where she left off. If your initially chosen bedtime turns out to be too late, and you always have to wake her in the morning, you can gradually move the bedtime earlier as long as she continues to fall asleep quickly.

Make Any Necessary Changes to Keep Your Child Safe

Children moving about at night may not be fully aware of their surroundings. Most negotiate stairways without trouble, but if your child sleepwalks, don't leave anything on the floor or stairs that she could slip on. If your child is young, you may need to install a gate at the top of the stairs, in the corridor, or in her bedroom doorway. If she sleeps in a bunk bed, put her in the lower bunk. If she tries to leave the house while sleepwalking, put an extra chain lock high up on the outside doors. If necessary, you can buy inexpensive alarms to alert you if doors are opened during the night. If your child walks to places other than your bedroom, you may want to attach a bell to her bedroom door or gate to notify you that she is up. Even a child who is old enough to open a gate by herself may benefit from one, if she wants to stop sleepwalking: in order to open the gate she has to stop and wake more fully, giving her a chance to realise what she is doing and to return to bed. Occasionally you might

have to lock windows and in extreme cases glass windows can be replaced with plastic.

Other Treatments to Consider

Try Relaxation Exercises

Progressive relaxation exercises have been used successfully by
some children seven years and older. Books on these techniques are
readily available. In bed, before going to sleep, children practise relaxing the different regions of their body one part after the other.
Concentrating on relaxation rather than on active behaviour at bedtime may diminish a child's drive to wake fully during night-time
arousals since, again, at night-time wakings people tend to pick up
what they were doing when they fell asleep. This practice will help
her to get right back to sleep instead of trying to wake up completely during the night.

Consider Counselling for Emotional Issues

A decision about counselling should be based on several factors.
As explained above, it's important to base your assessment mostly
on the child's behaviour during the day. Even frequent arousal
events do not necessarily mean a child needs psychotherapy, but
keep an open mind. If you are unsure, consultation with a mental
health professional may help you to decide.

Bear in mind, too, that therapy is a means to identify and treat
certain psychological problems, not a specific treatment for arousal
events. Improvement in sleep often follows progress in therapy very
slowly. It may take your child some time to learn new ways of
dealing with difficult feelings so that she can go to bed without
worrying about relaxing her emotional defences in sleep.

Try Medication if Necessary

Partial arousals in school-aged children and adolescents are usually easy to control with medication. Its effect in younger children

is less predictable. A small bedtime dose of clonazepam (Klonopin), a drug similar to diazepam (Valium), often works quite well, as do other related agents. If a small dose decreases the frequency and intensity of episodes, a slightly higher dose will probably eliminate them. However, nightly use of such agents in young children is generally not warranted. Even though the dose required is usually small, and thus the side effects are usually mild to nonexistent, I typically recommend medication for children only if they seem at risk of injuring themselves (unlikely in younger children) or if their partial arousals are particularly frequent, long-lasting, intense and disruptive, and only if other treatment measures were unsuccessful. Sometimes, once we have determined a dose that works satisfactorily, the child reserves its use for sleepovers, travel and camp. A few children must use medication nightly for several years.

It is not known just why this class of drugs is so effective, but they suppress physiological changes that usually accompany arousal (such as increases in heart rate and blood pressure), and they likely reduce the cognitive drive to wake as well by making a child less anxious or concerned about any job to do. Medication treats the symptom of partial wakings, but it usually does not cure the underlying problem, if there is one. However, occasionally a treatment course of several weeks seems to interrupt a pattern and the events do not re-start when the drug is stopped.

What to Do During an Event

Let Arousal Episodes Run Their Course

Once an arousal episode has begun, keep your distance, wait it out and intervene as little as possible; when the arousal subsides, let your child return to sleep. During a partial arousal, parents often (and understandably) feel that they should 'do something'. Unfortunately, except in very calm events, you will usually only make matters worse if you try to hold your child, restrain her or even touch her while the episode progresses. She will not recognise you, even though she may be calling for you, and she is likely to react to any intervention as a threat or attack. If she squirms, twists away, pushes you or hits you, your attempts to help will only make her more upset. Generally, no amount of stimulation will bring your child to full wakefulness, at least during a major confusional event. A parent who shakes a child and yells at her until she wakes fully may think he has finally succeeded in awakening her, but the truth is that the child woke on her own when the episode was over, and the extra stimulation may only have prolonged it. It is much better simply to watch your child, ensuring that she is safe but otherwise letting the episode run its course.

All episodes eventually end on their own fairly suddenly. You can learn to tell when your child reaches this point: she will begin to relax, then typically stretch and yawn. Soon she will be ready to return to sleep. You can help her back into bed, or lay her back down, but don't do anything else. Remember, she is awake now, and you do not want to encourage full extended wakings by playing with her or engaging in long conversations, or it could become a habit.

Even fully developed sleep terrors should be allowed to run their course, though you may have to step in if your child is about to hurt herself or others, or if she might damage the furniture or walls. If you must intervene, do so as gently as possible, and use as little physical restraint as you can. An attempt to restrain an agitated seventeen-year-old could end up with both of you getting hurt.

A child who is less agitated during a partial waking may be easier to handle. This is especially true of a calm sleepwalker, who can often be re-directed or even led back to bed (in contrast to an agitated sleepwalker, who does not like to be touched and must calm down before you can direct her anywhere). Often parents lead a sleepwalking child to the toilet before directing her back to bed, on the (typically inaccurate) assumption that it was a need to urinate that got her up in the first place. That is not always wise: the frequent act of getting up to use the toilet, even when there is no great need, may only further condition the child to try to wake up at that time. This attempt to wake can develop into such a habit that it actually becomes the cause of sleepwalking; in fact, sometimes a boy – less frequently, a girl – will even get up on his own to urinate, but do so in the wrong place, most likely in the corner of the room or into a rubbish bin or closet, as if he knows generally what he is trying to do but is not fully aware of the specifics. Since most children past the age of toilet-training do not need to use the toilet at all during the night, consider not taking her to the toilet unless she specifically asks to go, or unless you find that she inevitably wets the bed later if you don't.

Keep Calm: Control Your Own Worries and Curiosity

If you attempt to help your child through a confusional event and she pushes you aside, it may make you angry. If she thrashes wildly as if 'possessed', you may be frightened. Try to avoid these reactions. By now you understand what is happening during a partial waking, and you should be able to watch it without misinterpreting your child's actions or mistaking it for something more serious. Do your best not to overreact, and control the impulse to try to wake your child. When she wakes after the episode ends, don't question her about it – she will not remember the event, anyway. Just let her go back to sleep. If she sees you upset at this time, she may only become upset herself, which can further disrupt her sleep: she may have difficulty returning to sleep and start to worry about having similar events in the future.

She may also be embarrassed: she has been acting in a way that she has no control over and that her family may regard as bizarre. If so, she might become angry if you ask about it. If her personality is of the tightly self-controlled type, she may already worry about losing control during the day, and the knowledge that she has been quite out of her own control during the night could cause her even more anxiety, increasing her worries at bedtime and possibly even leading to more arousal events. As a result, it's usually best simply to let your child's episodes pass without comment, unless she asks about them or is old enough to participate in decisions concerning psychotherapy and medication.

HOW WE HELPED THE CHILDREN
DESCRIBED EARLIER

Now that we've covered the spectrum of night-time arousals and seen how to understand and treat them, we can go back to the children described at the beginning of the chapter to take a closer look and see how their problems were resolved.

Marcy was the four-year-old girl who talked in her sleep and moved restlessly early in the night. She did not really have a significant problem, but her parents were worried that her sleep was not calm enough; they wanted to know for certain whether they should be doing something about it. Once I explained that Marcy's behaviour was completely normal and just part of the pattern of sleep-cycling across the night, they relaxed. There was nothing they needed to do.

Lisa, one and a half, went to sleep easily at bedtime in her cot with her dummy, but she would seem to wake several hours later, crying and thrashing. She looked more uncomfortable or frustrated than frightened. Her mother or father would pick her up and try to comfort her to no avail, and she wouldn't take her dummy. Instead, she thrashed still more strongly, arching her back and kicking. At various times her parents tried walking her, talking to her and shaking her in an attempt to wake her. On a few occasions they tried cold compresses or even screamed at her. Eventually, after ten to thirty minutes, Lisa would begin to quieten down, stretch and yawn, and her parents would find that they could finally wake her fully and reassure themselves that she was all right. At this point she would take her dummy and go back to sleep, usually until morning. Her parents would hear her stir several more times, but they would only have to go to her when she needed their help to find the dummy.

I explained to Lisa's parents that Lisa was not awake during these episodes, nor was she frightened or in pain; if she were, she would want to be held and would allow herself to be comforted. I told them to keep an eye on her during these spells, but not to do anything else unless she was awake and clearly wanted something. Once she stopped crying, they could help her lie down and cover her, but there was no need to wake her fully or to replace the dummy if she hadn't missed it. They soon grew accustomed to letting her get through the episodes without intervening and without feeling guilty.

I also suggested that they stop letting Lisa sleep with the dummy in the first place. Even though she was better able than most children her age to replace it by herself in the middle of the night, she did have to wake enough to look for it, and that need was probably contributing to her partial arousals. She got used to the change within three nights, by which time she had even stopped asking for it at bedtime.

Lisa's parents noticed two improvements almost immediately: her partial wakings became shorter, and she began going right back to sleep after each episode now that her parents were not trying to wake her. By the second week, the wakings had ceased to be a problem. Most of the remaining ones were mild, with only a little whining and thrashing, and her parents didn't even find it necessary to go into her room. Most nights, they were no longer sure whether she even woke at all. After a few weeks more, the wakings had completely stopped.

Noah, almost three, was happy and well behaved during the day, but he had been waking frequently at night for a year. At his 7.30 bedtime he always stalled, running off, demanding extra stories and running off again. Once it got late enough, he stayed in bed and fell asleep easily, but that usually didn't happen until 9.00 or 10.00. Two to three hours later he would begin moaning and moving about, then screaming, crying and sweating profusely. He would toss, turn and thrash wildly, get caught in the sheets and bump into the wall. He appeared confused or, as his parents described him, 'out of it'. He sometimes muttered intelligible phrases – 'I don't want to', 'Go away' – but much of his speech could not be understood. To his parents' dismay, they were unable to comfort him: he did not seem to recognise them and he would push them away, which sometimes made them angry.

Still, they would keep calling his name and shaking him until the episode finally ended after fifteen to twenty minutes. Then he would relax, stretch, yawn and start returning to sleep. Sometimes he had another episode an hour or two later, but it was almost always shorter and less intense than the first. The rest of the night was usually quiet. Shortly before bringing Noah to see me, his parents had tried eliminating his nap in the hope of improving his nighttime sleep, but that had only made the wakings worse.

Noah's partial wakings were similar to Lisa's, just more intense: he was bigger than Lisa, so his thrashing could be more violent, and as he was nearly three his failure to respond or to talk clearly during these events seemed stranger and more worrisome to his parents than it would have if he were younger. I explained the partial arousals to Noah's parents and gave them the same advice I gave Lisa's parents, recommending that they keep their distance during the arousals and let him go back to sleep without questioning him – although I suggested that they go into his room when he was having an episode, just to be sure he didn't hurt himself. Now that they understood the events better, they got less upset, and his apparent rebuffs of their efforts to help no longer bothered them.

There was room for improvement in other ways as well. It seemed to me that Noah was not getting enough sleep: he was falling asleep too late, at least on some nights, and the loss of his nap was not helping. If he was overtired, it would make partial arousals more likely. I was also concerned by his constant attempts to find new ways of putting off going to bed, because I suspected that he was trying to resume that behaviour when he began to wake, worsening the problem.

At my suggestion, his parents reinstated the nap and put him on a later – but firmly controlled – bedtime schedule. We set 8.45 as the time for a story, and they were to say good night at 9.00. I helped them to learn strategies for setting limits and enforcing the new rules (see Chapter 5). Once Noah began falling asleep quickly and easily, moving his bedtime earlier again would be an option.

Noah's parents were successful on all counts. Bedtime began to go smoothly (soon they moved it thirty minutes earlier), and Noah fell asleep quickly; he was napping again, and he was now getting enough sleep on a regular and predictable schedule. He had stopped testing limits at bedtime, and when he started to wake at night he was no longer being overstimulated by his parents' well-meaning attempts to help. His night-time partial wakings soon grew much rarer and milder, and over the next month or so they disappeared almost completely.

Christopher, eight, had been having abnormal night-time wakings for almost two years. His sleep problems had started two months after his father's death, when he and his mother moved to a new neighbourhood. He began walking in his sleep two or three times a week, calmly and quietly, without crying, talking or showing any signs of agitation. He would have what his mother described as a 'strange look' on his face, and he wouldn't always respond to her questions. Usually he appeared to be wandering aimlessly, but sometimes he seemed to be looking for something. Although he seemed not to recognise his mother, he would allow her to lead him back to bed, usually after a stop at the toilet to urinate. On two occasions he urinated in his room, once into the rubbish bin and once into his closet. Twice he walked out of the house and was led back home by neighbours. These episodes continued unchanged for a year, through several stressful periods: his mother was away for two weeks for emergency surgery, and shortly after that she re-married and his family moved again.

Then his mother became pregnant. Shortly before the birth of his sister, Christopher's night-time episodes changed. They now occurred several times a night, and they followed a new pattern. About an hour after falling asleep, Christopher would sit up suddenly and cry out briefly, appearing frightened. He would not respond to his mother; he resisted being touched, and he muttered incoherently off and on throughout the episodes. He would calm down in a few minutes, at which point he could be coaxed to lie back down in bed and would fall asleep rapidly. The episode would repeat itself an hour later, and again an hour after that. After the third episode he would begin to walk about the house in his sleep as he had when he was younger, but now in a more agitated manner. His mother and stepfather couldn't understand why these things were happening, and since their own sleep was constantly being interrupted, they were resentful and angry about his behaviour.

Christopher was a quiet, pleasant youngster, but he seemed tense and anxious. I learned that both his late father and his stepfather were alcoholics and that his family had some trouble with domestic violence. He was angry at the people around him, but he was afraid to express those feelings. He was also frightened by his lack of control over the world around him, and he was no doubt distraught that his parents could not control themselves. He devoted much of his energy to rigid self-control, worried that if he did not control his feelings, his parents would become even angrier and possibly increase his punishments.

Christopher and his mother both needed counselling, which they began separately on my recommendation. In the meantime, I explained the details of night-time arousals to his mother and stepfather so that they wouldn't be so angry at him. To keep him from leaving the house again in his sleep, I suggested a lock high up on the front door.

Given Christopher's ability to hurt himself while sleepwalking, and because his mother and stepfather were not yet able to be supportive, I also chose to prescribe medication to control his partial arousals, at least until his counselling had progressed. With a small dose of clonazepam taken before bed, his night-time arousals disappeared almost completely. Meanwhile, in counselling he was allowed to express his fears and concerns in a safe and supportive setting, and his mother began to learn how to listen to him in a sympathetic, non-judgemental way. He became happier, more relaxed and less fearful.

After six months, Christopher and his mother had made real progress in therapy and tensions had eased at home, so we gradually stopped his medication. Some night-time arousals returned, but they were milder now. His sleepwalking was no longer agitated, and often, instead of sleepwalking at all, he merely sat up in bed; instead of screaming, he would only talk softly. The episodes were much less frequent than before, never happening more than once a night, and his mother now knew how to deal with them without getting angry. They diminished even further over the next several months, and by the time he was nine they occurred only occasionally.

Maria's night-time arousals were still more dramatic than

Christopher's, falling somewhere between angry, agitated sleep-walking and full sleep terrors. At age twelve, she had been having them for just over three years. About an hour and a half after going to sleep, she would sit up and let out a single long, guttural scream. Then she would get out of bed and run about frantically, fumbling along walls and furniture as if trying blindly to escape a burning room. Sometimes she would fall to the floor and thrash, kick and roll about. Occasionally she ran wildly out of her room and even down the stairs.

Although weeks sometimes passed between Maria's episodes, more often they happened once or twice a week. Sometimes she seemed frightened; other times she seemed angry, frantic and confused. She pushed people away when they tried to restrain her, and when spoken to she responded with apparent anger, replying, 'Go away' or 'Leave me alone'. Once or twice she tried unsuccessfully to leave the house. Occasionally she had milder episodes, during which she sat up in bed talking and showed few signs of agitation. Her mother had discovered that she could trigger an episode by disturbing Maria's sleep in any way between sixty and ninety minutes after Maria had fallen asleep; she had learned to stay out of Maria's room at those times, not even trying to cover her with a blanket. Maria had not had any major problems during sleepovers at friends' homes, but the possibility worried her mother.

When Maria was nine her confusional episodes had lasted as long as half an hour, but now, at age twelve, most of them ended within five or ten minutes. As an episode ended she would grow calm, wake up enough to use the toilet and go back to sleep. Her parents often let her spend the rest of the night in their room. Some mornings they found her sleeping in their room, but neither they nor Maria knew when she had come in. Maria herself had no memory of any of the events, either immediately after they occurred or in the morning.

Maria's family tried to be supportive, but her parents were preoccupied with their own marital problems, which they were working on with the help of a marriage counsellor. Maria had recently started seeing a psychologist, too. She did not seem to have any striking emotional problems, and she was extremely well-behaved, at least away from home. However, she was not an outgoing youngster. She was angry at her parents over the strained mood at home and what she experienced as a lack of warmth and nurturance. She had difficulty expressing these feelings, and she was afraid that if she did express them it would only make matters worse.

I was able to reassure Maria's parents that she was physically normal – as are most children who have confusional events at night – and that arousals like hers were common. They were relieved to learn that we could stop the episodes with medication, but since the episodes were brief and occurred early in the night while they were still awake, we decided not to put Maria on a regular prescription. It would always be available when she was sleeping away from home, or if the episodes worsened. I also suggested that Maria sleep in her own room all night, every night. If she never found it necessary to change rooms and always knew where she was when she woke up, some of the causes of the arousals would likely go away. Her parents put a chair by their door so that if she came into their room they would hear her and could guide her back to her own bed.

Our hope was that as Maria continued to work with her psychologist, as she got out of the habit of switching rooms and as her parents continued to resolve their own problems, her wakings would gradually become rarer and less severe. In fact, they did diminish significantly over the next several months.

David was seventeen; over the eight years before I met him, his parents had divorced and both had re-married. Before their separation, David was known to talk in his sleep frequently. That was the extent of his night-time arousals until he was twelve, when his father re-married; then they started to show more severe variations. About once a month, around midnight, he would suddenly leap out of bed and begin yelling. His mother would find him standing in his room, apparently upset and looking, she said, 'as if he was worried that something was going to happen to him'. He did not seem to be actually frightened, although he occasionally mumbled cryptic phrases like 'I've got to get him'.

When David was fifteen his mother re-married as well, and his arousals became even more intense. Now they began with what his mother described as a blood-curdling scream, after which David would jump out of bed, knock over furniture and run about as if trying to escape from something. In these episodes he appeared truly terrified. He injured himself a few times; although mostly he got away with minor scrapes and bruises, once he broke a window-pane and cut his hand. On another occasion, he leaned dangerously out of an open window in his room on the second floor. He woke fully at the end of each episode, embarrassed to find himself in a room in disarray with his family staring at him.

David's parents described him as 'very controlled', with a tendency to 'hold things in' and 'handle things too well'. He seemed not to be working to the best of his ability in school. I found him pleasant and co-operative, but he seemed somewhat depressed. He was easy to talk to and, in fact, he was able to express many of his feelings, though he was clearly not fully aware of all of them, particularly those involving sadness and anger.

Although David's partial arousals were infrequent, they were so severe that I feared he might seriously injure himself. I have treated adolescents who have jumped out of windows during episodes like his. I placed David on medication that effectively stopped the arousals, but that was only a stopgap to ensure his safety. We wanted him sleeping calmly and safely without drugs. Even apart from any impact on his sleep, his mild depression, suppressed anger and unsatisfactory school performance all needed attention. For these reasons, I recommended psychotherapy.

David and his family followed through on this suggestion, and he profited enormously. Over time I watched him emerge from his shell and become a happier young man and a more successful student. After several months, we considered stopping the medication. Because his night-time arousals had been potentially dangerous, I reduced his prescription slowly and carefully, watching for recurrences at each step. By the time he left for university, he had been off medication altogether for several months, but I asked his family to be sure he had a roommate to report the recurrence of any problems. The medication would always be available if it became necessary again.

FIGURE 15. PARTIAL WAKINGS: A SUMMARY OF THE MAJOR PATTERNS ACROSS CHILDHOOD AND GENERAL RECOMMENDATIONS FOR MANAGEMENT

Behaviour	Typical Age	What to Do	General Suggestions
Confusional arousals (Extended periods of crying, sobbing, moaning, with wild, bizarre thrashing)	6 months to 6 years, occasionally older	• Watch your child to be sure she does not injure herself. • Let the episode run its course. Keep your distance. Don't forcibly 'help'. Hold your child only if she recognises you and wants to be held. Do not shake her or otherwise try vigorously to wake her. • Watch for the relaxation and calm that signal the end of the episode. You can then help her to lie down and cover her. Let her go back to sleep. Do not wake her more fully or ask her what was wrong or what she was dreaming about. Don't question her in the morning. Don't make her feel strange or 'different'.	• Make sure your child gets sufficient sleep. • Reinstate a nap if it was given up without good reason. • Make sure that her sleep and daily schedules are fairly regular and consistent. • If necessary, move bedtime later (but only to the time she usually falls asleep), so she can fall asleep quickly. • Eliminate bedtime activities that might be repeated during the night. • Eliminate night-time 'jobs' that your child must do before going back to sleep.
Calm sleepwalking	Any age from the time the child learns to crawl or walk	• Talk quietly and calmly to your child. She may follow your instructions and return to bed on her own.	• For young children, ensure adequate sleep and a normal schedule. Occasionally, that will help older children as well.

Behaviour	Typical Age	What to Do	General Suggestions
		• If she does not seem upset when you touch her, you should be able to lead her gently back to bed. There is no reason to stop at the toilet unless she asks. • If she spontaneously wakes after the episodes (as older children and adolescents commonly do), she will likely be embarrassed. Do not make any negative or teasing comments. Don't make her feel peculiar or strange. Treat the sleepwalking matter-of-factly and let her go back to bed.	• Make the environment as safe as possible to avoid accidental injury. If necessary, put a bell on her door and an extra lock on the front door. A gate may help to keep young children safe and serve to alert older ones (and their parents) if they try to leave their room in their sleep. If she sleeps in a bunk bed, the bottom bunk is safest. • If necessary, move bedtime later and eliminate inappropriate bedtime activities and unnecessary middle-of-the-night 'jobs' (as for confusional arousals).
Agitated sleepwalking	Middle childhood through adolescence	• If the agitation is marked, restraint will only make the event longer and more intense. Keep your distance. Hold your child only if she starts to do something dangerous. • When she calms down, treat her as you would a calm sleepwalker.	• Same as for calm sleepwalking. • If events are frequent, or dangerous, or if you are worried or have any questions about how to manage the sleepwalking, consult your GP. Medication and/or counselling may be warranted.

Behaviour	Typical Age	What to Do	General Suggestions
Sleep terrors (Screaming, look of panic and fear, possibly wild running)	Late childhood, adolescence	• Do not try to wake your child. Let the screaming subside and then simply let her return to sleep. Do not question her, and do not embarrass her if she reaches full waking. • If she runs and exposes herself to a risk of injury you may have to intercede, but be careful. Both you and she could get hurt. Talk calmly and block her access to dangerous areas, but avoid actual restraint if possible.	• Same as for agitated sleepwalking. • Make the room, windows and doors as safe as possible. • Sleeping on the first level of the house or in a finished basement room may be safest if the child runs wildly.

CHAPTER 14

Nightmares

What Nightmares Are
and Why They Occur

Nightmares are dreams – very scary dreams that wake you and leave you frightened and full of dread. A nightmare begins as an ordinary dream, but then, towards the end, it turns frightening. A child might dream he is happily walking his dog in the park on a sunny day. Then it suddenly gets dark, he finds he is lost in the woods and a monster jumps at him – and he wakes frightened. When we speak of nightmares, we're concerned with dreams that are frightening enough to wake your child. Most dreams, even scary ones, are forgotten unless we wake at the end at least briefly.

Like all dreams, nightmares occur in REM sleep. Although newborn babies presumably have rudimentary dreams – since they spend a great deal of time in REM sleep, during which they show eye movements and little smiles – we do not know whether they experience what we generally consider to be true dreaming with complex images, sounds, feelings and thoughts. But dreams, including nightmares, unquestionably do occur during the second year of life, a fact that becomes progressively clearer as a child develops speech and hence the ability to describe his dreams.

The content of a one-year-old's nightmare is likely to be simple. Typically he will re-create and re-experience a recent frightening event. Even though a one-year-old cannot describe his dream well, he may have enough verbal ability to indicate that it concerned a recent blood test, car accident or bee sting. A child of this age does not understand the difference between a dream and reality, so, on waking, he will not understand that the dream is over. He may still be afraid, as if the threat from the dream were still present. If he dreamed of a bee, for instance, his continued behaviour (pointing) and words ('Buzz-buzz here') may further demonstrate his conviction that the bee is still in the room.

By the time a child is two, his dreams have become more symbolic, with monsters or wild animals typically representing his impulses and fears. By this time he has begun to understand the concept of a dream, but he cannot yet fully appreciate the difference between dreaming and reality. He may describe dreaming of a monster yet still insist that 'the monster hasn't gone yet'.

As the child grows, his dreams become more complex. At the same time, he becomes more and more capable of distinguishing dreams from the real world. By about age five, he is likely to wake from a dream with an immediate and full understanding that he has been dreaming. It will be harder for him to reach this point after waking from a nightmare. A child's ability to accept a dream as 'just a dream' continues to develop, so that by age seven he may be able to handle an occasional nightmare without waking anyone for support. Still, even in an older child, the feeling of fright on waking from a nightmare is very real. As one child said: 'Mom, I know what happened in the dream wasn't real, but the *dream* was real!' The rational knowledge that nightmares come out of one's own imagination may have limited power compared to the emotional impact of the experience. Thus Hannah, an eleven-year-old girl, got up during the night to check that her younger brother was all right after dreaming that he had died – even though she knew full well that it was only a dream.

Although nightmares occur during sleep, for the most part they are caused by, and reflect, emotional conflicts that arise from a child's waking life. These conflicts are just the usual struggles children face throughout their normal development. Partly for this reason, all children have nightmares at one time or another. Some nightmares have other causes, such as illness or medication, and some *seem* to happen for no particular reason at all (at least none that can be easily identified).

The specific content or 'story' of your child's nightmares depends on several factors: his stage of physical and emotional development, the particular emotional conflicts he faces at his current developmental stage and any particularly scary or threatening daytime events he's been exposed to recently. The anxieties that produce nightmares may also lead to fears at bedtime and during periods of wakefulness at night, possibly interfering with your child's ability to fall asleep or get back to sleep (these problems are discussed in Chapter 7).

Young toddlers commonly fear separation from their parents. Your child may have nightmares when he first goes to day care, when you go out of town or must be hospitalised or after he has briefly got lost in a shop. As he gets a little older, he becomes more concerned about losing your love than about temporary physical separation; for example, he may fear that he is losing you to a new brother or sister. Or, in his third year, during toilet-training, he may struggle with his own impulse to soil while at the same time wanting to please you and fearing your disapproval. His dreams at these times may well reflect these anxieties.

Children between the ages of three and six must resolve many aggressive and sexual impulses. Your child will discover that he enjoys touching his genitals, and he may be jealous of your attention to a new baby and want to hit him or her. But he may also be frightened by his desire to do such things, especially if he believes you won't help him to control his aggressive urges or thinks he will be punished for giving in to the sexual ones. If he isn't taught that such urges are normal, shown what kinds of behaviour are acceptable and helped to control temptations towards truly inappropriate or harmful behaviour, then the scary feelings associated with these impulses may take shape as 'monsters' that frighten him at bedtime and during dreams. A three- to six-year-old may also be disturbed if he witnesses violent behaviour or overhears loud arguments at home. He may sense that you cannot control your own behaviour and worry that you won't be able to help him to stay in control himself.

A child may also feel conflicts deriving from the desire to replace one parent as the other parent's partner. Such anxieties can be stimulated further if the child is allowed to act out these feelings. Daniel, a five-year-old boy I saw, came into his parents' bed every night and ordered his father to leave. If his father did not go immediately, Daniel would begin to hit him. At that point his father would always move to another room – it was easier to give in than to struggle, and he could at least get some sleep that way. But for Daniel, having this power over his father was frightening. He was not sleeping well at all during this time, and he had frequent nightmares in which he was threatened by monsters.

Children around this age are often also struggling to understand the concept of death, and they may be afraid of falling asleep and never waking again. Alexander, aged six, never had any difficulty sleeping until he went to his uncle's wake. He was told not to worry, because his uncle 'would look just like he was sleeping' – in fact, he learned, his uncle had died in his sleep. Alexander's nightmares after this experience were related to his concerns about death and his confusion between sleep and death.

Anything that a child finds frightening or cause for worry can trigger bad dreams. Lauren, a five-year-old girl, came to see me with her family after three weeks of night-time wakings that began after she saw a scary film – one she probably should not have been allowed to see. Since then she had been waking and screaming for her parents at about 3.00 a.m. several times a week. They would find her awake, alert and shaking, clearly very frightened. Her dreams were not identical from night to night, but their content resembled that of the film she had seen. Her parents would stay with her only briefly and refused to allow her into their bed because they did not want her to develop what they considered to be bad habits. But being unable to get help at night only scared Lauren more, and her nights got even worse. Soon she did not want to go to bed at all, and she fought with her parents to keep them from leaving her alone at night.

In children between seven and eleven years old, nightmares ordinarily occur only occasionally – generally less than once a month. The conflicts of the preceding years should have been largely resolved by then (or at least repressed until adolescence), and new stresses are likely to be taken more in stride. If you have a child who, at this age, still has frequent nightmares – perhaps several each month – he may be struggling with conflicts that were not successfully resolved at an earlier age, or he may be facing significant new or ongoing stresses.

During puberty and throughout adolescence, new conflicts and anxieties emerge. As your child becomes an adult physically, sexually, emotionally and cognitively, he has to face new stresses every day. Nightmares seem to become somewhat more common at this time, although it is often difficult to say for certain, because adolescents are less likely than younger children to talk to family members during the day about their dreams, and they are certainly less likely to wake their parents at night after having a bad dream.

How to Help Your Child If He Is Having Nightmares

If your child has nightmares only now and then, maybe one every few months, a straightforward approach is usually sufficient. If your child is less than two years old, remember that he does not yet understand that dreams are not reality – you won't have much success by trying to show him that 'it was just a dream'. He simply needs to be held and comforted just as he would after a frightening event in the daytime. For a two-year-old, soothing, reassuring words will also help. At this age he may also be comforted if you listen sympathetically while he describes his dream or fears to you.

If your child is three or four, it may be useful to remind him that he was dreaming, though you must still treat his fear with empathy and reassurance. Even if he did not find it important to sleep with a night light on or his door open when he was younger, he may now.

When he wakes from a dream, the night light lets him see around his room and remember that he is at home and not in the dream scene. With the door open, he will feel less shut off from the rest of the house and closer to other family members. It will be easier for him to orientate himself and accept that the dream is over and he is safe. After waking from a particularly frightening dream, he may even want an even brighter light turned on.

The main point to remember when your child wakes from a nightmare is that he is truly frightened and needs your full reassurance and support. If he is afraid to go back to sleep, you may have to stay with him for a considerable time. (The length of time it will take for him to calm down may vary. Younger children typically need more time than older children, and, of course, the more intensely frightened they are, the longer it will take.) Occasionally lying down with him or even taking him into your bed won't hurt, and, in fact, it's the most reasonable approach when your child is very upset. Be supportive in a calm and convincing way, showing that you are in control and able to keep him safe. This is not the time to be extremely firm: it is unwise to shut your child's door when he is already too afraid to be alone.

On the other hand, you should not feel obliged to grant all your child's requests in an effort to allay his fears. For instance (as discussed in Chapter 7), don't feel compelled to turn on lights all over the house, look under the bed, rifle through the closet, rearrange the furniture and lock the windows. Remember, rather than reassuring him, such actions ultimately only support beliefs that monsters may be real and somewhere in the house. Instead, respond to his true needs by letting him know calmly and clearly that you will take care of him and protect him. Often even a thirteen-year-old who feels too 'grown-up' to be hugged in the daytime will appreciate such reassurance when he wakes frightened after a nightmare, and while an older adolescent may not need the physical comfort, he may on occasion still want someone close by to talk to.

If your child is having frequent nightmares – several a month, say – you need to work with him during the day to solve the problem. Try to determine what is worrying him and see if you can help to relieve his anxiety. For example, if your one-year-old has difficulty leaving your side, activities that practise separation, such as peek-a-boo – which makes a game of your disappearance and re-appearance – might help your child to feel comfortable when he is apart from you. If your two-year-old is having nightmares during toilet-training, even when it has been going well, try relaxing the training efforts for a while and encourage messy play such as finger painting. For three- to six-year-olds, children's books about sleep and dreams may help; you can also begin to talk directly to your child at this age about his fears and concerns. Screen the books, films and television programmes that your child sees. It goes with-out saying that you will want to avoid very scary ones, but because so much sex and violence regularly appear on prime-time television and in adverts, you will also need to monitor the rest of his viewing. Even if your four- or five-year-old enjoys these programmes and does not seem frightened by them, they could still stimulate enough anxiety to cause nightmares.

By all means allow your child to express his feelings, whatever his age, but teach him appropriate limits. Avoid moral condemna-tion. Don't make him feel guilty about having angry or sexual feelings; instead, help him to learn acceptable ways to express them, such as by talking angrily but not hitting. He may be reassured to learn that you used to have fights with your sister or brother or that everyone finds that it feels good to touch his or her genitals. With an older child, foster open communication and frankness, and encour-age him to discuss his concerns, even if they have to do with diffi-cult issues such as divorce, sex or drugs.

Daniel was the five-year-old who kicked his father out of bed every night and struggled with frequent nightmares. When I dis-cussed the situation with his parents, they agreed that they should be the ones making the decisions about who slept where, not Daniel. But they also came to understand that by giving in to his nightly demands, they had unwittingly been depriving him of a sense of security. They began insisting that Daniel stay in his own bed at night, and despite his initial protests and struggles, Daniel was ultimately much more comfortable with this demonstration that his parents were in control. Before long, his nightmares disappeared altogether.

Alexander, whose nightmares began after he attended his uncle's wake, clearly needed to work through the fears that he had developed in its aftermath. With coaching, his parents began encouraging him to discuss his feelings openly about his uncle's death and funeral, and after they corrected some of his misconceptions and read him a children's book about death, his bad dreams went away.

Lauren's fears and frequent nightmares had started after she saw a scary film, and they didn't seem to reflect any deeper anxieties. Because she was so frightened when alone at night, I suggested that one of Lauren's parents temporarily sleep in her room all night until her fears and nightmares stopped. In the meantime, during the day, they would discuss the film with her to help her deal with the fear. Lauren was relieved by this show of support. Within two weeks she was going to bed happily, and the night-time wakings and scary dreams had stopped. She then agreed to try sleeping alone again, but with the promise that if she had another bad dream one of her parents would return and stay the rest of the night. She had one more nightmare the next week, and her mother came willingly. After that, the problem was gone.

Occasionally, nightmares are a symptom of severe emotional difficulties. Regardless of your child's age, if he has frequent nightmares – perhaps weekly or more – over a period of more than one or two months, and you can't identify the cause of the stress he is feeling and help him to resolve it, then you should consider seeking professional help. This is especially true if your child also is troubled by fears during the daytime that seem excessive for his age, such as marked difficulties being away from you, unreasonable fears of being in his bedroom alone, reluctance to go to school or major phobias. As a parent, you should expect to take some part in at least some of the counselling sessions. If your child's anxiety reflects things he has seen or heard and perhaps does not understand, you may merely need help learning to recognise and deal with the causes of his distress. But if the issues are more deep-seated, they will be less responsive to emotional support alone. In that case, longer-term therapy will likely be needed.

NIGHTMARES AND CONFUSIONAL EVENTS

Before you try to address your child's nightmares, you should first be sure that nightmares are in fact the problem. If he cries out in the middle of the night and seems frightened, or jumps out of bed appearing very upset, then you might assume he had a bad dream. But you should also be aware that he might have had a confusional event, specifically a sleep terror, confusional arousal or episode of agitated sleepwalking (as discussed in Chapter 13). It is important to determine which kind of event it is, because the appropriate responses are quite different. The two phenomena are easy to mistake for one another, and to further confuse matters, the terms 'nightmare' and 'sleep terror' have sometimes incorrectly been used interchangeably. Nightmares are frightening dreams that occur in REM sleep and are followed by full waking. Sleep terrors, on the other hand, like other confusional events, occur during a partial arousal from the deepest phase of nondreaming sleep. Although in principle it sounds easy to distinguish the two, in practice the distinction is not always so obvious, especially in a young child.

The differences between nightmares and sleep terrors (and other intense confusional events) are discussed here and summarised in Figure 16 on page 343. Chapter 13 deals with confusional events in detail. Nightmares usually occur towards the end of the night, when REM sleep is most intense; in contrast, confusional events happen during the first few hours after a child has fallen asleep, when non-REM sleep is deepest. After a nightmare, a child who is old enough can describe a dream, but after a confusional event there is no dream to report. When your child wakes from a nightmare, he will cry (if he is young) or he may call for you (if he is older). He recognises you immediately and wants you to hold him and comfort him. He remembers the dream then, and he will still remember it in the morning. A child in the midst of a confusional event, on the other hand, is not fully awake. He may cry out, regardless of his age, but the cry may sound more like a scream, or he may talk, moan and cry all at the same time in a confused and possibly unintelligible way. During the episode he will not recognise you or allow you to comfort him. If you try to hold him, he may push you away and become more agitated. If he does wake briefly at the end of the confusional event, he will not remember the preceding yelling and thrashing, and he will have no memory of a dream. In the morning, he may vaguely remember being awake and perhaps talking to you during the night – that is, the period after the confusional event – but no more.

A child who has been frightened by a nightmare will remain frightened even when fully awake. Often he will be reluctant to go back to sleep alone in his bed afterwards. He may even be afraid to go to bed for several nights following an especially scary dream. On fully waking after a confusional event, however, the child will relax; all signs of fear and agitation disappear and he will return to sleep rapidly. Since he is unaware of the episodes, he will not be reluctant to go to bed on following nights.

It is much more common for parents to misinterpret confusional events as nightmares than the other way round. If a child is too young to describe his dreams, his parents may simply assume he has had a bad dream whenever he wakes crying and upset. They may make the same assumption when an older child 'wakes' thrashing or screaming, even if he does not describe a dream after he quietens down. If a child calls out, 'Help me!' his parents may understandably jump to the conclusion that he is fully awake and reacting to a nightmare that he just had.

Parents struggling to wake their child from a sleep terror may be misled by his initial confusion and lack of receptiveness. If he pushes them away, they may conclude that he is still dreaming, 'fighting off monsters'. If they succeed in waking him as the event ends, their own anxious questions may make him fearful, as he would be after an actual nightmare; telling him about his bizarre behaviour may do the same, since until it's described to him, he'll be unaware that anything unusual had even happened. Now, instead of returning to sleep

FIGURE 16. NIGHTMARES VERSUS SLEEP TERRORS

	Nightmares	Sleep Terrors, Confusional Arousals and Agitated Sleepwalking
What are they?	Scary dreams. They take place within REM sleep and are followed by full waking.	Partial arousals from very deep nondreaming sleep (Stage IV, non-REM).
When do you become aware the child had one or is having one?	After the dream is over, when he wakes and cries or calls – not during the nightmare itself.	During the event itself, as he screams and thrashes. When he wakes afterwards, he is calm.
When do they occur?	Usually in the second half of the night, when dreams are most intense.	Usually one to four hours after falling asleep, when nondreaming sleep is deepest.
How does the child appear and behave?	Wide awake; younger children cry, and all children appear frightened, even though they are fully awake and the nightmare is over.	Not fully awake; poorly responsive at best. Initially he may sit up and then thrash or run about in a bizarre manner with eyes bulging, heart racing and profuse sweating. He may cry, scream, talk or moan and show apparent fright, anger and/or obvious confusion, which all *disappear* when he is fully awake.

How does the child respond to attempts to calm him?	He is aware of and reassured by your presence; you can comfort him, and he may hold you tightly.	He is not very aware of your presence, will not be comforted by you and may push you away and scream and thrash more if you try to hold or restrain him.
How quickly does the child return to sleep?	It depends upon the intensity of the nightmare, the age of the child and the degree of parental support offered when he wakes. Return to sleep can be considerably delayed if there is marked and persistent fear.	Usually rapidly, once he has awakened fully – though that may not occur for up to forty-five minutes.
Can the child describe a dream after waking or in the morning?	Yes (if old enough).	No memory of a dream or of yelling or thrashing.

rapidly as he otherwise would, he may be unable to or unwilling to try. Even if he isn't frightened, once he is fully awake he may enjoy the attention, and if his parents keep asking him what he was dreaming about, he may make up a story to satisfy them.

Remember, as we saw in the previous chapter, a sleep terror is more physical than mental. During a sleep terror a child experiences all the physical changes usually associated with fear – his heart is beating rapidly, he is sweating and his blood pressure rises – and he looks and acts frightened, but when he wakes fully there is nothing frightening to remember. After a nightmare, however, a child is truly frightened and remembers the dream, but physical changes, such as of heart rate and blood pressure, are relatively mild.

When an intense sleep terror begins suddenly and (as may happen in the adolescent) lasts only a minute or two, a child may wake spontaneously to find himself still sweating and his heart still pounding and racing. To explain these feelings to himself – ones typically associated with fear – he may attribute them to a vague threat and say, perhaps, 'It was going to get me'. By contrast, if a child has had a nightmare he will be able to give a full dream report, with a story line, characters and settings. After a sleep terror, although he may feel some of the physical effects associated with fear, they will usually fade rapidly and he will be able to return to sleep quickly if his parents remain calm.

However, even though a child waking from a nightmare will usually be normally responsive – reaching up to be lifted out of the cot as soon as you come into his room, clinging to you when you pick him up or, if he is old enough, even getting out of bed and running into your room for reassurance – occasionally he may behave at first almost as if he were having a sleep terror. He may appear confused and seem unresponsive to your efforts to comfort him for several minutes. He may point around the room and refer to animals or monsters, but be too upset to describe a coherent dream. This situation happens most often with a very young child who does not fully understand what a dream is, that the monsters are not real and that the dream is over and he is safe at home. Still, he will not thrash about as wildly, or be as unresponsive, as a child actually having a sleep terror.

Finally, although both sleep terrors and nightmares may occur frequently or occasionally, events that occur *very* frequently – several times a week, nightly or even several times a night – are not likely to be true nightmares, particularly when such frequent events continue for more than one or two weeks; these events are much more likely to be of a confusional nature.

NIGHTMARES OR '"NO"-MARES'?:
'I HAD A BAD DREAM'

As we saw in Chapter 7, children sometimes report having nightmares when in fact they have not. They call for their parents or come to their room at night, even every single night, saying 'I had a bad dream'. These children have simply learned that whenever they say those magic words, they get a big response. If they say 'I want to sleep in your bed', they will be sent back to their rooms, but if they say 'I had a bad dream', they are told, 'Come on in'.

Of course, you should comfort your child when he really has had a scary dream. So how do you know if the complaint is genuine? Generally, it's not very difficult to tell. Since a child waking from a nightmare is truly scared, he will look and act scared. If your child – like the child described in the section on 'How Severe Is Your Child's Anxiety?' in Chapter 7 – gathers up his blanket and teddy bear every night, walks calmly to your room and taps you on the shoulder before saying he had a bad dream, then you can be sure that he didn't. If he can't describe what happened in the dream, that is another sign that it didn't happen. If it had, he would have run to you, or clutched you tightly when you answered his call, and he would have a dream story to report. If you are in doubt, err on the side of leniency for a night or two, but remember that scary dreams almost never happen nightly. Whether your child is truly having nightmares should become clear very soon.

However, for some children the words 'I had a bad dream' really mean 'I'm scared'. In such cases, it makes little difference whether these children actually had a dream or not. If your child is truly frightened, then you must deal with his fears (as discussed in Chapter 7), whether they arose from wakeful thoughts or from dreams.

CHAPTER 15

Bed-wetting

Bed-wetting, or *nocturnal enuresis,* is a very common and frustrating childhood sleep problem that can upset parent and child alike. It occurs in all societies and has been recorded throughout history. Although figures differ somewhat among cultures and among groups within a culture, approximately 15 per cent of all five-year-olds, 5 per cent of all ten-year-olds and 1 to 2 per cent of all adolescents still wet their beds at least once a month. Almost two-thirds of enuretic children are boys. Although the causes of enuresis are only partially understood, several methods of treating the disorder have proven successful.

When a child wets the bed, it is not the urination itself but its aftermath that frustrates and annoys: the child's pyjamas and sheets get wet, she wakes up and her parents might have to get up to change the bedclothes. Even if a child urinated nightly, if somehow nothing got wet in the process, it would not be a problem at all. For that reason, enuresis does not make its appearance as a 'sleep problem' until a child is – or should be – out of nappies.

Many families aren't especially perturbed by enuresis, especially if the child is younger than about seven years old and the bed-wetting is infrequent. If that describes your family, you might choose to wait for it to stop on its own. Just be sure the wetting doesn't upset your child (as discussed below) more than you think. You should be aware, however, that although most children do outgrow the problem eventually, for an individual child this may not happen any time soon: only about 15 per cent of enuretic children, at each age from five to eighteen years, will spontaneously outgrow the problem over the next year. Furthermore, the older the child and the more frequent the wetting, the more likely both the child and her parents will be to want to find a solution.

The Impact of Enuresis

Enuresis can affect your relationship with your child, her own self-image and her interactions with other children. Although she will not remember actually wetting the bed when she wakes, the wet sheets make it clear what happened: she doesn't need you to tell her, as she would after a sleep terror or a sleepwalking episode. Also, since bed-wetting generally happens unobserved (again in contrast to sleep terrors and sleepwalking), parents sometimes incorrectly assume that their child was awake and urinated voluntarily, making them angry and resentful rather than sympathetic and concerned.

Your reactions are very important. Without your understanding and support, your child will surely suffer. But even if you are fully supportive, even if you really don't mind changing the sheets, your child may still feel ashamed and embarrassed, especially if she is at least four or five years old and still wearing nappies or pull-ups at night. She may be reluctant to have friends sleep over, to go to their sleepovers or to attend overnight camp. If her schoolmates find out that she wets the bed (or, worse, that she still wears nappies), she may be teased. These emotional effects often prove to be of greater consequence than the bed-wetting itself.

Although the frequency of bed-wetting can usually be reduced greatly (using the techniques described that follow), it is not always possible to prevent it entirely. Whether the wetting stops completely or not, if the child's view of herself and her relations with her family can be improved, both she and her parents will be much happier.

Antonio was a six-year-old boy who wet his bed almost every night, although he had been toilet-trained since the age of three. He did have occasional dry nights, but he had never remained dry for more than a week. His parents were frustrated and angry. Sometimes they punished him, often by denying him special privileges, hoping that that would bring about some control. They made him sleep on a small cot and wear a nappy to bed, saying they would not buy him a regular-sized bed until he stopped wetting. Antonio's parents were caring people and they loved their son, but they did not understand bed-wetting, and the situation was not improving. Besides, they hated imposing the punishments, even though they thought they were necessary, and it was making them feel guilty. Finally they realised they needed help.

When the family came to see me, Antonio was surprised and delighted to hear me explain that it was not his fault, that punishment would not help and that he should be required neither to wear nappies nor to sleep in a cot. I told him that many children his age still wet the bed – he had thought he must be one of only a few. His father admitted, with much embarrassment, that he himself had wet the bed as a youngster, something not even his wife had known.

Antonio's parents were anxious to correct their mistakes, and I supported their efforts carefully in frequent initial meetings. We embarked on a programme of behaviour modification (described at length later in this chapter). The results were fairly good: although Antonio's bed-wetting did not cease entirely, it did decrease significantly. And even before that happened, the family had begun functioning much better. Antonio no longer felt ashamed about wetting, and his parents no longer suffered the guilt that punishing him had caused them.

Even when parents are not terribly concerned about bed-wetting, the child herself can be. Rebecca was an eight-year-old girl who wet the bed several times a week. Her home was happy and stable, and her parents were sympathetic; they accepted her bed-wetting without complaint, and although they would have preferred that she be dry, they were not much disturbed by the problem. Rebecca's father had been enuretic until age ten and he had openly discussed his own history with her. The parents sought my help not because of their own concerns but because Rebecca was deeply troubled by the wetting. An intelligent girl who expressed her concerns forthrightly, Rebecca was anxious to begin a programme that would help her be dry at night. We started a behaviour modification programme, which she followed with determination, and to her delight it was successful.

Benjamin, twelve, still wet the bed at night, and like most older children and adolescents in his situation, he was very upset by it. In fact, it was affecting his whole life. His self-respect suffered badly. Children in the neighbourhood teased him cruelly, and he was becoming withdrawn. He never slept at a friend's house and never invited a friend to spend the night at his. He wanted to go away to summer camp but refused to do so until he stopped wetting. Benjamin urgently needed to get the problem under control. Simply knowing that there were other children his age who also wet their beds would not be enough. In his case behavioural treatments were unsuccessful, but he responded well to medication: his self-esteem was restored, and he was even able at last to go away to camp.

WHAT CAUSES ENURESIS?

Several factors may play a role in enuresis: heredity, maturation, small bladder capacity, night-time awareness of the need to urinate, depth of sleep, medical issues, food sensitivity, emotional factors and environmental and early childhood influences. (For only some of these factors is the relationship certain.) Each of these is discussed below. It may not always be possible to say which are the most important in a given child.

Heredity

Overall, heredity is probably the single most significant factor contributing to enuresis. Children whose parents were bed-wetters are much more likely than other children to wet their beds. While only 15 per cent of all children wet their bed, the figure increases to almost half if one parent used to wet the bed and three-quarters if both parents did. What specific inherited traits are responsible is unknown, but they may include one or more of the other factors described below, such as a small functional bladder capacity.

Maturation

For a child to be continent, that is to have control over her urination, the part of her nervous system that controls her bladder has to reach a certain degree of maturation. An infant has little awareness of her bladder filling or of the need to urinate. Her bladder empties when necessary by a reflex contraction. At some point between the ages of one and a half and two and a half, a child begins to recognise when her bladder is full. She may stop playing when she has this feeling, and her facial expression may indicate her awareness that a urination is coming. If she is being toilet-trained at that time, she will be able to get to the toilet and remove her clothing in time to use the toilet. At this stage, however, she still can't postpone the flow of urine. She will develop that ability over the next year. By age three or four she can urinate at will, even when her bladder is only partially full, and she can now interrupt her urinary stream after it has started. She can go to the toilet before leaving the house, even if she does not feel the urge to urinate and she can catch herself when she realises she is starting to urinate at the wrong time. At this level of maturation, she is now physically capable of staying dry at night as well. If she continues to wet the bed, other causes are probably responsible.

Most children are dry at night before age four, but of course the actual age varies. A child's bladder grows considerably between the ages of two and four and a half, making it easier for her to hold her urine all night. A few babies are even dry at night before their first birthday. By the age of two and a half about 50 per cent of all children are dry, and by age three about three out of four no longer wet their beds. Although 'delayed maturation' is often blamed for

ongoing enuresis, it is unlikely for children of five or older to continue to wet for that reason. If your child is toilet-trained in the
daytime, then she has the ability to recognise when she is about to
urinate and to hold it until she is in the toilet or until her bladder
stops contracting and the urge ceases. If she is dry at night even occasionally, it suggests that she has the ability to wake up from sleep
and do the same thing.

Small Bladder Capacity

Many bed-wetters urinate more frequently during the day than
nonbedwetters do, and in smaller amounts. Although that seems to
imply that their bladders are unusually small, when these children
are examined under anaesthesia, they are usually found to have
bladders of normal size. Because their bladder contractions begin
too soon, these children feel the *sensation* of a full bladder and need
to urinate before their bladders are actually full. Furthermore, these
early contractions can be very strong. At night, wetting may result.
The 'bladder training' techniques described later in this chapter are
based on these observations.

Night-time Awareness of the Need to Urinate

A child who wets during sleep may not yet have learned to recognise
the sensations from a full bladder, or from a partially full bladder
that is already contracting, as a signal important enough to trigger a
full waking. You will recall from the discussion of sleep stages in
Chapter 2 that a stimulus that is important to you (like your baby's
crying) is much more likely to wake you than an unimportant stimulus (like a bird chirping or the wind blowing). Somehow you have
learned to make this distinction, even when you are asleep. Your
child must learn the same. If she doesn't, then she will not interpret
the sensation of impending urination as an important enough signal
to cause her to wake up and hold the urine in until either the urge
passes or she gets to the toilet; instead, she will not wake and will
wet the bed. Conditioning and behaviour modification techniques

appear to work by helping your child learn to pay closer attention to these signals.

Depth of Sleep

Laboratory studies have shown that bed-wetting does not take place during dreams. If your child wakes describing a dream about water and her sheets are wet, it does not mean that she wet because of the dream; the wetting episode came first, rather, and the feeling of wetness from the sheets and pyjamas then stimulated the dream.

Many parents of enuretic children report that their child sleeps more deeply than most other children and thus is unusually difficult to wake. Those perceptions are probably inaccurate, arising, at least in part, because whenever the parents try to wake the child to use the toilet before they go to bed themselves, the child will still be in the period of very deep sleep that predominates in the first few hours of the night. But although the sleep of enuretic children has been shown to be no deeper than that of many other children, it may be that enuretics' sleep falls at the deep end of the normal range. Parents of enuretic children rarely if ever characterise their children's sleep as 'light'.

Because most bed-wetting occurs in the first third of the night, usually during or immediately following an arousal from non-REM sleep, it has some similarity to the arousal disorders described in Chapter 13. That might seem to suggest that the urination occurs during the confusion of a partial arousal from deep sleep (even though the partial arousal may be completely normal otherwise). It is true that bed-wetting does sometimes accompany sleep terrors and episodes of confused thrashing or sleepwalking. However, in most cases when a child has both confusional arousals and a tendency to wet the bed, the two behaviours do not occur at the same time of the night or even on the same nights. Furthermore, episodes of bed-wetting also commonly occur during arousals from periods of relatively light non-REM sleep, when sleepwalking and sleep terrors are particularly unlikely to happen. We do know, however, that some bed-wetters' bladders contract more during non-REM sleep than during REM. It may be that these contractions sometimes trigger a partial arousal and, at different times, an episode of bed-wetting.

Medical Factors

Most of this chapter discusses what is called 'functional' enuresis, meaning bed-wetting that is not related to any medical disorder. Although most bed-wetting is functional, you should not assume that your child's wetting has no medical cause. All enuretic children five years of age or older should have a thorough physical examination before nonmedical treatment begins, both to rule out medical causes and to check for related problems. A urine specimen should also be examined to be sure the child does not have an infection. Urinary tract abnormalities and certain neurological conditions can occasionally cause bed-wetting, but in these cases, as well as when there is a urinary tract infection, there will usually be other warning symptoms that occur in the daytime – dribbling urine, daytime incontinence, frequent strong urges to urinate or frequent or painful urination – which you or your child will notice and which your GP will recognise as important. Although urinary tract infections don't generally cause enuresis, they are more common in enuretic children, especially girls, and of course they should be treated.

Sometimes children begin to wet the bed after many months of dryness. This condition is called *secondary,* or *onset,* enuresis to distinguish it from *primary* enuresis, in which the child has never stayed dry at night for long. Medical factors are more likely to be involved in secondary enuresis. But if medical problems can be ruled out, a child with secondary enuresis should respond very well to the same techniques we use to treat primary enuresis.

Food Sensitivity

In recent years, there has been a great deal of interest in the role of food sensitivity in a number of childhood health problems, bed-wetting among them. In a few cases, night-time wetting reportedly has decreased when certain foods were removed from a child's diet. Although it is conceivable that particular foods irritate the bladder in some children, increasing contractions and decreasing bladder capacity, there is no good evidence to support this hypothesis. In any case, unfortunately, very few children respond at all to changes in their diet.

Emotional Factors

Bed-wetting is somewhat more frequent among children who are emotionally disturbed. However, fortunately, such disturbances are not the cause of most bed-wetting, and the vast majority of enuretic children are normally adjusted. Any related emotional problems are more likely the result of the bed-wetting than the cause.

Environmental Influences and Early Childhood Experience

A child's early experience may affect her ability to be dry at night by the usual age. For example, studies have shown that bed-wetting is slightly more frequent than average in middle children, children in lower-income families and children faced early in their lives with stresses such as chronic illness or their parents' divorce. Stress is particularly disruptive during the third year of life, when a child is usually being toilet-trained. If toilet-training is handled punitively, a child is also more likely to become a bed-wetter. But these differences are small. If your child wets her bed, rest assured that it's not because you haven't been a good enough parent or because you failed somehow to prevent it. At most, the early family environment can provide only a very small part of the explanation.

APPROACHES TO TREATING ENURESIS

Throughout history people have described enuresis and treatments for it. Nowadays there are humane and caring methods for treating bed-wetting, but in the past enuretic children were subjected to more questionable 'cures'. As early as AD 77, Pliny the Elder recommended an elixir made from 'boiled mice'; during the Byzantine Era, potions included a fragrant wine made of hares' testicles; and the nineteenth and twentieth centuries brought plenty of new elixirs and potions, most of which have been no more effective than the 'flowers of the white oxe' administered hundreds of years earlier. Special rituals have been tried as well: enuretic children in the Navajo tribe, for example, were forced to stand naked with legs apart over the burning nest of a phoebe, swallow or nighthawk, since it was believed that birds do not wet their nests.

Some parents, like Antonio's, still make the mistake of trying to stop the bed-wetting by means of punishment, ridicule and shame. Not only is it unhelpful to treat an enuretic child this way, but it may actually prolong or worsen the problem, and the child may suffer emotionally as well. George Orwell, one of the most famous self-admitted enuretics, described the dilemma eloquently:

> I knew that bed-wetting was (a) wicked, and (b) outside my control. The second fact I was personally aware of, and the first I did not question. It was possible, therefore, to commit a sin without knowing you committed it, without wanting to commit it and without being able to avoid it.

You and your child will be encouraged to know that most enuretic children can learn to wet the bed less often, and many are able to stop doing it entirely. But before you begin your treatment programme, you must understand that solving the problem will require patience, persistence and family co-operation. Results may be very slow in coming, and your child may relapse. The behavioural methods of treatment require a good deal of consistency, and they will work only if both you and your child are willing to accept some temporary inconveniences. Your child can't stop wetting without your full commitment, and you can't make it stop if she isn't interested in participating and doesn't understand what the treatments are doing and why.

For these reasons, start by explaining to her (and reviewing for yourself) just how the urinary system works, what is necessary to avoid wetting, and what the approaches you will be using are actually trying to accomplish. Guidelines and pictures to help explain your child's urinary system to her are shown in Figure 17 on page 358. Some of that information may be new to you, too. Include as much or as little detail as her age and interest require, and modify or adapt the technical language to fit her level of understanding. She should understand that her bladder continuously fills and intermittently empties, that bladder contractions and the automatic (reflex) opening of the muscle of the internal sphincter lead to a feeling of urgency (the 'need to go') and that the weak muscle of the external sphincter is then the only thing keeping her dry until she can get to the toilet or until the contractions stop and the internal sphincter closes again. If her bladder becomes capable of holding more urine before it tries to empty, it will become easier for her to get through the night dry. If her external sphincter gets stronger, she may be able to keep herself dry long enough to wake and use the toilet. These are the goals of bladder training and start-stop exercises.

We treat enuresis using four main techniques, discussed in detail below: reinforcement and responsibility training, bladder training, conditioning and medication. The first three are behavioural approaches and can be undertaken simultaneously or in succession. Many families start with reinforcement and bladder training methods, then try conditioning if the first two are unsuccessful. Medication therapy requires a doctor's supervision and is usually recommended only in certain circumstances. The techniques of 'lifting' and dietary change will also be described.

Do not restrict your child's fluid intake during the day – it will not help. It is, however, reasonable to avoid *large* amounts of liquid after dinner and especially near bedtime. Also keep in mind that an initial visit to a GP is important. Don't begin a programme of therapy until you are sure your child does not have a medical problem that needs attention.

Before trying any of the behavioural approaches, discuss your plans with the whole family. Everyone will need to feel comfortable

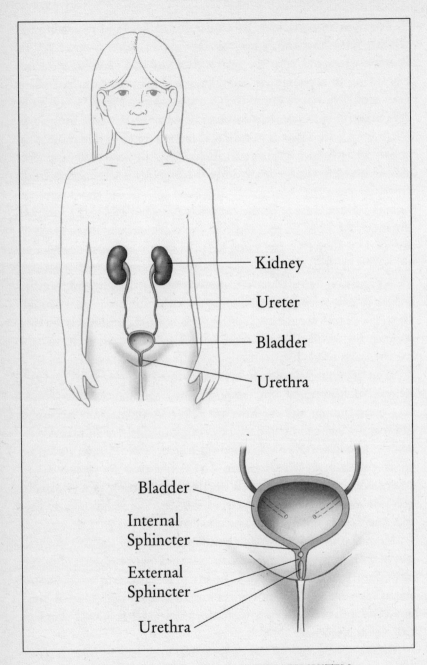

FIGURE 17. YOUR CHILD'S URINARY SYSTEM

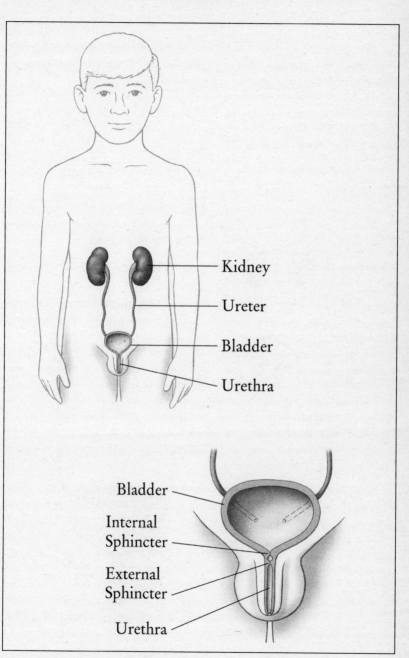

Kidney

Ureter

Bladder

Urethra

Bladder

Internal Sphincter

External Sphincter

Urethra

Use this text as a guide when going over the accompanying picture with your child. Depending upon your child's age, you may want to replace words like urine with the words you use at home to help your child to understand.

Kidney: These important organs are filters that remove unneeded chemicals from your blood. The filtered fluid (containing the unneeded chemicals) becomes urine.

Ureter: A soft tube down which your urine drips on its way from your kidney to your bladder.

Bladder: A storage container for your urine. It is actually a special kind of muscle. When it gets full it starts to contract, or squeeze closed, to push out the urine. When that starts to happen, you feel the need to go to the toilet.

Urethra: A short tube through which your urine passes [boys: through your penis] on its way out of your body.

Internal sphincter (often easier to describe to children as the 'first stopper'): This part of the urinary system is a muscle, too. It controls the flow of urine out of your bladder, the way a plug controls the flow of water out of a bathtub. Most of the time, it is automatically squeezed closed so that no urine can leave your bladder. When you go to the toilet, this stopper relaxes and opens so urine can come out. When you are at the toilet and want to urinate, it just seems to relax and open automatically, but only because you want it to. However, when your bladder gets very full and starts squeezing and trying to empty, this stopper starts to open on its own whether you want it to or not. When that happens, you feel the need to go to the toilet in a big hurry. The only thing keeping your urine inside of you now is your 'second stopper'.

External sphincter ('second stopper'): This stopper is another muscle that works to control your urine. It is usually relaxed and open, because the first stopper is closed and keeping your urine in your bladder. If the first stopper starts to open and you haven't got to the toilet yet, you have to close this second stopper to hold your urine in until you get there. This muscle does not work automatically: you can control it. When you hold your urine in, or stop urinating after you have started but before you are done, you can feel it tighten. But it is not a very strong muscle. If you have to go to the toilet badly and cannot get there quickly, it gets harder and harder to keep holding the urine in. If the muscle gets stronger, holding your urine will become easier.

When you practise your start-stop exercises (by starting to urinate, then stopping before you're done, then starting and stopping again repeatedly), you are strengthening the muscle of this second stopper and getting better at closing it even if you have already started to urinate. This is what you must do at night when you're sleeping. If your bladder starts to squeeze and your first stopper starts to open, you need to close your second stopper quickly and strongly so that you have enough time to wake and go to the toilet. By doing your exercises, you will get better at closing it quickly – you will hardly even need to be aware that you are doing it. If you are also doing bladder-stretching exercises (seeing how long you can hold your urine and how much urine you can hold), you are not only making the muscle of the second stopper stronger but also making your bladder able to hold more urine before it tries to squeeze and empty. That also makes it easier to get through the night without wetting.

about co-operating to solve this problem. If anyone resents the work or teases the bed-wetting child, it will be an obstacle. If you have been punishing or criticising your child for bed-wetting, explain to her that you have learned that you were wrong to do so and that you now understand that she wasn't to blame. Let her know that you want to work *with* her to help her control the problem and to feel better about herself. Don't treat her like a baby. You should probably not leave her in nappies at night if she is past her fourth birthday – definitely not if she is already five – and toilet trained in the daytime. She should sleep in a regular bed; you can use a waterproof pad under the sheet to protect the mattress. Don't restrict her in any way because of the bed-wetting. You will need to monitor your own behaviour carefully, too. Even the most well-meaning of parents can inadvertently show subtle disapproval when the bed-wetting continues.

Reinforcement and Responsibility Training

The first approach to treatment combines two related goals: first, helping your child learn to take on responsibility for dealing with her bed-wetting, and second, reinforcing her ability to stay dry.

The goal of the responsibility training is to help her learn to be more in control of herself in general. She should feel good about this endeavour, so present it as a privilege and an opportunity, *not* as a punishment. Once she becomes accustomed to responding promptly and automatically to her own needs, responsibilities and obligations during the day when she is awake, she will have an easier time doing the same at night when she is asleep. In particular, the sensation of needing to urinate may become significant enough to her to signal her to wake *herself* enough to prevent wetting and, if necessary, to walk to the toilet.

The reinforcement part of the treatment is intended to increase your child's motivation to react to these night-time signals and to help her learn to recognise night-time bladder sensations as important. You should use rewards for this purpose, not punishments: most people will work harder to earn a reward than to avoid a punishment. If parents and child work together in a spirit of co-operation, the treatment works even better.

Begin by discussing with your child how she can assume more general responsibility around the house, perhaps by taking on a job such as clearing the table, taking out the rubbish or feeding the dog. Above all, she must take on more responsibility concerning the bed-wetting itself. She should change her own pyjamas, and if she is old enough – usually about seven – she should help change the sheets and do the laundry. (But remember, this isn't a punishment: don't saddle a young child with the entire responsibility for these chores. Instead, give her extra privileges as she takes on the new responsibilities). These changes alone may lead to improvement. But even if they don't, you will be doing your child a service. Her view of herself, and you, will improve.

Next, set up a system for recording and rewarding dry nights. A sticker chart, specially drawn or kept on a calendar, is often successful, at least for children aged up to about ten. Give your child stars for dry nights, and award her special prizes after a certain number of stars. You can structure the system to suit your child's age and interests, but you may want to base it on the following example, which has worked well for many children. Choose one colour of stars to record dry nights, another colour to be used after every fourth dry night (consecutive or not) and a special sticker to mark any seven consecutive dry nights. Instead of stars, your child may prefer stickers with animals, cartoon characters or 3-D images – let her help to choose them. Agree in advance on a special (but inexpensive) treat or prize that she will earn for every two seven-day stickers. Have your child attach the stickers to the chart or calendar, and congratulate her when she has earned one. In the meantime, remember never to scold her or make her feel bad in any way after she has wet the bed.

Bladder Training and Start-Stop Exercises

The next approach is to help your child to develop the abilities to hold more urine and to exercise more control over her urination. You can begin bladder training at the same time as responsibility training, or postpone it for a while if you wish. Now would be a good time to (again) review with your child the nature of her urinary system and how it works (see Figure 17 on page 358).

Once a day, at the same time each day, have your child hold her urine as long as she can, at least to the point of some discomfort. Then, when she urinates (into a bottle, urinal or pan), measure the volume. Her efforts to beat her previous record will gradually increase her daytime bladder capacity. To pick a starting point, measure the volume each time she urinates at home for the first two days, and use the largest single volume of urine over the two-day period as the initial record to beat. Also note the amount of time between urinations: if your child urinates more often than once every three or four hours, have her try to wait fifteen to thirty minutes longer each day between urinations until she achieves a three- to four-hour minimum.

There is no specific volume that will guarantee night-time continence, but 300 to 360 millilitres, or at least 30 millilitres per year of age, is a reasonable goal. If that seems too ambitious, then try for at least a 50 per cent improvement over the initial record.

At least once a day, also have your child practise starting and stopping the stream of urine several times. She should stop the stream not just momentarily but long enough to get good control over it.

When your child has been dry at night for two consecutive weeks, reinforce the success with a programme of 'overlearning': encourage her to drink more and more fluid during the day and as much as two to four glasses just before bed so that she will keep getting better at controlling her bladder.

Conditioning

Conditioning systems have been very successful in treating enuresis. These devices rely on a sensor that fits into the child's underwear at night. When it gets wet, a loud alarm (usually attached to the child's pyjamas or wrist) is triggered. Several units are available commercially in the United States and can easily be ordered online. Although older versions of some of these devices posed slight risks of irritation or burns from the electrical current, modern designs have rendered them completely safe.

The object of conditioning is to wake your child as soon as she begins to wet the bed, on the theory that she will gradually come to unconsciously associate the sensations she feels just before urinating with the need to wake. To use this method successfully you will need your child's full co-operation and understanding, so it is unlikely to be much help before she is at least seven (although some younger children are able to profit from it). Both the parents and the child should understand how the mechanism works, but the child should take responsibility for testing it and turning it on when she gets into bed at night.

If the alarm rings at night and your child does not wake immediately, it is up to you to wake her as soon as possible. Leave the alarm ringing, however, until she gets up and turns it off herself. She should then go to the toilet to try to complete her urination there, then help to re-make the bed, if necessary, and re-set the alarm. If she wets so early in the night that she simply cannot wake when the alarm sounds, try 'lifting' her (see page 366) – take her to the toilet before the time when the first alarm of the night usually rings. Later in the night her sleep will be lighter, so she should wake more easily and will still learn to respond to the alarm (and eventually, if all goes well, to the bladder signals that occur before that). Whether or not she wets later, gradually move the time of lifting towards bedtime, and then stop lifting her altogether.

It is crucial that the system be used every night and that you keep accurate records of the results. The conditioning process can be slow. Be prepared to continue for four to five months, although most children respond sooner. In general, 25 per cent of children are dry within two to six weeks, 50 per cent within three months and 90 per cent within six months. When conditioning is unsuccessful, it is most often because the family used it inconsistently or incorrectly or because they stopped too soon.

After your child has been dry for two weeks, begin an 'over-learning' process, as described in the section above on bladder training: have her drink extra fluid during the day and two to four more glasses before bed, and continue to use the alarm until she has stayed dry for an additional twenty-one consecutive nights.

Be aware that when children stop using the alarm the first time, the bed-wetting often starts again. If that happens, simply use the alarm again exactly as you did before. Several courses of conditioning therapy are sometimes necessary when the problem is stubborn.

Medication

When enuresis is a major problem and behavioural approaches are unsuccessful, medication is occasionally necessary to help bring the problem under control. If you think your child may be a candidate for medication, discuss it with your paediatrician.

One medication commonly used is desmopressin. This drug, a synthetic hormone, resembles the naturally produced hormone vasopressin, also known as 'antidiuretic hormone'. Vasopressin is normally secreted at night and helps to draw water from the urine back into the bloodstream. The urine that remains is more concentrated; hence there is less of it, making it easier to stay dry through the night. Although there is evidence that some enuretic children produce less than the typically expected amount of vasopressin at night, it is not clear that their hormonal levels are abnormally low. Nevertheless, desmopressin taken at bedtime, as a nasal spray or a pill, may help to suppress night-time urination. It is generally not recommended for children under six years old. When it does work, it is often useful for special occasions such as overnight visits, travel and camp. It can also be used nightly, especially for older children who are distressed by frequent wetting and for whom other approaches haven't worked. Bear in mind that the medication itself usually does not cure the underlying problem, so the bed-wetting typically re-appears when the desmopressin is stopped.

Lifting

You may already be 'lifting' your child – that is, taking her to the toilet at some point after she has fallen asleep, probably when you are about to go to bed. This precaution *sometimes* prevents wetting, especially in children who wet only once a night at a regular, predictable hour that is not too late. However, it is unlikely to have any long-term benefits.

By rousing the child rather than letting her learn to wake on her own from bladder signals, lifting may actually delay night-time continence. Besides, the child may already be wet when the parents go in, or she may wet again later in the night. On the other hand, when it does work, at least the child is dry, everyone is less frustrated and there are fewer sheet and pyjama changes to deal with. If you do find lifting useful, I suggest that every three months you try going two weeks without lifting, to check your child's progress and to give her a chance to learn night-time control or to see if she has already attained it and whether the lifting even needs to be re-started.

Dietary Changes

Major dietary changes are rarely useful as a means to decrease wetting: they require a lot of work and improvements are rare. Although advocates of this approach can be persuasive, there is little evidence to support their claims. If you do want to try this method, follow the same diets that are described in books on dietary therapy for hyperactive children. Ask your librarian for help. But remember, any improvement you see may only be coincidental. In any case, don't keep your child on a severely restricted diet indefinitely. Gradually add back the foods you have taken out of her diet. Be sure that a particular food is responsible for increased wetting before you make your child do without it for more than a few weeks.

Final Words

Enuresis can be difficult to stop entirely, and persistent enuresis is certainly frustrating. Although the treatments described in this chapter do not guarantee success, when they are carried out diligently, most children's wetting diminishes significantly and many children stop wetting altogether. Although enuresis is only a minor sleep disorder in itself, it can still be seriously disruptive. It is important that you understand the problem and respond to your child's needs appropriately. Even if there is nothing you can do but wait until she outgrows the bed-wetting, she must see that you are waiting patiently and sympathetically. Work *with* her positively, as part of a team. If you do that, you will help her to avoid months or years of unnecessary suffering, her self-image will improve, your own relationship with her will remain unharmed and she will get along better with her friends – and your attempts to reduce wetting will be more likely to succeed.

CHAPTER 16

Head-Banging, Body-Rocking
and Head-Rolling

Some children exhibit rhythmic, seemingly strange behaviours at night. Such a child might rock back and forth, roll his head or bang his head repeatedly against a hard surface such as a headboard or wall. To parents, these behaviours can seem peculiar and even quite worrisome, especially if they do not understand their origin or significance.

Jason, for example, was a healthy and normal two-year-old boy. His parents had first become concerned when he was seven months old, when he began to rock back and forth vigorously on all fours for about twenty minutes every night before falling asleep. Soon this behaviour included banging his head against the end of his cot, and he was still doing so each night at age two. Although he still usually stopped within twenty minutes and fell asleep, some episodes lasted as long as an hour. Even worse, he had started banging in the middle of the night as well, once or twice each night for up to forty-five minutes at a time. The rocking and banging often moved the cot across the room. It was constantly being damaged and had had to be replaced twice. Worried that Jason would injure himself, his parents put padding at the end of the cot, but he would either push it aside or find another hard spot where he could bang his head. When his parents moved him to a mattress on the floor, he simply crawled over to the wall and began to bang his head there.

If your child has behaviours like Jason's, you no doubt share his parents' concerns. But there is usually little reason to worry. Many young children engage in some sort of repetitious, rhythmic behaviour in bed. They rock back and forth, roll their heads from side to side, bang their heads against a hard surface or repeatedly drop their heads onto their pillows or mattresses. Some children hum rhythmically or make other sounds at the same time.

When Do These Behaviours Occur?

Children who rock or bang in bed usually do so at bedtime, but they may also rock or bang in the morning after waking, before naps or as they try to return to sleep after night-time wakings. Some children show these behaviours *only* after waking during the night. When a child rocks or bangs his head at night, he is usually drowsy, just falling asleep or in very light sleep, and the behaviour generally stops once he is soundly asleep. If the behaviour occurs in the morning, it usually stops once the child is wide awake.

Though these instances can seem bizarre, rhythmic behaviours are in fact an entirely normal part of a child's development. Breathing, sucking and crying, for example, are rhythmic behaviours all children engage in. In addition, most toddlers at least occasionally rock back and forth for a few minutes during the day, usually sitting up and commonly while listening to music. About one out of five rock on all fours at least once a day and about half of those children rock in bed before going to sleep. About 5 per cent of children exhibit other rhythmic behaviours, particularly head-banging and head-rolling; these behaviours are most likely to occur at night or at nap time. Head-banging appears three times more often in boys than in girls, but body-rocking and head-rolling are equally common in both.

What Do These Behaviours Look Like?

A child who rocks in bed typically does so on all fours, although some prefer a sitting position (as do most children who rock during the day). Similarly, when the behaviour includes head-banging, the child usually gets on all fours and rocks back and forth, hitting his forehead or the top of his head on the headboard, wall or other hard surface, or he sits up in bed and bangs the back of his head repeatedly on the hard surface. Sometimes a child will lie face-down and lift his head, or his head and chest, then drop them back into the pillow or mattress again and again. Less commonly, a child still in the cot may grasp the side rail and hit his head against it, or contort himself so he can rock, bang his head, suck his thumb and hold on to a stuffed animal all at the same time. A child who head-rolls usually lies on his back and moves his head rhythmically from side to side; he may also bang his head or body on the bed rail, wall or side of the cot in the process.

Some children vocalise while they rock or bang. Usually they produce a loud, continuous humming or chanting sound that waxes and wanes in intensity and pitch in the same rhythm as the body movements:

UHHHuhhhUHHHuhhh

UMMMummmUMMMummm

For parents who have to listen to these sounds, especially for long periods, it can be torture. The sound of a child's head repeatedly banging into the wall or headboard can be similarly excruciating. The thud of a child dropping into his mattress or pillow is at least easier to listen to.

Is Head-Banging Dangerous?

Although head banging looks dangerous, neurologically normal children do not hurt themselves seriously in the process (unless, perhaps, they have a disorder such as haemophilia that increases the likelihood of bleeding). Although foreheads do occasionally get bruised and, very rarely, there can be a small amount of external bleeding, the banging almost never leads to concussions, fractured skulls or other head injuries. Any damage is mainly restricted to cots, beds and walls.

When Should You Be Concerned?

Rhythmic behaviours generally don't reflect any underlying emotional difficulty or neurological illness, particularly if they follow the usual pattern, beginning before the age of eighteen months and mostly disappearing by age three or four. Most children with these habits are healthy, with no discernible physical or mental problems and no unusual tensions in their families. It is true that these behaviours occur more frequently in children with certain neurological or psychiatric disorders; in particular, children who have learning difficulties, are blind or autistic are more inclined than other children to rock their bodies or bang their heads (although they tend to do it during the day when they are fully awake). But for many other reasons, major disorders like these are usually quite apparent. So if your child is developing normally in other respects, there is no reason to worry about a significant problem simply because he has begun to engage in rhythmic behaviours.

If such behaviours begin, persist, or recur past age four, they deserve even more attention since in the school-aged child such behaviours are more likely to require treatment. Bear in mind, however, that rhythmic behaviours present in the older child are still likely of little concern if they are short-lasting and not particularly intense – perhaps brief periods of gentle head-rolling or a few minutes of mild thumping into the pillow before sleep. These are probably merely habits the child has learned to associate with falling asleep and are not very important. Although habits of this sort in a school-aged child may be slow to resolve completely, they do tend to become progressively briefer and less vigorous over time.

But regardless of your child's age, you should be concerned if his rhythmic behaviours are intense, last longer than ten or fifteen minutes or recur repeatedly during the night. In all these cases you should investigate further because such prominent behaviours may have causes that you can identify and should address, as discussed below.

What Causes Rhythmic Behaviours?

Although most of the behaviours described in this chapter can occur in young children as part of their normal development, there are a number of other possible causes to consider. Some of these causes will seem familiar, since they also underlie problems we've seen in other chapters, and they require similar treatment here, for the same reasons. For example, your child's rocking may be a habit associated with falling asleep (as discussed in Chapter 4); his humming and thumping, if they get you to come into his room, may be his way of testing limits or dealing with anxiety (as described in Chapters 5 and 7); or his rocking or banging may be the way he fills up long periods awake caused by an inappropriate schedule (as explained in Chapter 11). Other causes, including neurological problems, familial predispositions and inherent sleep disturbances, must be handled differently. Also, several causes may be at work in the same child.

Normal Development

Having little ability to keep themselves occupied, infants and young children derive pleasure in whatever ways they can. Children naturally respond to rhythmic stimuli, which is why they like to be rocked or listen to lullabies. The rhythms provide them with a feeling of pleasure and comfort, much like an adult tapping his foot to music. Early in life, infants derive pleasure from rhythmic sucking on a dummy, thumb or nipple; later they may find similar comfort in rhythmic rocking or head-rolling. (It is less clear how head-banging can be soothing, but some children do apparently find the loud rhythmical sounds of the impacts, or even the impacts themselves, comforting.) In the course of normal development, all of these behaviours generally go away as the child develops new abilities to think, listen, attend and move.

The rhythmic behaviours typically begin very early in life, usually within the first year. On average, body-rocking generally starts at around six months of age, head-banging and head-rolling at about nine months. But there is a wide range of variation. Head-rolling and the beginnings of rocking can appear in children as young as a month or two; head-banging – if it occurs at all – can begin as early as four months, almost always by the beginning of the second year. Often body-rocking or head-rolling starts first, and head-banging begins weeks or months later. Humming usually does not start before age one.

The behaviours may last only a few weeks or months; they usually disappear within a year and a half of onset. It is uncommon to see them after a child reaches four years of age. Occasionally, rhythmic behaviours that start as normal developmental patterns persist as pre-sleep habits throughout childhood; even in adulthood, some people still roll one or both legs from side to side for a few minutes while falling asleep.

Head-banging and rocking often begin at about the same time as teething; when they do, the behaviours – if they are short-lived – might be a response to the temporary discomfort. But too many sleep disorders in infants are ascribed to teething; in any case, it's unlikely to be the cause of any behaviour that persists for more than a few weeks. Temporary head-banging or rocking may also appear (or re-appear) when a child is facing an important developmental hurdle, such as learning to stand or take his first steps. Perhaps it helps him to release tension he feels during the day, or to return to sleep after waking from stressful dreams. We do not know for sure.

Inappropriate Sleep Schedules

While an inappropriate schedule alone cannot cause rhythmic behaviours, certain schedule problems can allow the behaviours to continue for long periods each night, to persist over months and to progressively worsen, regardless of the underlying cause. Fixing the child's schedule is often crucial to successful intervention.

A schedule that has a youngster in bed before he is ready to fall asleep and for more hours than he can sleep will increase the time available to him for rocking or banging, since most such behaviour in bed takes place in wakefulness, drowsiness or transitional light sleep and disappears once the child is sound asleep. As described in Chapter 11, this extra time awake (or drowsy with only brief periods of very light sleep) can appear at bedtime, during the night or in the morning. As we have seen before (particularly in Chapters 5 and 11), there are a number of ways for a child to pass that time – mainly playing, talking, crying or repeatedly calling out or leaving his room. Rhythmic activities are another way.

Worse, the more waking time a child has to repeatedly practise a rhythmic behaviour, the more that behaviour will be reinforced, and the more likely it will be to become a progressively demanding habit.

Habit

Habits that provide comfort and distract us from fantasies or worries are powerfully learned behaviours, and they can become partly automatic. Adults exhibit them much as children do: they tap their feet, stroke their face or bounce their crossed legs while thinking or in conversation. You can stop those sorts of movements when you're aware of them, but as soon as your attention drifts, as a child's does when he becomes drowsy, the movements are likely to begin again.

At the same time, the more such movements are repeated, the more automatic they become and the harder it gets to suppress them. Eventually the child may feel uncomfortable if unable to do them, in the same way that the more a child uses a dummy, the more he will come to feel uncomfortable without it. If the movements occur while a child is going to sleep, he begins to associate them with falling asleep – just as if he were being rocked to sleep (see Chapter 4), except he is his own rocker. And if a child is used to rocking or banging until he falls asleep at night, he is especially likely to start up again if he has long wakings in the middle of the night, picking up where he left off (though some children do rock or bang only at these wakings and not at bedtime). Eventually the behaviours may become so automatic that, like sucking motions, they continue through drowsiness into light sleep itself.

Emotional Needs

Rhythmic behaviours sometimes occur in response to anxiety. While they cannot overcome severe anxiety, they may help with less intense worries and concerns. We saw in Chapters 7 and 11 that even a child without any significant anxiety could end up scaring himself if his bedtime is too early and he is left alone with his thoughts for too long before he can fall asleep. A child with more anxiety will have still more difficulty tolerating time awake in bed. An older child or an adult can turn to a book or the radio, or to focused activities such as progressive relaxation or pacing, to distract himself until he is sufficiently sleepy. A young child usually turns to his parents for this purpose. But some children try to handle these feelings by themselves, rolling around restlessly or rhythmically. Rocking, banging and humming require effort and focus and can thus also serve as distractions (all the more so if the behaviours are intense), and the resulting noise can be distracting as well. While a child is engaged in these actions, scary thoughts are less likely to intrude. However, again, with nightly repetition the behaviours may become increasingly habitual until the child begins to feel uncomfortable without them even when he is not anxious or frightened.

Rhythmic behaviour can also be a stratagem to get attention from parents, even though there may be no significant underlying anxiety. It will be successful if parents do not limit their responses appropriately. A child who deliberately rocks, hums or bangs noisily enough to get you to come in can argue truthfully that he is staying in bed and not calling out. If he is rocking or banging to get your attention and you respond by repeatedly going into his room or calling out to him to stop, you may be rewarding the behaviour and thus inadvertently reinforcing it.

Jessica was an eight-year-old girl who had gone through a brief period of rocking in bed during her first year but stopped soon thereafter. Six months before her mother brought her to see me, she had begun 'thumping' – lying in bed face-down, lifting her head, and letting it fall into her pillow – every night for thirty to sixty minutes before falling asleep. She was healthy and seemed happy enough, if a little withdrawn. But the previous year had been a time of great difficulty for her family. Her parents had separated and were working out the details of a divorce; Jessica and her mother had moved into a smaller flat and her mother had returned to work. I learned that Jessica believed she somehow had caused her parents' separation and thought they might be angry with her over it. She was afraid of causing her mother more unhappiness and losing her love as a result. Apparently, Jessica's head-banging had recurred in response to these emotional struggles, perhaps to help her to avoid unpleasant thoughts while she was going to sleep, or to get some extra needed attention. She did not actually need to thump her head to fall asleep: in fact, she stopped whenever someone came into her room, and if they stayed long enough, she fell asleep without any thumping at all. Later in this chapter I explain how our understanding of the cause of Jessica's head-banging allowed us to help her with this problem.

Neurodevelopmental Abnormalities

Children with neurodevelopmental delays, as are present in autism, learning difficulties and related conditions, often seem to get considerable pleasure out of rhythmic self-stimulation, even after the early years. That may be because, like a normal younger child or infant, their physical, sensory or cognitive limitations prevent them from finding other ways to distract or comfort themselves; the basic drive that produces these behaviours may be no different from that seen in normal children in the early months and years of life. However, whereas otherwise normal youngsters who head bang do not do so to the point of pain and serious injury, some developmentally disabled youngsters seem oblivious to pain caused by their intense behaviours, or even take pleasure in it. These children may need to be restrained or otherwise protected to keep them from injuring themselves.

Familial Predisposition

In some families, the tendency to engage in rhythmic behaviour in bed is particularly common, occurring in many individuals over several generations. In this situation – one that occurs only infrequently – an inherited trait is evidently involved, but we don't know what that trait is. (Just as musical aptitude is a trait that may be inherited, perhaps a similar genetic trait makes rhythmic behaviours particularly pleasurable or compelling.) The episodes in inherited cases are usually brief and not particularly intense, provided that the child's sleep schedule is appropriate. They may be slow to resolve completely, if they ever do, although they do tend to become less intense over time.

Inherent Sleep Disturbance

Rhythmic behaviours rarely persist through drowsiness and light sleep into the deeper stages of sleep; but, occasionally they do, and in some children they occur only in those stages. A child who exhibits this variation will rock or bang in his sleep no matter what the circumstances – in his parents' bed, at a grandparent's or friend's home or at home with a babysitter. If you go into your child's room when he is rocking and find that he seems unaware of you even when you speak to him, then he is probably asleep; if he responds only after you speak loudly or shake him and then seems briefly confused, then he was certainly asleep. The child, even an older child who finds reports of the behaviours embarrassing, cannot suppress them.

This variant seems to be a truly automatic behaviour of sleep, rather than just a habit. Although it might appear that a child whose deep sleep is interrupted by these movements would suffer the effects of sleep deprivation, in fact he does not; usually there are no apparent daytime consequences. This problem may be more difficult to treat than a simple habit associated only with drowsiness, and it may persist longer. Nevertheless, the behaviour will likely become less intense over the years, with episodes becoming shorter and shifting to periods of lighter sleep or drowsiness. Eventually it will almost certainly disappear.

If your child bangs or rocks both when awake and when asleep, the wakeful part at least is treatable. But when this is done, you may find that the rhythmic behaviours in sleep decrease as well, since they may have been a result of the waking habits in the first place. Just as habits practised repetitively can become so automatic that they persist into light sleep (as mentioned above), occasionally they also persist into deep sleep (where there isn't even the slightest conscious awareness of doing them).

Treating the Problem

Once you have an appreciation of the causes and significance of rhythmic behaviour in your child, you can decide what you should do about it. There are a number of choices to consider.

Decide If You Need to Do Anything

In an infant or young toddler, brief rhythmic behaviours that don't annoy anyone or disrupt the household do not call for intervention. They will likely disappear before long. But (as suggested above), if your child's rocking or head-banging is more severe and lasts more than a few minutes, keeps you up at night or annoys you (or the neighbours), or damages the bed or cot, then you may want to see if these behaviours can be lessened, especially if your child is already of school age. More importantly, even if your child seems to enjoy the behaviour, he shouldn't have to work so hard just to fall asleep. If he didn't need to bang, he might be able to fall asleep much faster; thus, the banging may leave him getting less sleep than he would get otherwise.

Adjust the Sleep Schedule

The best way to break any undesirable habits associated with getting to sleep is to have the child practise falling asleep without them, and that is easiest if his schedule is adjusted so that he will be too sleepy at bedtime and night-time wakings to stay awake for more than a few minutes even if he wants to. If things go well, he will soon be rocking very little, if at all, at bedtime and when he wakes briefly during the night. Before long, he should start to feel comfortable in bed without rocking even when he is less sleepy.

Usually the best starting point is to cut back on the child's excessive time in bed, just as you would for any other child who takes a long time to fall asleep or lies awake for long periods during the night (see Chapter 11). Add up the amount of time your child spends rocking at night and shorten his time in bed by at least that amount. Do the same for nap periods. If he rocks or bangs a great deal at bedtime, move his bedtime later, at least to the hour he usually stops banging and falls asleep. Don't let his morning waking drift later to compensate. If he rocks or bangs in the middle of the night for more than a few minutes, you may have to move his bedtime even later, or move his morning waking earlier. If he rocks or bangs in the morning, get up with him as soon as he wakes and before he has had much time to rock or bang. Remember, the goal is to cut out the habitual patterns and get him used to being in bed and going to sleep without rocking or banging.

It may be necessary at first to reduce his time in bed to a period shorter than his actual sleep requirement to make him sleepy enough. Once things are going well and he has had a chance to practise going to sleep without rocking or banging, you can gradually extend his time in bed, as discussed in Chapter 11. Your goal is to reach a permanent schedule that allows him to fall asleep quickly, with little or no night-time waking, rocking or banging, spontaneous (or at least easy) morning wakings and normal daytime functioning.

Address Your Child's Emotional Needs

In school-aged children, vigorous and long-lasting head-banging or rocking could be a sign of emotional issues that require your help. As discussed in other chapters, and, of course, depending on the needs of your child, you may have to set consistent limits or provide other emotional support. You should certainly respond to your child's appropriate needs for attention, but don't let him demand it through head-banging, or you will only reinforce the pattern. Once you have shortened his time in bed as described above, ignore any rocking or banging at night. Instead, spend extra time with him during the day; show him that you enjoy his company. The time before bed is especially important. Rather than waiting for him to demand attention, offer it in the form of an unhurried bedtime routine in his bedroom. It sometimes helps, too, if you offer to stay in a nearby room when you are done, checking in on him until he falls asleep (even if he is perfectly quiet at the time).

If anxiety is a major factor, as it was for Jessica, you will need to address it directly. If your child is concerned about fighting or illness in the family, or about a major issue such as an impending parental divorce, you will probably be aware of it. If you recognise that the behaviours began after the development of concerns or the occurrence of important family changes like these, try to discuss the situation with him openly and encourage him to express his anger or feelings of guilt. If his anxiety is relieved, his need to rock or bang will diminish. If he is too young for such complex discussions, be particularly attentive and loving so that he will know that his world is safe and caring and that he is not responsible for the problems. It is sometimes hard to provide all this support on your own. If your attempts to help meet with little success, or if you cannot determine the source of the problem or how to deal with it, then consider seeking guidance from a psychotherapist. But in the meantime, changing your child's sleep schedule will still help by eliminating extra time he can spend worrying in bed.

Tackle the Behaviours Directly

There are a few things you can do to make your child's rhythmic behaviours more difficult to carry out or less enjoyable to do, or to motivate him to stop. If your child is in a cot and rocks forcefully enough to shake the cot or even 'walk' it across the floor, you may want to have him sleep on a mattress on the floor. Unfortunately, this approach is less effective with a child who bangs his head into the headboard; even if you set his mattress in the middle of a room, he will probably only crawl over to the wall and bang his head there, at least at bedtime. (On waking in the middle of the night, however, he may settle for rocking instead of banging.)

Some paediatricians recommend putting a loudly ticking clock or metronome in your child's room. The metronome may be set to beat at the same tempo as the rocking or banging, on the theory that it will fulfill your child's need for rhythmic stimulation, or you may chose a slightly different rate, just far enough from his typical rhythm to be difficult to match, and close enough to it to be confusing and disruptive if he tries to rock at his usual tempo. I have not had great success with this method, but it is certainly harmless, and you may want to try it.

You may also try to make it more rewarding for your child *not* to rock or bang by trying to make stopping the goal he is working towards. With a child aged three or older, a good way to do that is through a mutually negotiated sticker chart with prizes for success, like those mentioned in Chapters 5 and 7. To get this programme off to a good start, begin with a later bedtime and a shorter night than usual, to help assure initial success.

During the day, meet your young child's need for rhythmic stimulation by encouraging him to use swings or rocking horses, listen to music or rock in a chair. With enough of this activity during the day, he may have less need for it at night.

Protection and Medication

Finally, children with autism and learning difficulties – especially those with other significant neurological abnormalities – may vigorously bang their heads to the point of actually injuring themselves. Such a child may have to wear a helmet or be restrained, or his sleep surroundings may need to be provided with extra padding. Even for these children, shortening the amount of time they spend in bed can be helpful. Sometimes medication can help if nothing else is working, even though drug treatments for head-banging are generally of little use in the 'normal' child. Consult your GP if you think helmets, restraints or medication might be called for.

OUTCOMES

How Jason and Jessica Were Helped

Even though Jason was only two years old and his head-banging would probably have stopped on its own within a year or so, his episodes of banging were so long, intense and frequent – up to two and a half hours in total some nights – that we felt it made sense to try to shorten them. I learned that Jason was going to bed at 7.00 p.m., waking at 7.00 a.m., and taking a two-hour nap – fourteen hours in all, two to three more hours than a typical two-year-old is able to sleep. We moved his bedtime to 9.00 p.m., moved his waking time to 6.00 a.m., and limited his nap to ninety minutes. Almost immediately, his head-banging decreased markedly, to less than ten minutes at bedtime and ten minutes again once or twice during the night. Over the next few weeks the episodes became even shorter and the head-banging became less intense. Some nights his parents heard only a few minutes of banging at bedtime. At that point they gradually lengthened his night to ten hours, 8.30 p.m., to 6.30 a.m., and set his nap back to two hours. Now that he was getting all the sleep he needed without being in bed any more than necessary, the head-banging remained brief and occasional and never recurred as a significant problem.

As for Jessica, her mother sought counselling for both of them, at my suggestion, and the tension at home began to ease quickly. She and Jessica spent more time talking, and together they found it easier to discuss feelings related to the divorce. Jessica's mother was surprised to discover how much Jessica had to say about her father's leaving, and Jessica admitted that she felt responsible. She hadn't spoken up before because her mother had always avoided the topic. Now that Jessica could express her feelings, her mother was able to correct her misconceptions and reassure her.

Jessica wanted to stop 'thumping', but breaking any long-standing habit can be very difficult. I recommended that her bed-time be moved temporarily half an hour later, and that together she and her mother should begin to keep a star chart in which she earned rewards for quiet nights. Working on the chart provided them with some special time together during the day, as Jessica added stars and they talked about her success. Jessica's mother was careful to ignore any thumping at night – she did not call out to Jessica or go into her room – to avoid reinforcing it, and she made it a priority to spend extra time with Jessica during the day.

Now that Jessica and her mother were working together, their daytime relationship improved and they both felt better. Jessica was proud of her success and worked on earning stars for her chart with real enthusiasm. Her thumping disappeared within four weeks, except for occasional brief episodes in the middle of the night that were of little concern.

Final Points

Rhythmic behaviours at night and at naps are not as strange as they may seem at first. The causes can usually be determined, and the behaviours generally do not imply worrisome underlying conditions. Most often, with understanding and proper planning, these behaviours can be satisfactorily reduced or eliminated using straightforward approaches.

PART V

THE SLEEPY CHILD

CHAPTER 17

Noisy Breathing, Snoring and Obstructive Sleep Apnoea

When a child snores loudly in her sleep, parents often dismiss it lightly, joking that no one would ever be able to share a room with her. But other parents worry. Watching and listening to your child each night, you may have come to believe that she is actually struggling to breathe – perhaps, at times, *unable* to breathe – rather than 'just snoring'. You may even sit by her bed or take her into yours when she has a cold to make sure that she doesn't stop breathing. Even if your friends or doctors have told you that snoring is nothing to worry about, you watch and listen, and worry anyway.

It is not unusual or abnormal for children to snore occasionally, such as when they have a cold, but they should not snore most nights, and they should not routinely struggle to breathe or even have to sleep with their mouths open.

Although snoring used to be dismissed as a mere annoyance, we now know that it is often associated with significant breathing problems in sleep. It can be a sign of a disorder called *obstructive sleep apnoea*, which requires medical attention. Even if she does not have the fully developed syndrome, a child who snores is not breathing freely and normally at night, and it could be disrupting her sleep, even to the extent of affecting her daytime behaviour and her ability to learn.

What Happens in Sleep Apnoea

Doctors have been aware of sleep apnoea for many years, but it is only since sleep laboratories appeared in the 1970s that we began to recognise just how common it is. Although the problem is especially prevalent in men over forty and in women after the menopause, a great many children suffer from it as well. Unfortunately, sleep apnoea in children has been largely overlooked, perhaps because children's daytime symptoms are often less obvious than those of adults, or because most sleep centres mainly see adult patients.

'Apnoea' means the absence of breathing. When a child with obstructive sleep apnoea is asleep, her upper airway narrows or closes off repeatedly, typically for periods of eight to thirty seconds at a time (why this happens is explained below). Little or no air can pass through the obstruction no matter how hard she tries to breathe. Sleep specialists distinguish between the syndromes of 'obstructive sleep apnoea' and 'upper airway resistance,' but the difference is really just a matter of how much obstruction there is and whether the blockage of airflow is nearly complete or only partial. For simplicity, I will use the single term *sleep apnoea* to describe the entire spectrum of disorders.

Sleep apnoea is a problem not only because of the repeated temporary loss of oxygen, but because the sleeper has to wake partially to start breathing again. Depending on the severity of the apnoea, that can happen up to several hundred times a night. With these frequent interruptions, good sleep becomes impossible. (Often these wakings are too small and too brief to observe directly and can only be detected in the laboratory, but they are nevertheless effective at disrupting sleep.)

If there is some airflow during an apnoea event, the sleeper snores. The sounds will be soft and squeaky if only a tiny amount of air gets through, loud and raspy if the airflow is a bit better and softer again if the airflow is even better still. If the airflow is temporarily blocked completely, there is no noise at all because the sleeper isn't breathing. While the airflow is reduced, oxygen levels in the bloodstream drop until, usually after eight to thirty seconds, the sleeper wakes slightly, semi-consciously adjusts the muscles of her tongue and throat to open her airway and takes in several relatively unobstructed breaths. If her breathing was completely blocked before this point, these breaths will be accompanied by loud snoring or snorting. Thus, a complete blockage produces periods of silence alternating with ones with loud snoring. But if the obstruction is not complete – and there is continuous snoring during the period of decreased breathing (or *hypopnoea*) – alternating periods of louder and softer snoring result. After a few good breaths have improved her oxygen level again, at the end of an apnoea event, the apnoea sufferer falls back asleep (unaware of the partial waking), only to have her breathing become obstructed once more. Her sleep, disrupted by these efforts to breathe, may be quite restless. In extreme cases, sufferers sleep sitting up or bent forward in an effort to improve respiration.

In sleep apnoea the actual obstruction usually occurs in the back of the throat, behind the base of the tongue. The walls of the throat are relatively floppy in this region; if they collapse and the tongue falls backward, the airway can be blocked. While awake, we are able to prevent this happening by holding our tongue sufficiently forward and our throat sufficiently taut so we can breathe. In sleep, however, we lose some of that ability, and this is why even people without any trouble breathing during the day can still suffer from sleep apnoea at night.

Certain conditions make collapse of the throat walls more likely – for example, an abnormal narrowing higher up in the airway, in or behind the nasal passages, that forces a person to breathe very hard. Think of your upper respiratory tract like a drinking straw that you breathe through, as shown in Figure 18 on page 39. As long as the straw is intact, you can breathe without difficulty. However, if you bend the straw in the middle several times so that it becomes less

FIGURE 18. OBSTRUCTIVE SLEEP APNOEA

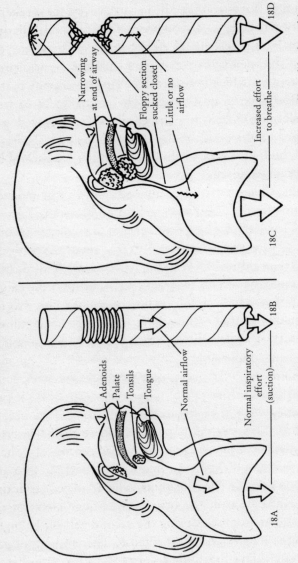

In Figure 18A, a girl with normal-sized tonsils and adenoids breathes well, with little effort, like breathing through a straw of sufficient width (Figure 18B).

In Figure 18C, the girl's air passages are narrowed by enlarged tonsils and adenoids. Now the girl must breathe in strenuously to get air past the narrowed region. But the floppy part of the airway just below the tonsils and adenoids is sucked closed by the increased force of the girl's breathing so that there is little or no airflow – like breathing through a straw that is pinched off at the end (Figure 18D) – and an obstructive apnoea event is produced.

rigid, you will find that if you breathe in too sharply, the weakened part of the straw will collapse. If you breathe slowly and regularly it will not. If now you pinch the far end of the straw between your fingers to make the opening narrower, you will have to suck harder than usual to breathe, which in turn will collapse the floppy part of the straw and produce an obstruction. This is analogous to what happens in a sleeping child whose upper airway is narrowed, perhaps by enlarged tonsils or adenoids. To get enough air, she has to breathe harder, but in the process the floppy area at the back of her throat may be sucked closed.

Unlike adults, children with sleep apnoea rarely have completely blocked airways – the child continues to breathe, but with difficulty. She must work harder to get air in, and even if this extra effort produces enough airflow, the struggle to breathe interferes with her sleep. The degree of difficulty breathing varies from child to child, and in a given child the severity may wax and wane over the course of a night. At one extreme is full-blown sleep apnoea. Towards the other end is mildly obstructed breathing, where the child still expends more effort than normal to get each breath in: her breathing will be mildly hampered, and probably open-mouthed. There may be heavy breathing, or intermittent soft snoring, with intervening periods of even greater difficulty or louder snoring. She may have particular trouble breathing when sleeping on her back, because the tongue falls back and blocks the air passage, and during REM sleep, in which the muscles of the head and face relax profoundly. She is likely to have less trouble, or even none, in non-REM sleep and when sleeping on her side. Her breathing is likely to be best during the deep non-REM sleep of the first three to four hours of the night, and most compromised during the second half of the night, when dreaming is longest and most intense. Therefore, if all you know about your child's breathing comes from looking in before you go to bed, you may not have a complete picture, since you may never see her when she's having the most difficulty.

In the past, doctors often failed to recognise sleep apnoea in children except in very severe cases where the strain from working so hard to breathe, coupled with low levels of oxygen in the blood, affected the functioning of the heart and the level of blood pressure. Fortunately, such problems are uncommon complications in children – unlike in adults – usually occurring only in cases of such severe obstruction that the child's breathing is impaired even when she is awake.

WHAT CAUSES THE OBSTRUCTION

Although we cannot always pinpoint the site of narrowing that causes sleep apnoea, any narrowing of the upper airway or unusual floppiness in the throat tissues can bring it about. Many adults with sleep apnoea have thick, short necks; usually they are also overweight, and excessive soft, fatty tissue deposited in the walls of the throat contributes to the narrowing. Obesity can likewise be a major factor in sleep apnoea in children. Children whose muscles are weak or who suffer from muscle-control problems (as in muscular dystrophy, spasticity and hypotonia) are also at risk.

Sleep apnoea can also be caused by oral or facial anomalies, especially an abnormally small, receding lower jaw (*micrognathia* or *retrognathia*), or a flattening of the middle region of the face. In some children the obstruction may be created intentionally, for instance when the roof of the mouth (palate) is surgically connected to the back of the throat (making a *pharyngeal flap*) to create a blockage. This procedure helps to correct speech problems caused by an inability to appropriately block airflow out of the nose – as is sometimes the case in children born with a cleft palate – but if too much obstruction is created, sleep apnoea can also result. Abnormalities of the nose, such as a deviated septum or a polyp, are only rarely causes of sleep apnoea. Nasal obstruction from allergies can lead to some snoring but is very unlikely to cause significant apnoea. For several reasons, children with Down's syndrome are prone to sleep apnoea: their tongues are often too large for their mouths, their nasal passages are relatively small, they often have enlarged and chronically infected adenoids with persistent nasal discharge and they may not have completely normal neurological control of their tongue and throat muscles.

In the vast majority of children with sleep apnoea, enlarged tonsils or adenoids are the source of the problem.

Enlarged Tonsils and Adenoids

The tonsils are pink, roundish glands that are easily seen at the back of the mouth just above the tongue and against either side of the throat. When infected, they can become quite swollen; afterwards, they usually shrink back to a normal size, but not always.

You can't easily see your child's adenoids, which lie against the back of her throat above the roof of her mouth, but they look much like the tonsils. Enlarged adenoids can block normal airflow through your child's nose, forcing her to breathe through her mouth. Her speech may take on a nasal quality and her nose may run constantly. Also, when adenoids are enlarged, the tube that normally drains her middle ear can become blocked: if that happens, fluid collects in the middle ear, and your child may suffer temporary hearing loss and repeated ear infections.

Not all children with enlarged tonsils or adenoids develop sleep apnoea. This is probably because of individual differences in respiratory control and anatomy. For instance, the size and shape of a child's throat may determine whether or not enlarged tonsils will significantly interfere with her breathing at night. And a child with large adenoids may still be able to breathe fairly well at night if she can automatically switch completely to mouth-breathing during sleep (although having to breathe through her mouth at night is far from ideal: her mouth dries out and sleep may still be disrupted).

Children who have difficulty breathing because of enlarged tonsils or adenoids often snore at night for many years. The snoring may or may not get worse over time. Occasionally symptoms begin suddenly in association with a bout of tonsillitis. Often breathing difficulties worsen in the winter months, when colds are more frequent.

Grace, a three-year-old girl, had a typical story. She was happy and alert during the day, except that she sometimes seemed unusually tired in the afternoon, despite a daily nap. She was well behaved and played co-operatively with her friends. When she was three months old she had begun snoring, and over the years her snoring had grown worse. She now snored most of the night, so loudly that she could be heard all over the house. As she slept, Grace seemed to struggle to breathe; her mouth would be open, and at times her chest would actually be pulled inward rather than expanding with each breath. Her parents noticed that sometimes her chest seemed to go in and out without any apparent airflow, and at these times they would shake her awake to help her start breathing normally again. After such episodes, Grace would shudder and make strange snorting sounds as air finally entered her lungs. When she had a cold, her breathing troubles were even worse.

Needless to say, Grace's parents were quite worried. They had discussed the problem with their paediatrician on several occasions. He noted that Grace's tonsils were large, and since she breathed mostly through her mouth, he believed that her adenoids were probably also enlarged. Nevertheless, he felt that removing her tonsils and adenoids was unnecessary, because (he said) 'snoring itself is nothing to be concerned about and will be outgrown', and because Grace had not suffered from repeated throat or ear infections.

To find out for certain what was happening to Grace when she slept, we had her spend one night in the sleep laboratory. Throughout the night we monitored her stages of sleep as well as the airflow into and out of her nose and mouth. We recorded her chest and abdominal movements as she attempted to breathe and, using one sensor clipped painlessly around her finger and another placed by her nose, we measured the amount of oxygen in her bloodstream and the carbon dioxide levels in her lungs. What we found was typical of many other children with similar stories, although Grace's problem was more serious than most.

During the night Grace experienced 350 episodes in which her breathing was either completely or partially obstructed for periods lasting between eight and fifty seconds, which is a huge number of obstructions; most normal children have none at all. She spent a full quarter of her sleep time struggling with these obstructions. She did sleep reasonably well in the early part of the night, during the deeper stages of non-REM sleep, when her breathing was fairly good and her snoring only moderate. But during the rest of the night, when her breathing was obstructed and she had to struggle to breathe, her sleep was severely disrupted. During most of the obstructive episodes, her blood oxygen level dropped significantly. As one would expect, the most severe obstructions occurred during REM sleep when Grace's throat muscles were most relaxed and her breathing was least automatic.

Watching Grace struggle to breathe all night was heartbreaking. Given the extent of her sleep disruption, it was surprising that she - wasn't more tired and irritable during the day. Grace's parents were relieved to learn that their concern had been justified and that we would be able to help her.

Jonathan was a five-year-old boy whose story was almost identical to Grace's. He, too, had enlarged tonsils and adenoids, and in the laboratory he also snored and slept with his mouth open. Nevertheless, we found his breathing troubles to be less severe than Grace's: he had only forty episodes of obstructed breathing, and each of those times his airflow was only mildly blocked for brief periods of time. Although Jonathan's oxygen and carbon dioxide levels did not change much, his snoring and mouth breathing took a toll. His sleep was broken by many brief wakings to swallow and moisten his dry mouth and to try to find a more comfortable position. Judging only by the number of obstructive events and his normal oxygen level, Jonathan had only a mild case of sleep apnoea. Taking into account the effect on his sleep, however, his problem was fairly severe.

Obesity

Sleep apnoea is common in children who are markedly obese. Most GPs are familiar with the so-called Pickwickian syndrome, which, generally speaking, refers to a child who is both very fat and chronically sleepy. The term derives from the character of Joe in Charles - Dickens's *The Pickwick Papers,* 'a fat and red-faced boy' who always seems to be 'in a state of somnolency'. When Mr. Pickwick is told that Joe 'goes on errands fast asleep, and snores as he waits at table', he responds, 'How very odd!' Perhaps, but these characteristics are common enough that we routinely perform a sleep study on almost every extremely obese youngster who is treated at the hospital where our sleep laboratory is located.

Justin was such a youngster. He was a twelve-year-old boy with two obvious problems: at almost 82 kilograms (12 stone, 9 pounds) he was quite obese, and he constantly fell asleep during the day even though he seemed to get enough sleep at night. He often fell asleep at his desk in school and at home while doing his homework. As a result he had had to repeat Year 6. His teachers and parents saw his sleepiness as laziness and reacted with anger instead of sympathy.

When they came to see me, Justin's family did not mention snoring; they were worried only about his sleepiness. But in response to my questions, they told me that for years Justin had snored loudly for much of each night. As it turned out, his sleep apnoea was even more severe than Grace's. He had over six hundred apneas in one night, each lasting between twenty and seventy seconds. He suffered profound oxygen deprivation, and often his oxygen levels did not completely return to normal during the arousals that followed each obstruction. Unlike Grace, he got no deep sleep at all, and few periods even of regular breathing. It was no wonder that he was so sleepy in the daytime.

TREATING SLEEP APNOEA

Naturally, the methods we use to treat a child with sleep apnoea depend on the cause of the disorder. At our centre we work closely with ear, nose and throat specialists as well as with doctors from other disciplines such as oral surgery, plastic surgery, pulmonary medicine, neurology, and nutrition. This co-operative approach enables us to diagnose and treat children who have apnoea regardless of the cause.

If enlarged tonsils and adenoids are responsible, as they are in most children with sleep apnoea, we usually recommend they be removed. For example, Grace's tonsils and adenoids were much too big; even though she had not had problems with ear or throat infections, we felt the severity of her sleep apnoea more than justified their removal. After the operation, Grace improved remarkably. Her breathing became completely quiet at night and her sleep returned to normal. Her mother, unused to the silence, went in periodically for the first few weeks after surgery to make sure Grace was really breathing. Although Grace had not seemed especially sleepy or irritable during the day, her parents nonetheless noticed a change for the better after the surgery. Grace's spirits improved, she complained less and she was full of energy, which she put to good use.

As for Jonathan, whose sleep was also badly disrupted, even though his sleep apnoea was otherwise less severe than Grace's, he underwent the same surgery. He, too, showed a great deal of improvement. When he returned to school, his teachers remarked that he had an easier time paying attention and learned his lessons more quickly than he had before.

If Grace and Jonathan had been born in the 1940s, it is unlikely that they would have suffered so long. Doctors are less inclined now than they once were to perform tonsillectomies. In the past, tonsils were often removed simply because they were large, but we now know that large tonsils (and adenoids) do not always cause problems. Nowadays, most paediatricians recommend their removal only if complications develop. The most common complications are chronic middle-ear disease, recurrent strep throat and sleep apnoea. Of these, only sleep apnoea is likely to go undetected.

If your child is obese, like Justin, treatment must include a programme of weight loss, which may cure the apnoea by itself. If other medical factors are contributing to the apnoea, they may need to be treated as well. For example, Justin's tonsils were considerably enlarged. After they were removed, a repeat sleep study showed a significant improvement in his breathing, though not yet to a fully normal or satisfactory pattern. Over six months of closely supervised dieting, Justin was able to lose 18 kilograms (2 stone, 12 pounds). He now experienced only a few obstructions at night, his sleep was fairly continuous and he was getting enough deep sleep. The result was that he was now able to stay awake all day without signs of sleepiness or 'laziness', and he was doing much better in school, to the delight of his parents, his teachers and most of all himself.

Although dieting is a straightforward solution, it is not easy. For very obese children, satisfactory weight loss is best accomplished under supervision, in a carefully run *medical* programme. Such programmes supply proper, individualised diets and close attention by a nutritionist, careful medical management and supervision by a doctor and essential counselling services and support groups. If your child has any medical condition causing or caused by obesity, that condition must be treated at the same time. Long-term hospitalisation with closely supervised dieting, or stomach or intestinal surgery, is recommended only in rare, extreme cases.

If the cause of sleep apnoea is an oral or facial abnormality, corrective surgery may be helpful. For example, if your child has a markedly recessed chin, it can be brought forward and her teeth readjusted. This is a major undertaking, however, and although a cosmetic improvement is fairly well assured, it is as yet impossible to be certain ahead of time that the apnoea will improve significantly (although newer techniques are continually improving our ability to predict results). If your child has apnoea caused by a surgically created pharyngeal flap, the flap may have to be removed or at least narrowed to allow more room for air to pass around it.

In some cases surgery is not an immediate option. This may be because there is no anatomical problem requiring surgery, or the surgical outcome will likely be of only limited value, or the child needs to grow further before surgery will be useful or practical, or the family prefers to try other approaches first, or other medical considerations make surgery too dangerous. In addition, if the child is not overweight, or the apnoea is too severe to wait for her to lose weight, or if other preferable interventions have failed, then *continuous positive airway pressure* (CPAP) can be used (see Figure 19 on page 399). At night, the child wears a mask over her nose. A hose connects the mask to a pump that blows air through the mask into the child's nasal passages. As long as the pressure blowing in is greater than the suction generated by the child breathing in – the pressure needed is determined in the sleep laboratory – the airway will stay open and

FIGURE 19. USE OF CPAP

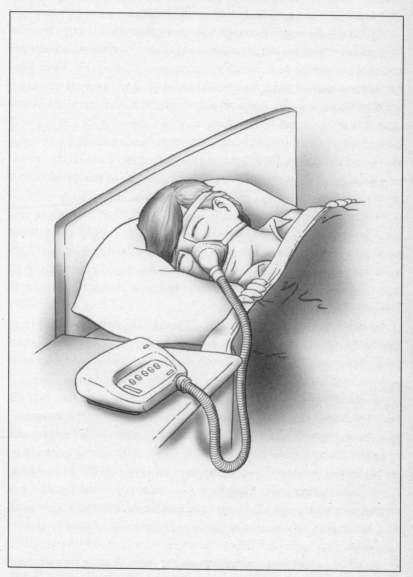

For some children with sleep apnoea, the best treatment is nightly use of continuous positive airway pressure, or CPAP. The child wears a mask over her nose, and the CPAP machine blows in air at a pressure sufficient to prevent obstruction and assure normal breathing.

the child will be able to breathe freely. (Remember the floppy straw analogy. Now imagine that, as you inhale through the straw, a machine blows air into the other end hard enough to keep it from collapsing.) Masks come in a variety of sizes and materials for comfort and proper fit, even for small children and infants. A humidifier can be attached to keep the airway from drying out. Still, getting a young child accustomed to sleeping with a mask on may take considerable effort. Usually, children start by practising in the daytime without the pump attached; most children eventually learn to wear the mask and sleep with it on without complaint.

Obviously, sleeping with such an apparatus is not ideal, but it does work very well. It can be used on a permanent basis or until the child grows and her airway enlarges sufficiently, until she undergoes planned surgery or (if she is overweight) until she loses the necessary weight. If Justin's tonsils had not been enlarged, or if surgery had not been chosen or recommended or had led to little or no improvement, we would have treated him with CPAP until he had achieved the needed weight loss.

In the past, it was necessary to perform a tracheostomy for children with severe sleep apnoea. In this procedure a tube is inserted into a hole made through the neck below the vocal cords (larynx) and into the trachea (windpipe) to provide for satisfactory breathing at night. Now such treatment is needed rarely, only for children who have very severe sleep apnoea and for whom other treatments, including other surgery and use of CPAP, have failed or are not possible. During the day, the tracheostomy tube can be plugged so air can pass through the vocal cords, allowing the child to speak normally. A child with a tracheostomy requires considerable care and, unless that can be provided in the school, the child may need to be placed in a new school setting where nursing help is always available.

Another procedure, *pharyngoplasty,* involves tightening the walls of the throat through surgery or laser treatments to make them less floppy. These techniques have been used with mixed results in adults but have not been very successful in children, probably because the walls of their throats are not very floppy to begin with. Finally, various devices that fit inside the mouth and hold the tongue or jaw forward have been used with some success in certain adults, but orthodontic and safety concerns make these devices less useful in children. Unfortunately, medication is not usually helpful in treating obstructive sleep apnoea.

Fortunately, most childhood apnoea can be treated by removing the tonsils and adenoids, by weight loss or both, with a smaller number being cured by other corrective oral or plastic surgery procedures. And, since CPAP has become available as a treatment, almost none require a tracheostomy. Tonsillectomy and adenoidectomy are relatively simple procedures and they are usually worth doing in children with sleep apnoea, even when the sleep apnoea is mild. However, if a child's tonsils and adenoids have been removed (or are very small) and she isn't overweight, it's not always clear how best to treat her if the sleep apnoea is very mild and daytime symptoms minimal. In such cases, CPAP may disrupt her sleep more than the apnoea did, and some doctors feel it may be best to leave mild sleep apnoea untreated – although if that course is chosen, they need to follow the child closely to be sure that no other problems develop and that the sleep apnoea does not grow worse. A trial period on CPAP may help with the final decision.

SOME WORDS OF CAUTION

The signs of sleep apnoea in children are generally obvious at night (if you watch carefully) with snoring, struggling and gasping, but symptoms in the daytime caused by the disrupted sleep are often not so apparent. Adults with sleep apnoea show more visible effects during the day, because their breathing may be so severely compromised that they get little deep sleep and have hundreds of full wakings. They are often very sleepy, and they are also much more likely than children to develop hypertension, headaches on waking in the morning and 'automatic behaviours' (which are periods of going about a routine activity without apparent awareness, as if sleepwalking). But since children usually have less severe breathing obstructions, their sleep (particularly their deep sleep) is less disrupted and, as a result, daytime symptoms may be absent or (as is the case with daytime sleepiness) at least not very obvious.

But these children may not be sufficiently rested, either, and their ability to learn, attend and control their behaviour may be affected. Carefully designed studies have revealed these deficits where they were once thought not to exist. Even a parent may not recognise subtle daytime symptoms, except by their absence after the problem has been treated. Sleepiness in a child may appear as any of a number of behavioural problems – hyperactivity, irritability, difficulty concentrating, forgetfulness, school problems or general 'laziness' – rather than as constant yawning and frequent napping. Children with sleep apnoea may also wet their beds and suffer from other sleep disruptions, such as nightmares, sleep terrors and sleepwalking. Rarely – when the sleep apnoea is very severe – an electrocardiogram (ECG) will show that the heart is working too hard; occasionally, a child's blood pressure may be elevated. Children who are very obese are more likely to have all of the symptoms usually seen in adults.

Sleep apnoea can be serious and should always be treated by a doctor experienced in its diagnosis and management. Sleep apnoea in the adult, if untreated, may cause considerable heart disease and occasionally may lead to death from a cardiac arrhythmia caused by low oxygen levels, or from an automobile accident caused by falling asleep at the wheel. Fortunately, since a child's heart is very resilient and children don't drive, the chances that sleep apnoea will lead to death in children is exceedingly small. It is not zero, however, especially if a child is taking any strong sedating medication that decreases the automatic drive to breathe and makes it harder to wake.

The *obstructive* sleep apnoea discussed in this chapter should not be confused with so-called *central* sleep apnoea seen mainly in infants, in which babies simply stop trying to breathe for periods of usually eight to thirty seconds with no obstruction present. Newborns, especially those born prematurely, may have long episodes of central apnoea that are truly life-threatening. Such episodes usually occur intermittently, not hundreds of times each night, and they may respond to respiratory stimulant medications. Despite much research trying to show that this phenomenon, or one like it, is a cause of Sudden Infant Death Syndrome ('cot death'), no definite conclusions can yet be drawn.

GETTING YOUR CHILD THE HELP SHE NEEDS

Even though you now have an understanding of the causes and treatments of obstructive sleep apnoea, you may have difficulty getting your child the proper evaluation and treatment. Not all doctors are aware of how common this syndrome is in children, and not all hospitals have facilities for studying children's sleep. Besides, few doctors have had the opportunity to watch a child with sleep apnoea during the night. This situation has improved considerably since the 1980s, and awareness of sleep apnoea as a problem in children is now much more widespread. Still, even if your paediatrician is well informed, he or she will probably only see your child during the day, when she is awake and probably breathing normally. You may have to work hard to persuade the doctor that your child has a problem at night that needs attention.

You may want to ask your paediatrician for a referral to a paediatric sleep specialist, or at least to a paediatrician or specialist in pulmonary or neurological disorders who is familiar with sleep apnoea in children. If there are no paediatric sleep centres in your area, try to find an adult sleep centre. Even if they mostly treat adults, they may still be able to evaluate (or properly refer) your child. If at the initial evaluation your child was not seen by a paediatric ear, nose and throat specialist, ask for a referral. If necessary, make a video or audio recording of your child's snoring so your doctor can actually listen to and perhaps even see your child having difficulty breathing.

Be persistent, and you will get the attention you need for your child. If necessary, ask your child's doctor to review the information in this chapter so that you can work together to solve your child's sleep disorder.

FIGURE 20. HOW TO TELL
WHETHER YOUR CHILD HAS SLEEP APNOEA

Main Symptoms

- Snoring
  - Loud, raspy, squeaky, snorting
  - Usually can be heard throughout the home (if you have to stand by the - child's bedside to hear it, sleep apnoea is less likely)
  - Present most nights (not just occasionally or only with a cold)
  - May be present more in the second half of the night
  - May only be a problem when the child sleeps on her back

- Difficulty Breathing
  - Child works hard or even struggles to breathe
  - Mouth may be kept open
  - Upper chest may be pulled inward rather than expanding when the child breathes in
  - Restless sleep
  - Repetitive pattern of obstruction: recurrent episodes of breathing difficulty followed by moving about (even 'shuddering') with partial waking and briefly improved breathing with loud snorting, snoring, gasping or heavy breathing
  - Episodes of completely blocked breathing: times when attempts to breathe are strong (the chest and abdomen move in and out) but actual breathing (airflow) seems completely, or almost completely, blocked

Associated Features Common in Children

- Enlarged tonsils or adenoids, or frequent sore throats or ear infections; obesity; abnormalities of the jaw, mouth or throat

- Overt daytime sleepiness is often mild; irritability, difficulty concentrating and school problems are more likely

- Presence of other sleep problems: bed-wetting; sleep terrors or confusional arousals

Other Symptoms, Seen Mainly in Adults and Less Commonly in Children

- Overwhelming daytime sleepiness

- Morning headaches

- 'Automatic behaviour' (carrying out routine daytime activities without apparent awareness)

- Cardiovascular problems (high blood pressure and electrocardiogram abnormalities)

Findings in Sleep Laboratory Study

- Recurrent respiratory obstructions

- Lowered oxygen values (usually)

- Elevated levels of carbon dioxide (often)

- Sleep disruption (of variable severity)

- Cardiac rhythm disturbances (uncommon in children)

CHAPTER 18

Narcolepsy and
Other Causes of Sleepiness

For the two years preceding his first visit to me, Brendan napped between forty and sixty minutes every afternoon. He usually went to bed after dinner, at about 7.00 p.m., and slept until 6.30 a.m. That may not seem unusual, but Brendan was ten years old. Sometimes he also fell asleep in school for ten or fifteen minutes, although he could usually fight off the sleepiness until he got home. He was in Year 5 when I saw him, and he was beginning to have both social and academic problems. His teacher was concerned and thought he should see a counsellor.

Jacqueline, eighteen, was also unusually sleepy for her age. She slept ten hours a night and usually took at least two twenty-minute naps during the day. Sometimes she would abruptly become so sleepy that it was almost impossible for her to stay awake, even when she wasn't sitting still. A year earlier, she had had a car accident – fortunately, a minor one – after falling asleep at the wheel. Since that time she had driven little and never alone. She quit university after her first year because she could not stay awake in class or complete her assignments. The excessive sleepiness had begun when she was fifteen, and by the time I saw her she had noticed two new symptoms. First, occasionally, just as she was about to fall asleep at night, she found herself unable to move at all, except to breathe and move her eyes; the paralysis continued for several minutes or until she fell asleep or someone touched her or talked to her. Second, when she laughed very hard, and sometimes when she felt angry, she became physically weak: she would have trouble holding her head up, or her knees would start to buckle, sometimes causing her to fall down. Both of these symptoms were frightening, and the episodes of weakness were often embarrassing; Jacqueline was reluctant to talk about them.

Both of these youngsters had a disorder called narcolepsy, whose main symptom is excessive sleepiness. Narcoleptic children usually develop other symptoms eventually as well: like Jacqueline, they may have sudden attacks of weakness during the day (*cataplexy*) and experience temporary paralysis and occasional hallucinations while falling asleep or on waking (*sleep paralysis* and *hypnagogic hallucinations*, respectively). In fact, cataplectic episodes such as Jacqueline's are a principal feature of this disorder. Brendan had not yet developed cataplexy, but he almost certainly would later on.

Although uncommon, narcolepsy is hardly rare. In the United Kingdom, about one in two thousand children will develop it – about half as many as will develop multiple sclerosis and five times as many as have cystic fibrosis. It occurs with equal frequency in boys and girls. If you attend a football game with forty thousand other fans, about twenty of them are already suffering from narcolepsy, or soon will be.

Narcolepsy usually does not appear before children are in their mid-teens, although, as in Brendan's case, it can happen. Both Brendan and Jacqueline had had symptoms for several years before their conditions were diagnosed and they began treatment. Most narcoleptic patients go eight to ten years or longer before being diagnosed, not because earlier diagnosis is impossible but because the symptoms are often misunderstood or unrecognised.

Not all overly sleepy children have narcolepsy. Sleepiness is also a symptom of other sleep disorders, various medical problems and depression. Abnormally sleepy children are often thought to be simply 'lazy' or 'sluggish', a potential error that GPs can make as easily as families. But sleepiness is a serious complaint that should not be dismissed lightly. If your child seems sleepier than he should be, be sure to investigate further. If he seems very sleepy day after day without an obvious cause, see that he gets medical attention.

Is Your Child Abnormally Sleepy?

If you suspect that your child might have narcolepsy or any of the other problems discussed in this chapter, the first question to ask is whether he really is excessively sleepy. Extreme cases are obvious, but the milder the sleepiness is, the harder it is to make this judgement. Approximate normal amounts of sleep for children of various ages are listed in Figure 1 on page 10. If your child sleeps up to two hours longer than the average for his age *but seems fine during the day,* then he probably just needs more sleep than most, which is usually nothing to worry about. If he averages more sleep than that, however, or seems tired during the day despite getting all the sleep he wants at night, there may be some cause for concern. For instance, an eight-year-old who sleeps fifteen hours every night should be seen by a GP, even if he is wide awake and cheerful during the day – he may simply be a long sleeper, but a need for that much sleep can be a sign of trouble. Napping that persists into primary school age is another sign of excessive sleepiness. Napping ordinarily decreases significantly by age four and it is uncommon by age five. Any child of age six or older who still takes regular naps or who starts napping regularly again, however short the naps, may well be abnormally sleepy.

It is harder to decide if your child is too sleepy if he *looks* tired but does not actually fall asleep, or perhaps falls asleep only when riding in the car. He may be irritable; he may yawn and seem low on energy. He may have difficulty sitting still and keeping his attention focused. (Parents, teachers and doctors often misdiagnose these symptoms of excessive sleepiness in a young child as hyperactivity, a learning difficulty or simple laziness.) Although there are ways of quantifying sleepiness in the laboratory, mild excessive sleepiness is often difficult to recognise with certainty by observation alone. So if your child has any of these symptoms, it would be wise for you to be suspicious.

CAUSES OF SLEEPINESS OTHER THAN NARCOLEPSY

Some causes of sleepiness are easy to identify; others are not. If you judge that your child is sleepier than he should be, the next questions to ask are whether he is getting a sufficient amount of sleep and whether the quality of the sleep is good. Without laboratory study it may be impossible to be certain about the quality, but you can make some important observations on your own.

First, consider the amount of sleep your child gets. Keep track of his sleep patterns for several weeks. Pay close attention at weekends and on holidays to determine how much sleep he gets when he does not have to wake up for school or day care. For example, if your ten-year-old is hard to wake for school after nine hours of sleep and remains sleepy during the day, but at the weekend he wakes spontaneously after eleven hours and stays alert all day, then nine hours is simply not enough sleep for him. Teenagers are especially likely to get too little sleep, because they often like to stay up late and because they are particularly prone to phase shifts (see Chapter 10). If your teenager goes to sleep at 2.00 a.m., wakes at 6.00 a.m. for school and naps every afternoon, it should be clear why he needs those naps. Some teenagers also seem to have a very long sleep requirement. Teenagers can binge on sleep at the weekends, especially if they do not get enough sleep during the week. When they get the chance, they can sleep fifteen hours at night and possibly nap during the day, too. But they should not do so seven days a week; if your teenager does, you should be concerned.

Second, try to determine whether your child is sleeping well once he goes to bed. This determination is quite difficult to make outside the laboratory, but if your child is very restless or seems to wake often during the night, even if only for short periods, or if he snores every night, especially if the snoring is loud and he gasps and struggles to breathe, his sleepiness could be coming from poor quality of sleep as well as from inadequate or insufficiently deep sleep.

If the problem is insufficient sleep, you may be able to correct it yourself. But if your child is sleepy despite appearing to get enough good sleep, or if his sleep appears to be of poor quality, or if you're just not sure of the cause, you should seek medical consultation.

Many medications cause daytime sleepiness, among them antihistamines used to treat allergies and many of the medications used to treat seizures. Illness of any sort can leave a child feeling fatigued and sleepy. Viral infections, especially mononucleosis and hepatitis, and any illness that produces a high fever are especially likely to cause fatigue. But the sleepiness should not last for months: it should go away soon after the fever does, or after no more than several weeks in the case of a slower-resolving viral infection. Children with anaemia, hypothyroidism and certain other chronic conditions tend to be tired, but truly excessive sleepiness is uncommon in these conditions. High and low blood sugar levels rarely cause significant sleepiness. Serious illnesses, including cancer, can certainly make a child appear run-down and, to some extent, cause him to sleep more.

If your child is *never* wide awake, you should be greatly concerned. If he sleeps long hours at night, naps repeatedly during the day and is still never fully alert between naps, he certainly needs medical attention. If this behaviour is not the temporary consequence of an acute illness or a recently started medication, he must be evaluated for serious medical and psychological conditions as well as for basic sleep disorders such as narcolepsy and sleep apnoea.

Treating Simpler Causes of Sleepiness

If your child is mildly sleepy due to inadequate sleep at night, you need to help him to increase his sleep time according to the methods outlined in other chapters of this book. In these cases the main problem is the insufficient sleep, and the daytime sleepiness is only a consequence.

If it seems that your child simply has a long sleep requirement, your family may have to make a few adjustments to allow for it. That may not always be easy or practicable. An adolescent who requires eleven hours of sleep and needs to get up at 6.30 a.m. for school would have to go to sleep at 7.30 p.m. to get enough sleep every night. You will have to arrive at a compromise. Perhaps your child can have a relatively early bedtime on weekdays, maybe 9.00 or 9.30, and make up the missing sleep by sleeping late at the weekend or taking naps. (However, the amount of morning and daytime sleep must not be so great that he becomes unable to fall asleep early enough at night.) Although such a remedy is less than ideal, it may be workable and it can be enough to produce an improvement. If your child has been going to bed at 11.30 p.m. until now, the extra two hours of sleep each night could make a big difference.

If your child's sleepiness results from illness, medication or a medical condition, work with your doctor to find ways of alleviating his symptoms. A change in medication or in dosage regimens may be helpful, for example.

EVALUATION AT A SLEEP DISORDERS CENTRE

If neither inadequate sleep nor known medical factors seem to explain your child's sleepiness, then a full evaluation is crucial. It may reveal an undiagnosed medical disorder, an emotional problem such as depression or a primary sleep disorder – that is, one involving basic sleep mechanisms.

If at all possible, your child's sleep should be evaluated in a sleep laboratory. Not all medical centres have the facilities to carry out sleep studies, especially in children. However, sleep disorder centres are growing in number, and even if the one nearest you mainly sees adults, its staff can probably test your child or at least refer you elsewhere.

Two kinds of sleep study are useful in evaluating a sleepy child. In the first, a sleep study or polysomnogram (PSG), the child is monitored during the night. This study aims to answer questions including:

- How long does it take the child to fall asleep? (A truly sleepy child is unlikely to lie awake for a long time, even in the laboratory.)
- Does the child get a normal amount of sleep, too much or too little?
- Does he go through all the normal sleep stages, and do they last the expected lengths of time? In particular, are the deepest phases of non-REM sleep, Stages III and IV, present and sufficiently long? (These stages contribute the most to feeling well rested.)
- Are sleep stages well maintained, or is sleep broken by frequent arousals? (Fragmented sleep, even if it adds up to a normal amount, can cause sleepiness.)
- Does the child show the normal pattern of cycling from one stage to the next?
- Does the beginning of REM sleep occur at the expected time, or does it start too early? (In narcolepsy, and to a lesser extent in depression, REM tends to appear very soon after the start of sleep. Children with narcolepsy often enter REM sleep within ten minutes of falling asleep at night, and even faster during naps.)
- Does the child have sleep apnoea, and if so, how severe is it?
- Are there any brain wave (EEG) abnormalities, especially patterns that suggest epileptic seizures or tumours?

A second study, the Multiple Sleep Latency Test (MSLT), is carried out on the day after the initial sleep study, if possible. It measures a child's actual degree of sleepiness and his tendency to enter the REM state rapidly. The child is monitored, as he was at night, but this time not continuously. Instead, every two hours he is allowed to lie down in a dark, quiet room and given twenty minutes to fall asleep. If the child does fall asleep, he is allowed to sleep for fifteen minutes. This procedure is repeated four or five times at two-hour intervals. (Special modifications of this routine may be required for young children, when some napping is still normal.)

Most children fall asleep only occasionally during this test, and it will usually take them more than twelve minutes to fall asleep, averaged over all the trials. Abnormally sleepy children will fall asleep in most of the trials and in only five to ten minutes. Narcoleptic children usually fall asleep within two or three minutes in all or almost all of the trials, and at least two of the naps will include extremely rapid transitions into REM sleep, called *sleep-onset REM periods*, or *REM onsets*.

If the results of a sleep study and MSLT are normal, then it is unlikely that your child is abnormally sleepy. That doesn't mean he isn't physically tired in the daytime. (You could be tired after a game of tennis or running round the neighbourhood, yet not feel at all sleepy.) His fatigue may still have a medical or an emotional basis.

If testing confirms that your child is very sleepy, but he does not appear to have narcolepsy (that is, if he falls asleep rapidly or deeply in the MSLT but never enters REM), and his sleep both at night and during the day is normal, then, once medical factors are eliminated, psychological causes and another sleep disorder (similar to narcolepsy but without the REM abnormalities) must be considered.

While adults suffering from depression usually sleep poorly, youngsters, especially adolescents, sometimes react to depression quite differently, withdrawing into their inner world of sleep as a way of escaping problems that seem too difficult to face. How they do that is unknown, but the sleep is genuine and long-lasting. They may sleep deeply at night and have repeated naps during the day. They may even spend most of the day in bed. If your child is exhibiting this behaviour, *don't* wait for the problem to pass on its own. Seek medical and psychological help.

Finally, the child who is sleepy, but for whom a specific medical or psychological cause cannot be identified, is said to have *idiopathic hypersomnolence* – that is, we know he is sleepy, but we don't know why. Idiopathic hypersomnolence may reflect several different disorders that happen to have the same symptoms, but because the pattern of difficulties is often quite similar from one child to the next, it is thought that most people with this problem probably have the same disorder, or perhaps one of a few closely related disorders. These problems tend to run in families. For instance, it's fairly common for one parent and several children in a family to have the symptoms, often almost from birth. Children with idiopathic hypersomnolence tend to be long sleepers and long or frequent nappers, but otherwise they are normal. Often there is no need to treat them until they start school, when their sleepiness starts to interfere with learning and socialisation.

NARCOLEPSY

Although insufficient sleep is the most common cause of daytime sleepiness, narcolepsy, idiopathic hypersomnolence and sleep apnoea are the three main sleep *disorders* that cause it. You will recall that in sleep apnoea the problem is an inability to breathe normally while asleep, which in turn causes the sleep disruption (see Chapter 17). Although children with sleep apnoea are often sleepy during the day, the signs of that sleepiness are often subtle. In narcolepsy and idiopathic hypersomnolence, the daytime sleepiness is more evident. In these disorders, the brain systems responsible for controlling sleep are directly affected.

Narcolepsy usually appears starting in adolescence or early adulthood, but it can begin in the primary-school years and occasionally even earlier. About 50 per cent of narcoleptics show symptoms by age sixteen. The symptom of excessive sleepiness, once present, never leaves. If symptoms start in early childhood, they may worsen as the child goes through adolescence. Patterns of sleepiness sometimes change temporarily during pregnancy, either improving or worsening. Otherwise, after adolescence these patterns tend to remain fairly constant for years. The symptoms of sleep paralysis, hypnagogic hallucinations and cataplexy, on the other hand, are more variable and tend to wax and wane in frequency and severity over time.

The condition has no known cure, though the sleepiness may eventually decrease as the narcoleptic adult reaches middle age, and some of the other symptoms may even disappear. All of the symptoms can be treated with naps and medication. Often treatment is very successful, but both the severity of the disease and the response to therapy vary widely.

Narcolepsy is often confused with epilepsy. It is in fact a completely different disorder, although some of its symptoms occasionally resemble certain forms of epileptic seizures. In narcolepsy, sleep systems turn on inappropriately during the day, and they don't always work as they should at night. Although both REM and non-REM sleep are affected, most often it is the REM system that becomes active at the wrong time, accounting for most of the symptoms.

Sleep Disturbances in Narcolepsy

Despite the common misconception, most narcoleptic patients are not truly 'hypersomniac' – that is, the amount of sleep they get each twenty-four-hour period is actually normal or nearly normal, and their sleep is not unusually deep. Often their night-time sleep is broken by many brief wakings and a few longer ones, just as their daytime waking is broken by naps. Sleep is thus distributed across the twenty-four-hour day rather than consolidated into a single block at night. (When the disorder first appears in childhood, the pattern is often different. Affected children often go to bed early – possibly right after school, even skipping dinner – and sleep through until the next morning, getting eleven to sixteen hours of sleep. By stretching out the night in this way, they seem to be able to avoid sleeping during the rest of the daytime hours. The quality of narcoleptic children's sleep is generally good, unlike in adults. When narcoleptic children do nap, they may sleep for two or three hours. By contrast, adult narcoleptics generally take brief, refreshing naps of about twenty minutes.

As mentioned above, the other main characteristics of sleep in narcoleptics is that REM sleep frequently occurs immediately upon falling asleep, or at most within ten minutes. In normal infants older than three months, REM does not ordinarily occur until a full cycle of non-REM sleep has completed. Older children may even have two non-REM cycles before their first REM period. Outside of narcolepsy, REM onsets are seen only under a few conditions: during withdrawal from a medication that decreases REM sleep (which leads to a 'REM rebound'); on returning to sleep in the morning soon after waking; when going to sleep at the wrong time, such as after a large and abrupt time-zone change or when on a very irregular sleep schedule; and, possibly, after a period of sleep deprivation.

Because not all of a narcoleptic's sleep periods begin with REM, a study of one nap or one night's sleep may not be sufficient to diagnose the disorder. But the repeated naps of the MSLT can be decisive: if a child takes only a few minutes to fall asleep during the tests, and if he goes right into REM sleep in at least two of the naps, we can usually confirm the diagnosis of narcolepsy.

Partial Activation of the REM System

Sometimes narcoleptics have episodes in which REM systems are functioning but REM sleep is not fully established. As described below, this unusual phenomenon can happen at bedtime, on waking or during the day, and it accounts for the other symptoms of narcolepsy: cataplexy, hypnagogic hallucinations and sleep paralysis. In these conditions, certain features of the REM state, namely dreaming or paralysis or both, seem to be activated while the patient is still fully awake or only partly asleep.

The Major Symptoms of Narcolepsy

Sleepiness and cataplexy are the hallmarks of the narcolepsy syndrome. If your child has both of them, then a diagnosis of narcolepsy is fairly certain.

The Sleepiness of Narcolepsy

Narcoleptic children are continually sleepy. They will fall asleep quickly whenever there is nothing happening to keep them awake. However, when they are up and about and not in monotonous or tedious settings, most narcoleptics can stay awake. Most of them feel very sleepy from time to time during the day – and these periods of marked sleepiness can come on fairly rapidly – but with a strong enough motivation to stay awake and an ability to move about, narcoleptics can fight off sleep, at least for a while. If they do fall asleep, they can be wakened.

Narcoleptics do not really fall asleep suddenly and without warning, as is often believed. We all feel irresistibly sleepy on occasion, but narcoleptics feel that way every day, and their desire to sleep is much more overwhelming. To give you an idea of how a narcoleptic person feels, imagine watching a dull programme on television in a very warm room after a big dinner. Your eyelids feel heavy; you know that you will not be able to stay awake unless you get up and go for a walk. It feels good just to let yourself fall asleep. Trying to fight off sleep is difficult and unpleasant. If you do fall asleep, you will probably wake after a short nap feeling much better. The overwhelming sleepiness will be gone.

What narcoleptics experience is no different, except that the urge to sleep can come on at any time during the day, though most commonly and most intensely in settings where anyone might find it hard to stay awake. Without physical activity, narcoleptics find it almost impossible to fight off sleep. Even if they do manage to stay awake, they feel groggy and their ability to concentrate is greatly diminished.

Typically an adolescent or adult narcoleptic's naps are short – sometimes only a few minutes, occasionally up to an hour, but rarely much longer. And the naps often do seem to be considerably refreshing. At school, for example, a narcoleptic adolescent can often resume productive work if he is allowed to nap for twenty minutes. If he has to fight off sleep instead, he may be unable to concentrate for hours, finding it impossible to remain still, listen quietly and stay awake at the same time. He must move about and talk, or else he will fall asleep. Either way, he will probably wind up in trouble with the teacher. (Remember, younger children with narcolepsy may sleep long hours at night and not seem particularly sleepy during the day. Any naps they do take tend to be long; if the children are wakened after twenty or thirty minutes – which may be difficult – they will probably seem groggy rather than refreshed.)

Cataplexy

Cataplexy is a sudden muscle weakness, or even temporary total paralysis, triggered by strong emotion. This dramatic symptom is very disconcerting and even dangerous to the narcoleptic, although it may strike an uninformed observer as funny. Laughter and anger are typical triggers, but any strong emotion or excitement can initiate a cataplectic event. Cataplectic adults often learn to control their emotions rigidly, avoiding all expressions of laughter, anger or excitement. Children in the family, however, may delight in provoking them to laughter just to watch them fall over at the dinner table.

Cataplectic attacks vary from person to person in frequency, severity and length. Your child's cataplectic weakness may be very mild – his knees may buckle briefly, his jaw may sag or he may have a moment's difficulty holding his head up – or it may be so severe that he falls to the ground, unable to move any muscles except those that control breathing and eye movements. Most cataplectic attacks last between a few seconds and one minute. Less often, attacks last several minutes, and on rare occasions they can last up to half an hour. An episode that continues for several minutes may lead into a period of sleep. Most untreated narcoleptics with cataplexy have between one and four cataplectic attacks each day. Some patients have them less often; others experience cataplexy many times each day with very little provocation.

Severe, frequent cataplexy is crippling if untreated. Even infrequent attacks can be very dangerous if the weakness is pronounced. Although serious injuries are uncommon, an unfortunately timed attack can cause a person to drop a pot of boiling water or fall down the stairs. Outside the home, the dangers can be even greater: a child might fall down in the street if he is startled by an approaching vehicle, and an adolescent or adult can have a cataplectic attack while driving a car.

Like the attacks of sleepiness in narcolepsy, cataplexy is entirely distinct from epilepsy, despite some superficial similarities. Although it can be tempting for observers to assume the weakness is imagined or 'hysterical', especially when it is precipitated by unusual circumstances, for example, when the sufferer is frightened or sexually aroused, it is very real. Cataplexy is a true weakness, identical to the paralysis that occurs during normal REM sleep (see Chapter 2). The system controlling REM paralysis seemingly turns on suddenly and inappropriately during the day instead of confining itself to periods of REM sleep. Why cataplexy can be triggered by emotion is not yet known.

The age at which cataplexy first appears in narcoleptics varies greatly. Cataplexy and sleepiness may or may not begin at the same time; even several years can elapse between the onsets of the two symptoms. Most often, sleepiness appears first. Cataplexy usually follows within five years, but much longer delays are seen occasionally. It is rare for cataplexy to appear in a child of five or younger. By early adolescence it is seen more often, but roughly 85 per cent of narcoleptics do not develop the symptom until after the age of fifteen.

Cataplexy can be difficult to recognise. Many children have trouble describing the weakness they feel during mild episodes. Even if you see your child drop to the floor when laughing hard, you are unlikely to be alarmed. Many normal children fall to the ground or flop down onto the table when they are laughing hard and feeling silly. But you should be concerned if your child seems frightened by his weakness at these times, has difficulty getting back up once he has stopped laughing or experiences a similar weakness when he is angry or startled. Cataplexy in older children is usually easier to recognise, at least in part because they can describe their own perceptions of the weakness better than younger children can.

The Minor Symptoms of Narcolepsy

The two other important symptoms often present in narcoleptic patients are sleep paralysis and hypnagogic hallucinations. These symptoms are not required for a narcolepsy diagnosis, since they aren't present in all patients with narcolepsy and they *are* present in some people without the disorder. Like cataplexy, they reflect a partial activation of the REM system.

Sleep Paralysis

Children who have sleep paralysis find themselves alert but unable to move. This phenomenon is similar to cataplexy, but it does not occur during full waking. It happens during the transition to or from sleep, most frequently just when a narcoleptic child is about to go to sleep, less often just as he wakes. As in cataplexy, sleep paralysis involves the paralysis of REM sleep occurring an inappropriate time, in this case just before or just after actual sleep and dreaming. Most episodes last only a few minutes. They end either spontaneously or when broken by some outside stimulation, typically touch or sound. Generally, sleep paralysis occurs only a few times a month. In rare patients it happens almost nightly.

Sleep paralysis can begin at any point in the development of narcolepsy. About two-thirds of narcoleptic patients have at least occasional episodes of sleep paralysis, and about half of all patients have repeated episodes; one out of four develops the symptom by age sixteen. Not surprisingly, sleep paralysis can be frightening to children, especially the first time it occurs.

Hypnagogic Hallucinations

Occasionally, just as a narcoleptic child is drifting off to sleep, he may see or hear something imaginary that seems very real. This is called a hypnagogic hallucination. (The senses of smell, taste and touch are less commonly involved in the hallucinatory experience.) These visual or auditory hallucinations can be pleasant or scary. A child might see only moving coloured blobs or hear meaningless noises, but more often, the images are better formed. The child may visualise scenes that appear to him to be believable or bizarre. He may hear music or voices. He may see burglars, strangely shaped or oddly coloured animals or threatening monsters. The theme of intrusion and threat is common, and the imagery can be quite realistic. Whether a child recognises these visions or sounds as unreal may depend on his age and how close to sleep he is. The child may also hallucinate that he is doing something, perhaps running away or trying to fight back an attack. If he has sleep paralysis at the same time as a hypnagogic hallucination and is thus truly unable to move at all, he may understandably find the experience particularly frightening.

Hypnagogic hallucinations occur just before falling asleep. They reflect a partial activation of the REM system in which a dream has begun while sleep and (generally) paralysis have not. (Similar phenomena, so-called *hypnopompic* hallucinations, may occur on waking in both normal children and narcoleptics and reflect the continued activity of part of the dream system for a few minutes after waking.) Although about half of all narcoleptics eventually develop hypnagogic hallucinations, only 15 per cent have them by age sixteen.

Since hypnagogic hallucinations can be scary, a child who often experiences them may resist going to bed. Young children may have difficulty describing these experiences, while older children are often afraid to talk about them for fear of being thought crazy, especially if the images they experience are very bizarre. (You should not think, however, that all children complaining of 'seeing' monsters at night are having hypnagogic hallucinations; most are not. Monsters that are the products of a normal, vivid, waking imagination are far more common than those produced by an abnormal activation of the dream system.)

The occurrence of hypnagogic hallucinations may simply be a consequence of the fact that the transition from wakefulness to sleep takes time – as wakefulness only gradually gives way to sleep. Normally this transition is directly into non-REM sleep, and if we are at all aware that non-REM is starting, we will only notice that we are getting very sleepy or that our thoughts are starting to wander and we are starting to daydream. But in the narcoleptic, the transition is from waking directly into REM sleep, and if it is gradual enough, the person may be aware that true dreaming has started before he is completely asleep. Not only that, but the dream imagery present is often quite intense. (The intensity of the dream imagery may well be part of the abnormality of the REM sleep system in narcolepsy; the same abnormality probably also accounts for the fact that narcoleptics have more frightening nightmares than most people.) The narcoleptic's awareness of the unreal nature of these hallucinations depends on how early in the transition to sleep the dream actually began.

Many narcoleptic patients find that their best course is not to fight off the hallucinations but just to let full sleep overtake them. That probably doesn't end the dream, but conscious awareness gradually slips away.

The Importance of an Early Diagnosis

Although in narcolepsy any of the four characteristic symptoms can be the first to appear, in nine out of ten affected children the initial problem is sleepiness. Cataplexy usually follows within a few years. Hypnagogic hallucinations and sleep paralysis, if they appear, may begin at any point.

Sometimes symptoms start abruptly, possibly following an important incident in the child's life. Emotional trauma, for example, is occasionally associated with the onset of sleepiness. In these cases, the initial diagnosis may incorrectly identify the sleepiness as a psychological problem, and the true cause of the symptoms may not be recognised for a long time. Other times, when the sleepiness starts gradually, the parents and child might blame it on insufficient sleep or increased school demands.

Cataplexy, on the other hand, is unmistakably abnormal in clear-cut cases, and once it has become noticeable it is usually brought to medical attention. Narcolepsy is the most likely diagnosis and it will probably at least be suspected, although sometimes the symptom is misinterpreted as a form of epilepsy or hysteria. If the cataplexy is less pronounced, if the child is not yet showing excessive sleepiness, or if the doctor doesn't know enough about narcolepsy, the disorder can go undiagnosed for years.

Whether the initial symptom is sleepiness or cataplexy, the personal cost of a delay in diagnosis and treatment can be enormous. A child's academic performance and self-esteem may suffer tremendously as he goes through school with an undiagnosed disability. In perhaps one-third of all narcoleptic patients, sleepiness begins early enough to interfere with performance in primary school or secondary school. Later on, it can cause people to unnecessarily change their plans for further education or even a career. In older children it can be the cause of significant social problems. People may assume the child is lazy or has 'psychological problems'. Undiagnosed narcoleptics sometime enter psychotherapy in an attempt to treat the symptoms, an effort which will not be successful because the real problem is not being treated. (A therapist can, however, help a patient learn to cope with the symptoms of narcolepsy once it has been properly diagnosed.)

For these reasons, it is important to recognise narcoleptic symptoms as early as possible. Many parents don't seek help for their child immediately unless the symptoms are dramatic, which they often are not. Even when sleepiness is so excessive that it is impossible to ignore, parents may well assume that it will pass. (And sometimes it does, for example, if it was the result of a low-grade viral infection or some emotional struggle rather than narcolepsy.) Prominent sleepiness that persists more than a week and mild sleepiness that lasts over a month or two should definitely be evaluated.

Although we cannot predict which children will eventually develop narcolepsy, at least not yet, there is some evidence that these youngsters' sleep habits may be unusual even before major symptoms emerge. Retrospective studies on adult narcoleptics suggest that many of them continued napping into primary school. Over 10 per cent of them were also misdiagnosed as hyperactive in childhood and treated with stimulants because they could not sit still and pay attention. (This may be a case of the right drug for the wrong reason, since narcolepsy and hyperactivity respond well to some of the same medications; see below). You should be especially suspicious if your child seems overactive yet still naps inappropriately.

Sleep Paralysis, Hypnagogic Hallucinations and Cataplexy Without Narcolepsy

Although the symptoms of sleep paralysis and hypnagogic hallucinations are characteristic of narcolepsy, both can occur independently as well, not as part of the narcolepsy syndrome. In fact, many people without sleep disorders experience one or the other from time to time.

When they are not accompanied by excessive sleepiness or cataplexy, sleep paralysis and hypnagogic hallucinations present no cause for alarm. Independent sleep paralysis in children occurs most often as the child is waking, as might be expected, since children (like adults) commonly wake directly from REM sleep, whereas sleep-onset REM periods usually occur only in narcoleptics. Independent hypnagogic hallucinations occur as a child is falling asleep, and they can be quite intense and even frightening. However, they happen only occasionally.

Independent cataplexy is much rarer than independent sleep paralysis or hypnagogic hallucinations. Some researchers believe that cataplexy is always a sign of narcolepsy and that it only appears to be independent when the symptom of sleepiness is not yet apparent. This theory is plausible, since cataplexy does sometimes precede the onset of sleepiness by many years. In any case, if your child experiences cataplexy, he should see a doctor. Cataplexy can be dangerous in and of itself, and symptoms resembling cataplexy can also be caused by other disorders.

THE CAUSE OF NARCOLEPSY

In recent years, research into the cause of narcolepsy has made outstanding progress. Some facts are now certain. But research continues advancing rapidly, with new theories constantly emerging or being disproved. What we know so far is that a previously unknown neurotransmitter (a chemical that nerve cells release to stimulate other nerve cells) called *hypocretin* or *orexin* has been found in the lateral hypothalamus, a region of the brain known to be important in the control of certain basic body functions such as appetite. Dogs with a certain inherited form of narcolepsy have a defect in the nerve cell sites that are supposed to respond to this chemical, and mice that lack the gene necessary to produce it exhibit a similar syndrome. While most humans with narcolepsy do not show either of these genetic defects, they do have markedly reduced levels of hypocretin, and some evidence points to a loss of the nerve cells that produce it. It may be that these cells are normal at birth and become damaged later in life, which would explain why narcolepsy does not usually start until the second or third decade of life and why it does not grow worse over time. (Symptoms may actually become milder over many years, but it is not known whether this is because damaged cells regain some function or whether another mechanism is involved.)

Most narcolepsy is *sporadic,* which is to say that the condition is not a straightforward inherited trait. Furthermore, there is only a 1 in 4 chance that the identical twin of a narcoleptic patient will also develop narcolepsy, and no more than a 1 in 50 chance that the child of a narcoleptic parent will. If narcolepsy were simply a genetic disease, then if one identical twin developed narcolepsy, the other twin always would too. But if genetics had nothing to do with it, the risk to the twin would be only about 1 in 2,000, the same as the risk to the population in general. The implication is that some trait is inherited that increases the risk of narcolepsy but is not by itself enough to cause the disorder.

In that light, another discovery is extremely important: nearly 90 per cent of all narcoleptic patients with both sleepiness and cataplexy have a characteristic gene in the so-called HLA region of one chromosome. Since genes in this region are known to be important to the immune system, which recognises viruses and bacteria as foreign and attacks them, and since most diseases associated with HLA genes are autoimmune in nature – that is, the body attacks its own cells – this finding suggests that narcolepsy might be an autoimmune disease as well. The trigger may be a virus that, due to the defective gene, the immune system cannot distinguish from the brain's normal hypocretin-producing cells: the response to the infection damages or destroys these cells along with the virus. Although studies have found some support for this idea, to date all attempts to confirm this hypothesis have failed.

In a small number of families narcolepsy is clearly genetic, passed consistently from generation to generation. However, in these families the disorder is slightly atypical: often it starts earlier, takes a milder form and has no association with a specific HLA gene. There is evidence suggesting that at least some of these families have genetic defects similar to those found in affected dogs or mice, although the defect may not be the same in all families affected.

These developments are exciting, because they suggest that soon, for the first time, we may be able to start designing treatments aimed at correcting a specific chemical abnormality rather than simply treating the resulting symptoms.

THE TREATMENT OF NARCOLEPSY

The majority of people with narcolepsy can expect that, with treatment, most of their symptoms will be brought under control. Usually, the patient can achieve a normal life. Though children who develop narcolepsy will always have the disorder, it need not interfere seriously with their schooling, work or social life. These children should not plan to become aeroplane pilots or long-haul lorry drivers, but there are few other limitations on their life choices.

We treat narcolepsy with medication, judicious napping, appropriate schedules that allow for sufficient sleep, education and common sense. Treatment must be supervised by a doctor. And we handle the different symptoms of narcolepsy in a variety of different ways.

Sleepiness

The sleepiness of narcolepsy can be lessened with medication and a carefully maintained schedule. A short regular nap after lunch or at other times can help a child stay alert and use less medication during the day. In primary school, that can often be managed without upsetting the child's overall schedule; for example, the child may be able to nap in the nurse's office. In addition, when we are treating a young narcoleptic child at our clinic, we (and the family) contact the child's school and discuss the disorder with his teachers and counsellors. If a nap is necessary, we set up a place and time that prevent embarrassment. Teachers must understand that they should never punish or ridicule the child for falling asleep in class, and they should help educate the child's classmates about the disorder and discourage them from teasing.

Adolescents often have a harder time fitting naps into their schedule, especially naps that occur on a regular and predictable basis. It may mean missing classes, and leaving class to nap may make an adolescent feel different from his peers and uncomfortable. (Although adult narcoleptics can often manage a short nap during their lunch hour every day, teenage patients usually cannot fit a nap into the typical half-hour lunch period.) However, a child of any age can take a short nap after school before beginning his homework, at least if after-school activities and jobs do not interfere.

While parents can usually control the schedule of a child in primary school, adolescents can present more of a problem: some try to keep up the (possibly unreasonable) schedule of their peers, even to the extent of denying that they have narcolepsy, and alcohol can become a factor, since it causes drowsiness. However, most adolescents are willing to acknowledge the disorder and accept limitations on their late-evening activities and alcohol consumption.

A proper medication regimen should keep a child needing as few naps as possible during school and allow him to participate in after-school activities and do his homework. There are a few kinds of drug available for this purpose. Often one preparation works better for a given child than another. Rules for the use of certain drugs in children vary from country to country and from time to time, including the agents mentioned below. The advisability and even ability to use these drugs in your own child should be discussed with your doctor. Stimulants such as methylphenidate (Ritalin, Concerta XL, Equasym XL, Medikinet XL) and the amphetamines (dexamphetamine, for example) have proven useful for many children. These drugs do have potential for abuse, but that is not a major worry in childhood, when parents control the dosage; significant side effects (like loss of appetite and weight loss, abdominal pain, nervousness and tics) can be a concern, though, particularly at high doses.

Modafinil (Provigil) and armodafinil (Nuvigil) are newer drugs that seem to help narcoleptic patients stay awake without many of the problems often seen with stimulants. These drugs seem to affect only a very small area of the brain (possibly directly affecting the hypocretin/orexin system that has been implicated in the cause of narcolepsy), without causing the more widespread brain stimulation seen with other wakefulness-promoting agents. Patients on these drugs don't 'crash' as the medication wears off or get a buzz from an effective dose, and there seems to be little or no potential for abuse. At this writing, neither modafinil nor armodafinil has been formally approved for use in children.

Another drug even more recently approved is sodium oxybate (Xyrem). Although approved specifically for the treatment of cataplexy, studies have shown it to also improve the quality of a narcoleptic's sleep at night and possibly to decrease sleepiness during the day. Its mechanism of action is uncertain, and to date there is relatively little experience of its use in children.

Depending upon how severe the symptoms are and which drug is being used, a child may need medicine once or several times a day (or, in the case of sodium oxybate, at bedtime and once during the night). He should be followed closely by a doctor knowledgeable about narcolepsy, and dosage decisions should be reviewed frequently.

If the teenager is old enough to drive, the physician should be involved in decisions about that as well. Generally, a teenager should be allowed to drive only if his sleepiness – and cataplexy, as described below – are satisfactorily controlled and the child is felt to be mature and reliable. The teenager should never drive late at night or alone for long periods.

Once sleepiness is properly controlled, the child often shows dramatic changes. There are usually major improvements at school, at home and in the child's social life. With Brendan, we were able to significantly reduce his daytime sleepiness by allowing him to nap after school (also during school on occasion) and putting him on a daily dose of methylphenidate. He felt much better about himself, and his schoolwork improved considerably. He continued to do well when I later switched him to modafinil. He no longer slept overly long hours at night; instead, he spent the time after dinner with his family or doing homework. Jacqueline, too, responded to medication (methylphenidate early on then modafinil when it became available), and she was able to finish university.

Cataplexy, Hypnagogic Hallucinations and Sleep Paralysis

Cataplexy, hypnagogic hallucinations and sleep paralysis usually respond well to medications ordinarily used in the treatment of depression, namely the tricyclics and the selective serotonin re-uptake inhibitors (SSRIs). Sodium oxybate given at night, although not an antidepressant, also decreases cataplexy significantly, perhaps because of its known effect of improving sleep and decreasing REM onsets (though how it does that is unknown).

The symptoms of hypnagogic hallucinations and sleep paralysis, if they are present at all, don't always need to be treated, especially if they are mild and occasional. They are annoying and somewhat frightening, but they are not dangerous, and once children understand why these symptoms occur they often learn to accept them. If a child's cataplexy is very mild and episodes are rare, treatment may also be postponed. But if the cataplexy is dangerous, embarrassing or frightening, it should be treated.

Jacqueline's cataplexy was moderately severe, and besides, it was important to her that she be able to laugh freely in public without

fear of embarrassment or of injuring herself. So her medication programme included treatment for cataplexy, and both that symptom
and her sleep paralysis were easily controlled. If Brendan required
similar treatment, it probably would not be for several years, but he
and his family knew what to look for and would understand the
symptoms if and when they appeared.

Future Treatments

A number of drugs to treat the symptoms of narcolepsy are in varying stages of development, including some that mimic the effects of
the deficient hypocretin molecule itself. It is hoped that such research will lead not only to better treatment of symptoms but also
to treatments directed at the cause of the disease itself, and thus
effectively to a cure.

Index

active sleep, 22
Adam (sleep phase), 222, 224, 225, 243
Adderall (amphetamine), 187, 428
adenoids, and sleep apnoea, 390,
   393–95, 401
adolescents:
   anxious, 153
   irregular schedules of, 32
   narcolepsy of, 414, 427
   nightmares of, 338
   routines for, 37
   sleep deprivation of, 12, 208–10,
     231, 409
   sleeping pills for, 184
   sleep patterns of, 57, 204
   sleep phase delay of, 209
   sleep phase shifts of, 230–40
   sleep requirements of, 30
   sleep terrors of, 294
adults:
   deep sleep of, 24, 27
   naps of, 201
   sleep associations of, 65
   sleep-wake patterns of, 57
advanced sleep phase, 220–22,
   230–31
alertness, 200, 201–2

Alexa (sleep associations), 69–70, 88,
   89–90
Alexander (nightmares), 336,
   340
Allison (night feedings), 138–39,
   147–48
alpha waves, 17
Alupent (metaproterenol), 187
Anna (sleep phase), 238–39
antibiotics, 187
antidiuretic hormone, 365–66
antihistamines, 191, 204
Antonio (bed-wetting), 349
anxiety, 94–95, 151–53, 204
   and confusional events, 308–10
   generalised, 174
   and nightmares, 335, 339
   pseudo, 157
   and rhythmic behaviours, 375–76,
     380–81
   separation, 48–49, 94, 152, 160–61,
     173–75, 335, 339
   see also fears
apnoea, meaning of term, 388
Ashley (limits), 134–35
asthma, 181, 187
automatic behaviours, 169, 401

babies:
    bedtime routines for, 34–35
    central sleep apnoea of, 402–3
    colicky, 178–81
    continuous night-time sleep of, 29
    dummies of, 40, 87, 149–50
    feeding patterns of, 54–55
    naps of, *see* naps
    non-REM sleep of, 23, 24
    partial wakings of, 293–94
    REM sleep of, 22, 23, 97
    settled, 29, 35
    SIDS of, 37–41, 45–46, 87
    sleep environment of, 39–41
    sleep patterns developed in, 21–23,
        28–29, 53–57, 58, 97, 264–65
    sleep positions of, 37–39
barriers:
    doors as, 119–23
    gates as, 117–19
    setting limits via, 114–23
    and siblings, 128–29
basic rest-activity cycle, 200
bedding, inappropriate, 40, 45
bedroom:
    enjoyable time in, 167
    learning to stay in, 121–23
    shared with child, 123–24
bedtime:
    appropriate, 317
    difficulty falling asleep at, 8, 243,
        245
    early, 159
    late, 126–28, 167–68
    negative associations with, 35
    putting child down awake, 35
    routines for, 34–37, 113, 316–17
bed-wetting, 8, 347–67
    awareness of need to urinate,
        352–53, 362
    and bladder capacity, 352
    conditioning in, 364–65
    and confusional arousals, 353
    and depth of sleep, 353–54
    and dreaming, 353
    environmental influences on, 355
    and food sensitivity, 354–55, 366–67
    and heredity, 350–51
    impact of, 348–50

    and maturation, 351–52
    medical factors in, 354
    as reflex contraction, 351, 357
    start-stop exercises, 360–61, 363–64
    treatments for, 355–67
    and urinary system, 357–60, 361
behaviour:
    automatic, 169, 401
    and sleepiness, 402
    wild, 117–19
Benadryl (diphenhydramine), 185
Benjamin (bed-wetting), 350, 356
Betsy (sleep association), 63–64,
        67–68, 71, 73, 78–80, 81
biological clock, 14, 28, 31, 56, 197,
        204–5, 236, 299
biological rhythms, 31–32, 196–99
bladder training, 357, 363–64
blanket, favourite, 52–53
blinds and curtains, 251
body temperature, 31, 137
brain:
    abnormal functioning of, 188–92
    and biological clock, 197
    blood flows to, 18
    during sleep, 14–15
    maturation of, 22
brain waves, 16, 17, 18, 22
breastfeeding, and dummies, 40, 144
breathing:
    regular, 16
    in REM sleep, 18, 19
    and sleep apnoea, 391, 404
Brendan (sleepiness), 406, 407, 429
Brethine, Bricanyl (terbutaline), 187

car accidents, 208–9
Caroline (ear infections), 183
cataplexy, 407, 418–19, 422, 424, 428,
        429
Catapres (clonidine), 185
checking, 170–71
children:
    anxious, 152–53
    bedtime routines for, 36–37
    confusional events of, 291–96,
        308–11, 312
    eliminating naps of, 30
    restless sleepers, 46, 47

sleep pattern development in,
   23–28, 29–30, 57, 58, 265–66, 299
with special needs, 85
spoiling v comforting, 82, 99
chloral hydrate, 185
Christopher (sleepwalking), 287,
   325–26
circadian biology, 196
circadian drive, 202, 203, 260, 298
circadian rhythms, 31–32, 196–99
   and forbidden zone for sleep,
      200–4
   and sleep phases, 199–200, 203
cleft palate, 392
colic, 178–81
Concerta XL (methylphenidate), 187,
   428
confusional arousal, 95, 288,
   291–311
   and bed-wetting, 353
   biological factors of, 304
   evaluating, 312–15
   general advice, 316–18
   having a job to do, 305–11
   and nightmares, 341–45
   safety factors for, 317–18
   and sleep terrors, 294, 297–98
   and sleepwalking, 30, 292, 308
   spectrum of behaviour in, 295
   summary chart, 330–32
   treatment of, 315–33
   variability of, 311–12
   what to do during, 319–21
   what it feels like, 296–97
   why it happens, 297–311
   wild thrashing in, 24, 293, 321
Connor (sleep phase), 231–34
continuous positive airway pressure
   (CPAP), 398, 399, 400
co-sleeping, 39, 41–49
   adult v child sleep cycles, 46–47
   benefits and drawbacks of, 44–45
   embarrassment or shame of, 48
   H pattern in, 46
   parents separated by, 42–43, 46–47
   and sleep associations, 87–91
   stopping, 43, 48–49
cot death (SIDS), 37–41, 45–46, 87,
   403

crying, colicky babies, 180
curtains and blinds, 251

Daniel (nightmares), 336, 339–40
darkness:
   and biological clock, 31, 55
   fear of, 156, 163–64
David (sleep terrors), 288, 328–29
daydreams, 16
day-night reversal, 54
death, and sleep, 336, 340
deep sleep, 16, 17, 18, 24, 26, 27–28,
   289–91
delayed maturation, 351–52
delayed sleep phase, 222–28, 230,
   231–35
delta waves, 16, 17
depression, 204, 413
desmopressin, 365–66
Desyrel (trazodone), 185
dexamphetamine (amphetamine), 187,
   428
diet therapy, 366–67
digestive system, 137
door:
   closed, as cause of fear, 164
   setting limits via, 119–23
dreaming, 19–20
   and bed-wetting, 353
   and brain waves, 17
   every night, 20
dreams:
   bad, *see* nightmares
   developing complexity of, 334
   distinguished from real world, 334,
      337
   in REM state, 26, 333
drifting tendency, 205, 207
drowsiness, 15–16, 17

ear infections, 41, 149–50, 182–83,
   397
electronic distractions, 208, 253–55
Emily (bedtime routine), 37
entrapment, 39, 45
enuresis, *see* bed-wetting
epilepsy, 187, 415, 419
Equasym XL (methylphenidate), 428
Eustachian tube, 149–50

family differences, 33
fears, 151–77
  the anxious child, 151–53, 157
  bedtime, 153–56
  control of, 154
  coping with, 165–67
  of the dark, 156, 163–64
  day v night, 160
  evaluating, 156–65
  and fantasies, 152, 154, 162–63
  of going to bed alone, 35
  identifiable cause of, 161–62
  intensity of, 159–60
  and night-lights, 170, 338
  and nightmares, 157–58, 335,
    337–39
  physical symptoms of, 344
  self-reinforcing pattern of, 164–65
  separation anxiety, 160–61
  short- v long-term, 161
  and siblings or pets, 175
  specific v general, 162
  talking about, 36–37, 166, 169
  techniques for, 167–75
  testing limits v, 158–59
  transient, 161
feeding patterns, 54–55, 56
feedings, 136–50
  bedtime, 85–86, 96
  diluting with water, 147
  medical issues with, 149–50
  and naps, 149
  night-time, 29, 83, 84–86
  reduction or elimination of,
    140–48
  sleep problems caused by,
    139–40
foetus, REM sleep in, 21, 23
food sensitivity, and bed-wetting,
    354–55, 366–67
forbidden zone for sleep, 200–204
functional enuresis, 354

Gabriella (naps), 275–76
gas, and colic, 179
gastro-oesophageal reflux, 183–84
gates, 90, 91, 114–19, 128–29
Grace (tonsils), 393–95, 396–97
guilt, from setting limits, 108, 109–10

head, flattening, 38–39
headaches, 181
head-banging, *see* rhythmic
    behaviours
head-rolling, *see* rhythmic behaviours
heartburn, 183–84
heredity:
  and bed-wetting, 350–51
  and rhythmic behaviours, 377
homeostatic drive, 202, 203, 204, 251,
    260, 298
humidifiers, 400
hunger:
  sucking habit v, 144
  timing of, 137, 198, 200
hypnagogic hallucinations, 407,
    420–22, 424, 429–30
hypnagogic startle, 16
hypnopompic hallucinations, 421
hypocretin, 425
hypopnoea, 389
hypothalamus, 14, 197, 425

idiopathic hypersomnolence, 413
illness, and sleep disruption, 181,
    303–4
infants, *see* babies
inhibitory system, 19
insomnia, 300
internal clock, 14, 28
Isabella (limits), 129–30
itching, 181

Jacob (sleep associations), 71, 80, 86
Jacqueline (sleepiness), 406–7, 429,
    430
James (sleep cycle), 257–60
Jason (rocking), 368–69, 382
Jessica (rhythmic behaviours), 376,
    383
jet lag, 32, 198
job to do, 305–11
Jonathan (tonsils), 395, 397
Joshua (sleeping pills), 186
Justin (obese), 396, 397–98, 400

Kaitlyn (sleep associations), 71–72, 80
Kayla (night feedings), 137–38, 148
K-complex waves, 16, 17, 22

Klonopin (clonazepam), 319
Kyle (limits), 131–34

language, of dreams, 20
larks and owls, 206–7
Lauren (night-time wakings), 336–37, 340
lifting, 366
light:
    blocking, 251
    exposure to, 31, 55, 197–98, 204–5, 207–8, 235
limits, setting, 35–36, 105–35
    difficulty with, 108–10
    door, 119–23
    gates, 114–19, 128–29
    importance of, 109
    in late bedtime, 126–28
    at night, 112–14, 165–66, 170
    overlapping syndromes, 111–12
    problem examples, 129–35
    reward system for, 124–26
    with siblings, 128–29
    testing of, 158–59
    when child shares your bedroom, 123–24
    who's in charge?, 106–8, 113–14
Lindsey (sleep phase), 224–25, 227, 245
Lisa (partial wakings), 287, 322–23

Marcy (partial wakings), 287, 288, 291, 322
Maria (confusional arousals), 288, 326–28
Mark (sleep phase), 224, 225–27, 243
maturation, and bed-wetting, 351–52
medication:
    for bed-wetting problems, 365–66
    for confusional events, 318–19
    sleeping pills, 184–88, 236
    sleep problems affected by, 187–88, 303–4
Medikinet XL (methylphenidate), 428
Megan (limits), 107
melatonin, 197, 236
metronome, 381
Michael (limits), 130–31
micrognathia, 392

middle-ear infections, 41, 149–50, 182–83, 397
migraines, 181
monsters, fear of, 162–63, 335, 421
motivation, reward system as, 124–26, 168–69
motor development, 39
multiple births, 49–52
Multiple Sleep Latency Test (MSLT), 412–13

naps, 264–83
    accepting what works, 283
    of adults, 201
    changing, 198
    developing pattern of, 28, 29–30, 264–65
    drifting/splitting, 278–80
    elimination of, 30, 275–76, 280–81
    and feedings, 149
    hidden, 267–68
    at home and day care, 282–83
    inconsistent schedules, 278
    interrupted, 276–77
    long, 271–72
    short, 270–71, 272–74
    and sleep associations, 98, 281–82
    and sleep patterns, 54, 56, 204, 242, 265, 268–70
    and sleep phases, 218–19
    too early or too late, 274–75
narcolepsy, 8, 30, 406–30
    as abnormal sleepiness, 408–10
    and cataplectic attacks, 418–19
    cause of, 424–26
    early diagnosis of, 422–24
    evaluation of, 411–14
    and hypnagogic hallucinations, 420–22
    onset of, 414
    sleep disturbances in, 415–16
    and sleep paralysis, 420
    sporadic nature of, 425
    symptoms of, 416–22
    treatment of, 414–15, 426–30
nerve impulses, blocking of, 19
neurological disorders, 188–92, 376–77
neurophysiology, 14–15

Nicholas (birth injury), 190–91
night-day reversal, 54
night lights, 163, 164, 170, 338
nightmares, 157–58, 164–65, 333–46
  and confusional events, 341–45
  and emotional difficulties, 340–41
  false alarms, 345–46
  helping child with, 337–41
  story of, 335
  what they are, 333–34
  why they occur, 334–37
Noah (confusional arousals), 287, 288,
  323–25
nocturnal enuresis, *see* bed-wetting
noise, external cues of, 55
noise disturbances, 251–53
non-REM sleep, 15–18
  cycles of, 27
  development of, 21, 23, 301
  partial wakings from, 288, 289, 341
  restorative function of, 21
  stages I-III, 15–16, 17
  stage IV, 16–18, 24, 27, 301
nursing:
  and let-down response, 145–46
  at nap time, 146
  night, 85, 137, 145
Nuvigil (armodafinil), 428

obesity, and sleep apnoea, 392,
  395–96
obstructive sleep apnoea, *see* sleep
  apnoea
oesophagus, 184
onset (secondary) enuresis, 354
orexin, 425
Orwell, George, 356
otitis media (middle-ear infection),
  150
overheating, and SIDS, 40
overlearning, 364, 365
overlying, danger of, 39
overstimulation, 179
owls and larks, 206–7

pacifiers:
  bottle used as, 147
  breast used as, 144
  and SIDS, 87

sleeping with dummies, 40
  and middle-ear infections, 41,
  149–50
  and progressive-waiting approach,
  86–87
pain, 95, 181, 182, 204
palate, 392
paralysis, in sleep, 19, 407, 420, 424,
  429–30
partial wakings, 24, 287–333
  as confusional events, 291–311
  evaluating, 312–15
  as normal transitions, 289–91
  summary chart, 330–32
  treatment for, 315–33
  variability of, 311–12
  what to do during, 319–21
  what they are, 287–89
Paul (bedtime routine), 36
peek-a-boo, 339
pets, sharing rooms with, 175
pharyngeal flap, 392, 398
pharyngoplasty, 400–1
phenobarbital, 187
Phyllocontin (aminophylline), 187
Pickwickian syndrome, 395–96
Pliny the Elder, 355–56
point charts, 124–26, 168–69
polysomnogram (PSG), 411–12
poor sleepers, natural, 6–7
preadolescence, sleep needs in, 30
prenatal care, and SIDS, 38
primary enuresis, 354
progressive-waiting approach, 72–83
  cold turkey v, 80, 82, 87
  consistency in, 92–93
  for night-time feedings, 83, 84–86
  with dummy, 86–87
  procedure of, 73, 74–76
  schedule considerations in, 93–94
  sleep chart, 77
  when to start, 96–97
prone (face-down) sleep position, 38
Proventil (albuterol), 187
Provigil (modafinil), 428
puberty, *see* adolescents

quiet sleep, 22

Rachel (fear), 155–56
Rebecca (bed-wetting), 349–50
reflux, 183–84
relaxation, 18, 19, 318
REM (rapid-eye-movement) onsets, 413, 415
REM (rapid-eye-movement) sleep, 15, 17, 18–21
  brain waves in, 17
  development of, 22, 23
  dreaming in, 26, 333
  elimination of, 20
  of foetus, 21
  narcolepsy in, 415–16, 421
  near-paralysis of, 289
  nightmares in, 333, 341
  partial activation of, 416
  rebound, 416
  sleep-onset periods, 413, 424
  waking from, 20, 97
responsibility training, 360–61, 362
rest-activity cycle, 200
retrognathia, 392
reward system, 90, 124–26, 168–69
rhythmic behaviours, 368–83
  alternative activities to, 381
  causes of, 372–78
  as concern, 371–72
  as habit, 374–75, 383
  protection in, 382
  treatment of, 378–82
  and vocalisation, 370
  what they look like, 370–71
  when they occur, 369
rhythms, sleep-wake, 196–99
Ritalin (methylphenidate), 187, 428
rituals and routines, bedtime, 34–37, 113, 316–17
rocking, *see* rhythmic behaviours
rocking your child to sleep, 34
room, learning to stay in, 121–23
room dividers, 89
room temperature, 40
rotations, head-to-toe, 46
rubbing your child's back, 34
rules, 35–36, 90

Sam (sleep associations), 70, 91
Sarah (muscular dystrophy), 189–90

scary films, 152, 161, 164–65
schedules, 53–58, 195–213, 241–55
  consistent, 57, 316
  electronic 24/7, 208, 253–55
  inconsistent, 32, 195, 255–60, 278, 303
  of larks and owls, 206–7
  and progressive-waiting approach, 93–94
  and rhythms, 196–99
  and setting limits, 109
  short sleep requirements, 249–51
  sleep phases in, *see* sleep phases
  and travel, 260–61
school, avoiding, 239
secondary (onset) enuresis, 354
secondary gain, 108, 110
second wind, 202, 260
sedatives, 185, 204
sensory overstimulation, 179, 302–3
separation anxiety, 48, 94, 152, 160–61, 173–75, 335, 339
Seth (night-time wakings), 246–48
settled:
  inability to become, 62, 98–99
  learning new ways to be, 84
  use of term, 29, 35
  without help, 61
sex, separate room for, 47
sexual impulses, 335
short sleep requirements, 249–51
siblings, 128–29, 175
SIDS (sudden death in infants), 37–41
  and co-sleeping, 45–46
  and dummies, 87
  and sleep apnoea, 403
siestas, 201
sleep, 14–32
  average amounts of, 9, 10–11
  biological rhythms of, 31–32
  brain wave patterns in, 17
  changing position in, 26
  conditions for, *see* sleep associations
  and death, 336, 340
  developmental patterns of, 28–31
  enough, 9, 30–31, 250, 316
  inability to return to, 8, 64
  irregular schedules of, 32, 195, 255–60, 278, 303

non-REM, 15–18, 27
patterns of, 21–23, 28–32
purposes of, 15
REM, 15, 17, 18–21
requirements for, 202, 249–51
sleep (*cont.*)
  restorative function of, 15, 21
  through the night, 12, 29, 34, 97
sleep apnoea, 387–405
  causes of, 392–96
  central, 402–3
  getting help for, 403
  and sleeping pills, 185
  and snoring, 388–89
  tonsils and adenoids in, 390,
    393–95, 401
  treatment of, 396–401
  what happens in, 388–92, 404–5
  words of caution about, 401–3
sleep associations, 61–104
  anxiety, 94–95
  and babysitter, 102–3
  bedtime feedings, 85–86, 96
  confusional v habitual wakings, 95
  consistency in, 100
  and co-sleeping, 87–91
  crying or screaming child, 82, 102
  disruptions in process, 103–4
  dummies, 86–87
  general observations, 95–104
  help in settling, 98–99
  importance of, 65–67
  learning, 99–100
  making changes in, 83–85, 96
  medical considerations, 95
  for naps v night, 98, 281–82
  and other children, 102
  procedural considerations, 92–93
  progressive-waiting approach,
    72–83, 96–97
  schedule considerations, 93–94
  sharing parental responsibilities in,
    101
  spoiling v comforting a child, 82, 99
  and trust, 96
  typical problems, 63–64, 67–72
  variations in, 98
  and vomiting, 101–2
  waiting schedule, 101

when to begin, 100
sleep chart, 77, 219
sleep cycle:
  in children, 23–28, 299
  deep sleep in, 27–28
  irregular, 32, 255–60, 303
  length of, 23
  rhythms of, 196–99
  transitions in, 289
  variable, 299
sleep debt, 204
sleep deprivation, 12, 207–10, 231,
    301–2, 409
sleep environment, and SIDS, 39–41
sleep habit development, 33–58
  bedtime routines in, 34–37
  co-sleeping, 41–49
  family differences in, 33
  favourite blanket or toy, 52–53
  reducing SIDS risk, 37–41
  schedules for, 53–58
  of twins and triplets, 49–52
sleepiness:
  and behavioural problems, 402
  causes of, 409–10
  excessive, 8, 408–10
  fighting off, 199–200
  and homeostatic drive, 202
  relieved by sleep, 15
  treatment of, 410–11, 427–29
  unpredictable, 198
  see also narcolepsy
sleeping pills, 184–88, 236
sleeping through the night, 12, 29, 34,
    97
sleep laboratory, 411
sleep-onset REM periods, 413, 424
sleep paralysis, 19, 407, 420, 424,
    429–30
sleep patterns:
  in adolescence, 57, 204
  in adults, 57
  in babies, 21–23, 28–29, 53–57, 58,
    97, 264–65
  changing, 55–56, 204
  chart of, 77, 219
  in children, 23–28, 29–30, 57, 58,
    265–66, 299
  disruptions in, 58, 303

and feeding patterns, 54–55
and naps, 53, 56, 204, 242, 265, 268–70
sleep phase delay, 31, 204, 209
sleep phases, 199–200, 202, 203, 204–5, 214–19
  early (advanced), 220–22, 223
  guidelines, 228–29
  how to identify, 216–18
  late (delayed), 222–28, 230
  naps, 218–19
  shifts in, 219–29, 230–40, 409
  weekends and holidays, 218
sleep position:
  and middle-ear infections, 149–50
  and SIDS, 37–39
sleep problems, 8–9
  causes of, 211–13
  day v night, 266
  electronic disruptions, 253–55
  environmental disturbances, 251–53
  inconsistent schedules, 255–60
  too-long-in-bed problem, 242–43, 244
  travel, 260–63
  trouble falling asleep, 243, 245
  waking in middle of night, 246–48
  waking too early, 245
sleep readiness, 199
sleep spindles, 16, 17, 22
sleep talking, 288, 291
sleep terrors, 8, 20, 332
  and confusional events, 95, 294, 297–98
  and nightmares, 341, 343–45
  and partial wakings, 24, 288, 293
  what to do during, 320
sleep-wake rhythm, *see* sleep cycle
sleepwalking, 8, 20, 298, 330–31
  and confusional events, 292, 308, 310
  and nightmares, 343–44
  and partial wakings, 24, 288, 292
  safety factors for, 317–18
  what to do during, 320–21
sleep zone, 199
Slo-Phyllin, Slo-Bid (theophyline), 187
smoking, and SIDS, 38, 39, 45

snoring, 8–9, 388–89
special needs, children with, 85
sphincter muscles, 360
sprinkle technique, 71
stage IV sleep, 16–18, 24, 27, 301
startles, 22
start-stop exercises, 360–61, 363–64
sticker charts, 124–26, 168–69
stimulants, 204, 236, 428
strep throat, recurrent, 397
stress:
  and anxiety, 152
  and confusional events, 309, 312
  and nightmares, 337
sucking habit, 144
suffocation, risk of, 39, 45
supine (face-up) sleep position, 38–39, 46, 149
sweating, 16

teenagers, *see* adolescents
teething, and rhythmic behaviours, 373
television, 253–55, 339
thunder, fear of, 154–55
time zones, 32, 197, 198, 204–5, 260–63
toilet-training, 152, 321, 362–63
tonsils, and sleep apnoea, 390, 393–95, 401
too-long-in-bed problem, 242–43, 244
tooth decay, 150
toy, favourite, 52–53
trachea (windpipe), 184
tracheostomy, 400, 401
tranquillisers, 185
transitional objects, 52–53
travel, and time zones, 32, 205, 260–63
Truphylline (aminophylline), 187
twenty-five-hour day, 31, 56
twenty-four-hour sleep schedule, 54, 56
twins and triplets, 49–52
twitching, 16, 19, 20
Tyler (fear), 154–55, 162, 175–77

upper airway resistance, 388
urinary system, 357–62

urination, *see* bed-wetting

Valium (diazepam), 185, 319
vasopressin, 365–66
Ventolin (albuterol), 187
Victoria (sleep phase), 220–21
vocalisation, 370
vomiting, 101–2, 184

wake zone, 199
waking:
   biological rhythms of, 31–32
   brain waves in, 17
   in dream state, 19
   drowsiness as transitional state in,
    16
   habitual, 95
   and hunger, 137
   and inability to go back to sleep,
    8, 64

night-time, 12, 246–48
   partial, *see* partial wakings
   patterns of, 28–31
   from REM sleep, 20, 97
   in sleep cycle, 27, 199
   from stage IV sleep, 27
   stimulus for, 352–53
   too early or too late, 8, 245
   transition stage to, 289–91
waterproof pads, 362
weaning, 85, 148–49
white-noise generators, 251
William (sleep associations), 68–69,
   91
windpipe (trachea), 184
worries, talking about, 36–37

Xyrem (sodium oxybate), 428, 429

About the Author

DR RICHARD FERBER is widely recognised as the leading international authority in the field of children's sleep problems. He is a paediatrician, founding director of the Center for Pediatric Sleep Disorders at Children's Hospital Boston, Massachusetts, and an associate professor of neurology at Harvard Medical School. He lives in Washington DC, and is the proud father of two grown-up children and has two much-loved grandchildren.